# Plagues, Politics, and Policy

# Plagues, Politics, and Policy

## *A Chronicle of the Indian Health Service, 1955–2008*

David H. DeJong

LEXINGTON BOOKS
A division of
ROWMAN & LITTLEFIELD PUBLISHERS, INC.
*Lanham • Boulder • New York • Toronto • Plymouth, UK*

Published by Lexington Books
A division of Rowman & Littlefield Publishers, Inc.
A wholly owned subsidiary of The Rowman & Littlefield Publishing Group, Inc.
4501 Forbes Boulevard, Suite 200, Lanham, Maryland 20706
www.lexingtonbooks.com

Estover Road, Plymouth PL6 7PY, United Kingdom

British Library Cataloguing in Publication Information Available

**Library of Congress Cataloging-in-Publication Data**

DeJong, David H.
  Plagues, politics, and policy : a chronicle of the Indian Health Service, 1955-2008 /
David H. DeJong.
      p. cm.
  Includes bibliographical references and index.
  ISBN 978-0-7391-4603-3 (cloth : alk. paper)
 1.  United States. Indian Health Service—History. 2.  Indians of North America—
Medical care—History. 3.  Alaska Natives—Medical care—History. 4.  Indians of North
America—Health and hygiene—History. 5.  Alaska Natives—Health and hygiene—
History. 6.  Indians of North America—Government relations—1934- 7.  Alaska
Natives—Government relations. 8.  Public health—United States—History. I. Title.
  RA448.5.I5D456 2011
  362.1089'97—dc22                                                  2010040046

Printed in the United States of America

# CONTENTS

# TABLES

Tables

# ACKNOWLEDGMENTS

It has taken nearly twenty years to complete this study of the Indian Health Service and its companion volume on the Indian medical service. The former is now being published while the latter was published by Lexington Books in 2008. Many people have assisted me in this endeavor and I would be remiss if I did not recognize them. Dr. Jennie Joe, of the University of Arizona's Native American Research and Training Center, was instrumental in piquing my interest in Indian healthcare and her guidance has made this study a better one. I also appreciate the support and documents provided me by the late Dr. James "Ray" Shaw, who was the last director of the Indian medical service (1952-1955) and the first director of the Indian Health Service (1955-1962). I met with Dr. Shaw at his Tucson home in 1990 and was struck by his keen sense of history. I acknowledge the input of Dr. Stanley Stitt (retired) of the Indian Health Service, and the first American Indian director of the Indian Health Service, Everett R. Rhoades, both of whom answered questions and provided insight into the operations of the agency during the 1980s.

The Government Documents librarians at the University of Arizona and Arizona State University were most helpful and rendered valuable assistance when I researched hard-to-find documents. The librarians of the Commissioned Corps Centennial Archives, History of Medicine Division, in National Library of Medicine in Bethesda, Maryland, were supportive and provided valuable assistance. I recognize the friendship and support of my former Indian Health Service colleague, William Katzel. Finally, I acknowledge the support of my family. My wife Cindy encouraged me to persevere. I had no children when I began this endeavor; now I have five, so I must acknowledge the sacrifice of time that Rachelle, Rebecca, Joshua, Ralissa, and RaeAnna made that allowed me to devote the resources necessary to complete this chronicle on the Indian Health Service.

# INTRODUCTION

Over the past century, American Indians and Alaska Natives have experienced a ~~AND~~ *[handwritten: AND COVID-19]* remarkable decline in pandemic and epidemic diseases such as smallpox, typhus, trachoma, tuberculosis, influenza, and others. These diseases once decimated American Indians and Alaska Natives, reducing many tribal nations to a fraction of their former strength. For those American Indians and Alaska Natives who survived, ill-health became, and in many instances remains, a fact of life and adversely affected their physical, spiritual, social, and mental well-being.

In the twentieth century, contagious and infectious diseases gave way to diseases and ill-health caused by an aging population and behavioral choices. In 1908, the United States Indian Service (now Bureau of Indian Affairs) initiated formal medical services when it hired Joseph Murphy as the first Chief Medical Director of the Indian medical service. Until 1955, the Bureau of Indian Affairs (BIA) provided curative services to American Indians and Alaska Natives. At mid-twentieth century, Congress, intent on terminating Indian-only services, transferred the Indian medical service to the United States Public Health Service (PHS).

The dispensation of medical services under the Bureau of Indian Affairs was chronicled in *"If You Knew the Conditions": A Chronicle of the Indian Medical Service and American Indian Healthcare, 1908-1955*, in which I covered the first half century of Indian medical care by evaluating the challenges facing American Indians and Alaska Natives. In *Plagues, Politics, and Policy: A Chronicle of the Indian Health Service, 1955-2008*, I examine the history of the Indian Health Service (IHS) since it was relocated from the Bureau of Indian Affairs into the Public Health Service. This covers the period of time from the Indian Health Transfer Act of 1954 to the election of Barack Obama as president of the United States and the appointment of Yvette Roubideaux as the first woman director of the Indian Health Service.

Curative medicine has long been the norm in Indian Country, although the Indian Health Service, in consultation with tribal nations, has made progress in establishing preventative medicine. As this transformation occurred, critics have argued that the Indian Health Service has become an "acculturating agent" by

1

encouraging American Indians and Alaska Natives to view disease as rooted in "ecological adaptation and social organization" and requiring medical treatment.[1]

## The Indian Health Service Today

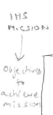

Since 1955, Congress has charged the Indian Health Service with administering a health program for American Indians and Alaska Natives. The agency is responsible for not only working with tribal nations and organizations to elevate the health status of the eligible American Indian and Alaska Native population, but it is also responsible for providing the opportunities and assistance necessary for them to assume full control over those programs designed for them. To achieve this mission, the Indian Health Service works to accomplish three objectives. It designs, operates, and maintains, in cooperation with tribal communities, a comprehensive healthcare system. It also secures and manages the financial and professional resources to support the healthcare system. Finally, it provides the technical assistance necessary for tribal nations to exercise self-governance in the field of healthcare services.

Table I.1

*Directors of the Indian Health Service, 1955-2009*

| Name | Years |
|------|-------|
| James R. Shaw | 1955-1962 |
| Carruth J. Wagner | 1963-1965 |
| Erwin S. Rabeau | 1966-1969 |
| Emery Johnson | 1969-1981 |
| Everett R. Rhoades (Kiowa) | 1982-1993 |
| Michael Trujillo (Laguna Pueblo) | 1994-2002 |
| Charles W. Grim (Cherokee) | 2002-2007 |
| Robert McSwain (North Fork Mono) | 2007-2009 |
| Yvette Roubideaux (Cheyenne River Sioux) | 2009- |

The Indian Health Service carries out its responsibilities through the operation of a health service delivery system that provides preventive, curative, rehabilitative, and environmental services. This system integrates direct care services provided in Indian Health Service or tribal health programs, along with contract care services provided in private and state and/or local health facilities. American Indians and Alaska Natives are also free to take advantage of other healthcare resources, including Medicare and Medicaid. In addition, the Indian Health Service partners with federal and state agencies, as well as other public and private organizations, to develop more effective methods of providing needed services to American Indians and Alaska Natives.

The Indian Health Service is comprised of eleven area offices that administer the program within specific geographic areas. The Tucson Office of Health Program Research and Development, although technically a headquarters office, is often referred to as the twelfth area office. The agency provides services through four distinct methods: IHS facilities, tribal health programs, contract facilities, and urban Indian programs. The area offices are subsequently divided into 155 service units, which are the basic administrative units at the local level. Of these service units, 92 are controlled by the tribal community they serve. Tribes also control 13 of 49 hospitals, 172 of 231 health centers, 260 of 309 health stations, and 3 of 5 school health centers. There are also 34 urban Indian programs.[2] The Indian Health Service and the tribal health programs it funds operate facilities in 33 states, as shown in the Table I.2.

Table I.2

*Reservation States with Indian Health Service Responsibilities*

| State | State | State |
|---|---|---|
| Alabama | Maine | North Dakota |
| Alaska | Massachusetts | Oklahoma |
| Arizona | Michigan | Oregon |
| California | Minnesota | Pennsylvania |
| Colorado | Mississippi | Rhode Island |
| Connecticut | Montana | South Dakota |
| Florida | Nebraska | Texas |
| Idaho | Nevada | Utah |
| Iowa | New Mexico | Washington |
| Kansas | New York | Wisconsin |
| Louisiana | North Carolina | Wyoming |

(Indian Health Service, 2001)

Many American Indians and Alaska Natives continue to face health challenges that result from the consequences of poverty, geographic and social isolation, inadequate sanitation facilities, poor economic opportunities, and discrimination. Among the more severe challenges are accidental injuries, alcoholism, mental health, nutritional deficiencies and inadequate dental care. Chronic challenges include diabetes, cancer, heart disease, and liver disease, with maternal and child healthcare an acute challenge in some communities.

The Indian Health Service has had an important and positive impact on the health status of American Indians and Alaska Natives, particularly since the 1970s. Infant and maternal mortality, pneumonia, gastrointestinal diseases, tuberculosis, and other infectious disease incidence rates have all declined. Despite such reductions, the rate of alcoholism is six and a half times the non-Indian rate. Accidental deaths and diabetes are nearly triple the national average and homicide and suicide rates are considerably higher. While life expectancy at birth among American Indians and Alaska Natives has increased to 72.3 years, it is still below the 76.9 years of life expectancy among the U.S. general population.

Congressional parsimony adds to the difficulty of providing meaningful service. While the Indian Health Service has a defined mission of elevating the spiritual, physical, mental, and social well-being of American Indians and Alaska Natives to the highest level, it continues to experience high turnover rates among professional staff, even among American Indian and Alaska Native healthcare providers. This makes program continuity all but impossible. Despite President Obama's proposed $4.03 billion budget for fiscal year 2010 (in addition to $500 million in American Recovery and Reinvestment Act funding for fiscal years 2009-2010), the Indian Health Service constant budget increased just 26 percent between 1990 and 2002.[3]

While the Indian Health Service is funded by discretionary appropriations, its services are provided as a result of a 200 year-old federal Indian trust relationship. Based on treaties, acts of Congress, Presidential Executive Orders, and judicial interpretations (and the cession of more than a billion acres of land), the trust relationship extends to federally recognized tribal nations a unique political relationship that results in American Indians and Alaska Natives being citizens of the United States and citizens of their own sovereign tribal nation. In return for land cessions and the protection of the United States, tribal nations were promised a myriad of services, including medical care. Thus, the Indian Health Service is unique in all the federal bureaucracy, particularly in the field of healthcare. It represents the federal government's largest and most ambitious—albeit less than stellar—effort of providing a comprehensive healthcare system to a categorical population group in the United States. No other people group can claim such a system of services.[4]

## Guiding Questions

In *Plagues, Politics, and Policy: The Indian Health Service, 1955-2008* I seek to answer several broad policy questions: Have American Indians and Alaska Natives received appreciably better care since the Indian medical service transferred into the Public Health Service in 1955? Have community-based programs been successful in providing culturally relevant and community-oriented approaches to well-being? Can American Indians and Alaska Natives expect Congress and the Administration to fully fund a program that will allow them to achieve health parity with other Americans? In seeking answers to these questions, I provide a comprehensive chronicle of the Indian Health Service. In each chapter, I provide an overview of the health program, including administrative policies and functions within the program. Furthermore, I examine the impact of federal-Indian health policy and the status of American Indian and Alaska Native health and the priorities of each director of the agency.

In so doing, several conclusions can be reached. First, in the initial decades of Public Health Service control of the Indian Health Service, infectious diseases were largely eliminated, although they were replaced by a rising incidence of disease rooted in social and behavioral issues. These diseases are reflected in high rates of mental illness, alcoholism, accidental injuries, and accidental deaths. Furthermore, as American Indians and Alaska Natives live longer, there has been an increase in the incidence of chronic diseases associated with geriatrics. Many American Indians and Alaska Natives face public health challenges rooted in the social and political history of the federal Indian relationship. More than any other Americans, American Indians and Alaska Natives continue to be affected by hundreds of laws, thousands of court rulings, and countless administrative actions.

From its beginnings in 1955 through 2008, the Indian Health Service has pla[y]ed an important role in elevating the status of American Indian and Alaska
N               of the once malign diseases no longer plague Indian
C                       :ing American Indians and Alaska Natives.
T                       al leaders to work together to come up with
s                       d Alaska Native people live longer, chronic
c                       evalent. Improvement in the future will to a
                       inges among American Indians and Alaska
                       Congress. Consequently, the Indian Health
                       inue to seek new ways of dealing with illness

ie present study is and is not. This study is a
ice; it is not a definitive analysis or exhaustive
s an overview of the major health issues
l Alaska Natives over the past fifty years; it is
challenges facing American Indians and Alaska
eral government's attempt to provide medical
people in the United States; it is not a detailed
lthcare should or should not look like. And,
ie major issues affecting the delivery of services
ka Natives, not an evolutionary history of the

# Notes

1. Stephen J. Kunitz, *Disease Change and the Role of Medicine: The Navajo*

*Experience* (Berkley: University of California Press, 1989), 3-4.

2 *Trends in Indian Health, 2000-2001* (Health and Human Services, Indian Health Service, Washington, D.C.: Government Printing Office, 2002), 25. All Indian Health Service hospitals, health centers, and health clinic labs are accredited.

3 "President Proposes 13 Percent Increase in FY 2010 Budget for Indian Health Service," www.ihs.gov/publicaffairs, *Trends in Indian Health*, 2002, 26. The ARRA funds are scheduled to be used for: $227 million for health facilities; $100 million for maintenance and improvements; $85 million for health information technology; $68 million for sanitation facilities construction; and $20 million for health equipment. "IHS Releases $500 million in Recovery Act Funds to Improve Health care and Boost Economy in Indian Country," www.ihs.gov/publicaffairs.

4 Robert Kane and Rosalie Kane, *Federal Health Care (With Reservations!)* (New York: Springer Publishing Company, 1972) xi.

# CHAPTER ONE

## Now That You Know the Conditions

By all accounts, American Indians were a relatively healthy people prior to contact with Europeans. But they were also unprepared for the biological impact of European pathogens. Diseases and epidemics to which the American Indians had little or no immunity devastated tribal nations across the continent, and throughout the sixteenth, seventeenth, and eighteenth centuries, disease struck in successive waves, mortally wounding millions of American Indians. Colonial governments could do little to alleviate the suffering and consequences of disease. As more colonists arrived and the frontier advanced, disease and epidemics spread farther into the interior of the continent. Smallpox, influenza, typhus, dysentery, plague, and a host of other diseases spread inland, with American Indians "succumb[ing] to every infection that came [their] way."[1]

President Thomas Jefferson authorized vaccinations for visiting tribal delegations to Washington, D.C.[2] By 1803, the United States Army took measures to combat smallpox along the frontier military posts, but did so more to protect soldiers than to ensure the survival of American Indians. Congress did not appropriate any revenue for Indian healthcare until 1819, when it provided funds to prevent "the further decline and final extinction of the Indian tribes." Most of the funds were dispensed to missionary organizations for education and "such other duties as may be enjoined" to protect and preserve the American Indians adjoining the frontier settlements of the United States. Superintendent of Indian Trade Thomas McKenney administered these funds and, in 1824, established an Office of Indian Affairs under the direction of the secretary of war.[3]

Under the auspices of the War Department, the dispensation of medical services and the application of sanitary regulations applied only to those American Indians living adjacent to military posts. Not believing it was a federal responsibility to provide healthcare to American Indians, Congress appropriated minimal funds for Indian medical services. While Indian agents increasingly requested through the War Department that Congress appropriate funds for medical supplies, they rarely received them.

The first specific order of the Office of Indian Affairs concerning the health of American Indians was a Congressional directive requiring the Indian Service to guard "the health of the Indians" during the era of Indian removal. When the U.S. Army removed the Creek Nation from Georgia and Alabama in the 1830s, the United States agreed to provide a surgeon for each emigrating party of 1,000 people for the purpose of attending the ill. Despite such measures, smallpox devastated the Creek, Cherokee, Choctaw, Chickasaw, and Seminole nations en route to and upon arrival in Indian Territory.[4]

It was not until 1832 that Congress made funds available for vaccinating American Indians, and then only in response to an epidemic sweeping the Old Northwest. Congress appropriated $12,000 for smallpox vaccinations to save American Indians "from the destructive ravages of that disease," and conferred upon Secretary of War Lewis Cass authority to employ physicians and surgeons to execute the charge. Congress also charged Cass with supplying "genuine vaccine matter" to all Indian agents for the purpose of "arresting the progress of smallpox."[5]

With Congressional authorization and appropriations, Commissioner of Indian Affairs Elbert Herring paid surgeons $6 per diem or $6 per hundred vaccinations to inoculate the Indians in the Missouri River Valley. Herring informed Cass in 1833 that reports indicated when the Indians were "properly influenced" they accepted the vaccine and "appreciated the object of the Government." Some tribes, especially those in Kansas and along the Upper Missouri River, resisted vaccinations because of the influences of Indian traders who cultivated a lack of government trust among the Indians. Despite limited appropriations, 10,000 Indians were vaccinated by February 1833.[6]

## Treaty Provisions Related to Healthcare

Treaty-making was the primary vehicle by which the United States dealt with tribal nations until the latter nineteenth century. Treaties not only were recognition of the limited sovereignty of tribal governments by the United States but they were also the method of providing goods and services to tribes in exchange for cessions of land, federal protection, and peace and friendship. Of the 382 ratified Indian treaties, 31, or 12 percent, contained provisions related to medical care. Of these, 28 provided for physicians and 9 for hospitals.[7]

The first treaty to specifically address the health of American Indians was the 1832 treaty with the Winnebago (Ho Chunk) Nation, made at Rock Island, Illinois. Article 5 of the treaty committed the United States to provide "for the service and attendance of a physician at Prairie du Chien, and of one at Fort Winnebago."[8] In 1854-1855, the United States consummated fourteen treaties containing medical provisions with the tribes in the Pacific Northwest. In 1867-1868, seven of the Peace Commission treaties, signed with the tribal nations on the Great Plains and in the Southwest, contained medical provisions.

Medical facilities and physicians were increasingly important to tribes by the middle of the nineteenth century. In the 1854 Chasta, Scoton, and Umpqua treaty talks, for example, treaty commissioner Joel Palmer reported to Commissioner of Indian Affairs George Manypenny that, while retaining certain parcels of land was important to the Northwest Coastal Indians in consideration of the treaties, the federal pledge to establish schools and a hospital among them "contributed very much to overcome their objections." In the 1855 Nisqually and Puyallup treaty, Washington Territorial Governor Isaac Stevens informed the Indians: "This paper . . . gives you mechanics and a Doctor to teach you and cure you. Is that not fatherly?"[9]

Despite treaty provisions for hospitals and medical services, the United States often failed to fulfill its obligations and, when it did fulfill them it usually did so many years later. In an 1855 treaty with the United States, the Nez Perce ceded land lying between the Cascade and Bitter Root Mountains in exchange for, among other provisions, a federal promise "to erect a hospital, keeping the same in repair, and provided with the necessary medicines and furniture, and to employ a physician." At the time of the 1863 Nez Perce treaty, the United States had yet to fulfill its earlier obligation. "I took pains to ascertain what had been promised to, and what had been done for the Nez Perce nation," the agency superintendent wrote the commissioner. "I found there was not as much as you had the right to expect, not as much as the U.S. Govt supposed. . . . I was surprised to see so little improvements made, in view of the large appropriations, which I know have been made. . . . I found no hospital built."[10]

Consummation of a federal treaty did not guarantee continued medical services or health professionals. The 1867 Medicine Lodge Treaty with the Cheyenne and Arapaho tribes included a provision furnishing a physician. However, "at any time after ten years from the making of this treaty" the United States had the right to withdraw the physician.[11] Although most treaties included such stipulations, usually not to exceed twenty years, the United States adopted the policy of extending such services under general appropriations.[12]

## Initiating Medical Services

Many American Indians maintained faith in traditional healing practices rather than accepting the "white man's" medicine. Congress, nonetheless, encouraged the Indian Service to use all efforts to persuade American Indians to accept Western medicine as one step in the assimilating process. On ration days and special occasions, for instance, agency physicians were encouraged to demonstrate their medical skill in front of the Indians, showing how quickly they could extract teeth, lance boils, or perform surgical procedures. If successful, a physician might win over a few converts who "would want the white doctor."[13]

In the post-Civil War years the need for medical care among American Indians increased. A Senate Committee chaired by Senator James Doolittle (D-WI) in the wake of the Sand Creek (Southern Cheyenne) Massacre in eastern Colorado in

1864, concluded that, with the exception of the Five Civilized Tribes in Indian Territory, American Indians were "rapidly decreasing in numbers," principally from disease, intemperance, and war. Army Major General John Pope opined that the Plains Indians were "rapidly decreasing" as a result of disease. Brigadier General George Wright concurred, adding that tribes in the Far West were "rapidly diminishing by death and disease."[14]

It was not until 1873 that the Indian Service organized the first medical services for tribal nations by establishing the Medical and Education Division. Ely Parker, the first American Indian Commissioner of Indian Affairs, established central administrative control of the heretofore uncoordinated medical services by initiating standardized reporting and distribution systems. President Rutherford B. Hayes discontinued the division four years later before it was fully organized and placed responsibility for medical reporting and distribution of supplies in the Civilization Division. Medical services were strictly controlled by local Indian agents.

As tribes were confined to reservations, the need for medical care increased. "The Kaws," agent Cyrus Beade wrote to commissioner Ezra Hayt in 1877, "are decreasing in number from year to year. Disease contracted with dissolute whites before their removal to Indian Territory permeates the tribe, and seems to be incurable." Henry Mizner, agent at the Hoopa Agency in northern California, observed that the Hoopa, too, were "fast being swept by disease from the face of the earth." Annual agency reports to the commissioner of Indian affairs teemed with similar observations, with requests for hospitals, physicians, and medical supplies dominating the reports. In 1876-1877, ten agencies requested funds for hospitals, with appropriations made for one. Between 1893 and 1895, sixteen additional requests were made, most of which referred to the "imperative necessity" or "urgent necessity" of establishing hospitals and medical services.[15]

The delivery of basic healthcare in the latter nineteenth century was hampered by the several states rejecting any responsibility for Indian affairs and the federal government limiting its role despite treaty obligations. As a practical matter, prior to 1878 medical degrees were not a prerequisite for employment as a physician in the Indian Service. This brought challenges, as C. A. Ruffee, agent at the White Earth Chippewa Agency, explained. Because of unqualified doctors, American Indians were losing faith in the "white man's medicine" and returning to their traditional healing methods. Ruffee urged Hayt to hire only medical school graduates who proved they were competent. "Hereafter persons employed as physicians on Indian reservations [should] be graduates of some medical school and have the necessary diplomas." Without this policy change, physicians were sure to meet "with poor success in keeping down sickness."[16]

Limited remuneration also affected the quality of healthcare. Inadequate salaries meant agencies faced difficulties in hiring and maintaining personnel. Mizner reported in 1879 that he had "been unable to secure the services of a citizen physician for the salary offered ($900)."[17] As late as 1890, physicians in the Indian

Service earned 40 percent of what their colleagues in the Army and Navy earned (see table 1.1).[18]

Owing to the low physician pay and high patient loads, the Indian Service experienced a chronic shortage of doctors. In 1879, 59 Indian Service physicians treated 67,352 Indians, an average of 1,142 patients per physician. A decade later, 81 physicians treated the same number of patients, although they were responsible for nearly 200,000 Indians. This responsibility excluded the "Five Civilized tribes" in Indian Territory, which maintained their own health facilities.[19] As a result of heavy physician caseloads, the Indian Service did little more than provide crisis-oriented services and prescribe drugs.

Table 1.1

*Salaries and Patient Loads for Select Federal Physician Pools, 1890*

| Agency | Physicians | Annual Pay* | Eligible Patients | No. Treated | Per Physician |
|--------|-----------|------|-----------|---------|-----------|
| Indian | 82 | $1,028 | 180,184 | 68,165 | 831 |
| Navy | 160 | $2,622 | 9,955 | 11,499 | 72 |
| Army | 192 | $2,823 | 26,739 | 31,420 | 164 |

* Average annual salary

(Source: Commissioner of Indian Affairs, *Annual Report*, 1890, p. xxi)

To compound matters, Indian Service physicians lacked professional associations, faced infrequent salary increases, and were prohibited from maintaining a side practice. The Indian Service feared, correctly in some instances, that if physicians maintained a private practice, they would pay more attention to their non-Indian clients than to their Indian charges. Consequently, retention of physicians and other competent employees was an elusive goal. Commissioner Thomas J. Morgan suggested to his superiors that the barriers of practicing medicine in Indian Country might be overcome, but only with supervision by a medical expert and recognition of good service.

Congressional parsimony also hampered healthcare, as physicians found it futile to dispense drugs when there were no resources to purchase them. Most physicians made do without hospitals and basic medical instruments, and rarely had access to medical journals. Transportation, especially on expansive western reservations, was a constant challenge. Congress failed to provide any resources for wagons and teams, with some agents grumbling that lawmakers operated under the assumption that "street cars and elevated railroad lines" traversed reservations.[20]

It was not until 1882 that Congress authorized construction of the first permanent hospital for American Indians.[21] During the 1880s nearly every agency physician recommended the construction of a hospital for his agency. The agent at the Kiowa, Comanche, and Apache Agency appealed to commissioner Hiram Price that the treatment of American Indians in their homes was less than ideal because the Indians rarely took their medicine as prescribed. The common theme was the unavailability of hospitals impacted the effectiveness of physicians.

Physicians also saw hospitals as a means of assimilation. "The influence [of the medicine man] is still very great," the agent at the Kiowa, Comanche, and Apache Agency told Price, "and the agency physician finds it opposing him in all his practices." This was especially pronounced in those instances where physicians were "called to treat in the camps, when . . . the patient is subjected to the severe treatment of the Indian doctor at the same time that the agency physician is prescribing for him." The promised cure for such challenges: "the building of a hospital." Not only would physicians be able to treat patients more successfully, but every patient "brought from the camp to the hospital would be thrown directly under civilizing and Christianizing influences."[22]

In 1885, the commissioner of Indian affairs received eight new requests for hospitals. Congress appropriated funds for two, one among the Osage in Indian Territory and one among the Menominee in Wisconsin. By 1889, there were still just four Indian hospitals, leading commissioner Thomas Morgan to opine that it was time to improve the medical branch of the Indian Service and place it "on an equal footing with the medical departments of other branches of the public service." Morgan set high objectives to accomplish this goal, recommending the development of a training program in all Indian schools to instruct children in the art of nursing. He further urged the construction of a hospital at every boarding school so that children could receive proper medical care.[23]

Although the Indian Service constructed additional hospitals in the 1890s, it spent most of the decade requesting additional resources to meet the exigencies in Indian Country. Unless Congress appropriated funds to construct hospitals, Morgan was "powerless to remedy a great evil."[24] While the need for hospitals was great, there were Indians who still refused to utilize such facilities for cultural reasons. Z. T. Daniel, physician at the Pine Ridge Agency in 1894, lamented this fact.

In old times [the Sioux] destroyed all buildings and tepees in which a death occurred, which idea they still adhere to but seldom execute now. . . . They have an aversion to being sick in a house where a corpse has lain. Then, too, they are intensely social, and in a hospital their visitors are not so numerous, nor are the patients and visitors allowed to gormandize, as is their custom in the camp. The patient is put on a sick diet, which, to him, is synonymous with starvation. They are under restraint in everything in a hospital. There can be no drumming, incantations, songs, etc . . . no vociferous proclamations of the sickness . . . no wailing by old crooning women. . . . It is too quiet, too still, too mysterious; it is another world to them, and they dislike everything about a hospital; their attention is continuously fixed on the deaths and failures. An Indian policeman one day was sick and applied for treatment. I suggested that he go into the hospital: He replied, "No, that is the dead home."[25]

Consequently, it was children who presented the Indian Service with its greatest hope. T. D. Howard, physician at the Menominee Agency, boasted that "it is with the children that we get our best results, since they are easily managed and respond more quickly." To this end, the Indian Service focused its attention on educating children. The result was that through the children Indian hospitals gained wider acceptance.[26]

## The Ravages of Disease

With Congress slow to appropriate funds to establish hospitals, disease ravaged tribal communities. Smallpox, for instance, struck the Pueblo Indians in New Mexico, claiming 249 lives among the Zuni. The spread of disease illustrates one of the diverse challenges facing American Indians and the Indian Service in the latter nineteenth century. When the disease was first detected in 1897, the Pueblo agent received and distributed 3,000 smallpox vaccine points, later requesting an additional 5,000 points. Most of the vaccine points proved to be useless, with only a handful of the 1,000 vaccinations in Zuni Pueblo proving effective.[27]

To prevent the spread of disease, the agent ordered each Pueblo governor to prohibit tribal members from visiting other pueblos. Any person traveling without authorization was arrested. Despite such prohibitions, smallpox spread west to the Hopi villages, where in December 1898, it surfaced at the First Mesa village of Walpi. Although the Indian Service used vaccinations and quarantines to prevent the spread of the disease, it spread in rapid succession to all the villages on First and Second Mesas. With the more traditional Hopis refusing assistance, and with transportation up to Second Mesa nearly impossible, the disease spread quickly. By the time it ran its course, 187 Hopis died. Of 632 cases on First and Second Mesas, 412 patients accepted the vaccine. Of these, 24 (6 percent) died. Of the 220 traditionalists who refused treatment, 163 (74 percent) died.[28]

By 1900 it was increasingly difficult to overlook the deficiencies in Indian health, with critics charging the Indian Service with neglecting Indian health. Inspector William J. McConnell, who spent most of his four-year term (1897-1901) investigating Indian health conditions, lamented the Indian Service policy of filling Indian schools at all costs, even if it meant admitting diseased children. McConnell informed Interior Secretary Ethan Allen Hitchcock in 1899 that the United States declared war on Spain because of its harshness towards the Cubans. "Yet," McConnell asserted, "I venture to say that upon every one of our Indian Reservations in the Northwest there are conditions as bad or worse than any which were exposed in Cuba."[29]

Spurred on by McConnell and others like him, the Indian Service slowly expanded its medical facilities and paid better attention to the unhealthful overcrowding of boarding schools. While there were only five Indian hospitals in 1900, there were 50 by 1911 and 87 by 1918. Physicians, which numbered 85 in 1900, increased to 196 by 1918 (see Table 1.2).

Table 1.2

*Hospitals and Medical Personal, Select Years, 1888-1918*

| Year | Hospitals | Physicians | Nurses | Matrons |
|------|-----------|-----------|--------|---------|
| 1888 | 4 | 81 | 0 | 0 |
| 1895 | 4 | 74 | 8 | 3 |
| 1900 | 5 | 83 | 27 | 21 |
| 1918 | 87 | 196 | 99 | 87 |

(Source: *The Indian Service Health Activities*, 1922)

In the latter nineteenth and early twentieth centuries, the Indian Service aggressively allotted in severalty tribal lands and "emancipated" American Indians from the "bonds" of tribalism. To accomplish this goal, the Indian Service instructed its agents to construct "civilized" houses in place of traditional dwellings. This spatial aspect of civilization began with ornately and stately designed schools and continued with home-building. In 1905, commissioner Francis Leupp ordered Indian agents and missionaries to encourage home-building among the Indians. "Indians who set up tepees," Leupp opined, "have no feeling of the American word 'home'."[30]

Most American Indians did not live in permanent homes, making the transition from traditional to modern homes difficult and, in some cases, deadly. While sanitation and hygiene were not new concepts—traditional homes were frequently moved or burned for cultural and hygienic reasons—the adoption of permanent homes often entailed sanitary deficiencies. Physician George M. Kober noted that during his twenty-year tenure in the United States Army (1874-1894) he had never encountered a case of pulmonary tuberculosis among the Paiutes near Fort McDermott, Nevada, until after 1884, "and then only among Indians who had exchanged their tepees for badly constructed and insanitary dwellings."[31]

Dr. George E. Bushnell noted that those Sioux who resided near the agency were prone to disease and illness. "Here was the mingling of two streams, the one kept free of the diseases of the whites, by enforced separation through continuous warfare; the other contaminated by the diseases and vices of civilization." Bushnell frequently witnessed

scrofulous youths from the agency, their fleshless limbs fully clad, looking on wistfully at the dances of the warriors in the summer twilight, where braves, stripped to the breech-clout, danced on the grass to the music of the tom-tom, reproducing, in pantomime, their exploits in border warfare, or in some horse stealing, and revealing in many instances a magnificent physique and a boundless vitality, which contrasted cruelly with the listless aspect of some of their spectators. The two streams became one, when the Indians abandoned their tepees and took up their residence in houses under guidance of the agency officials.[32]

By the turn of the century, the situation was desperate. "That the Indians of the present are in a deplorable condition as to health," Indian Service critic Warren K. Moorehead opined, "no person familiar with Indian affairs will deny. It is incomprehensible to me that appropriations for combating disease are so meagre, and the appropriations for allotting and education so lavish." An anonymous friend of Moorehead's went to the heart of the situation: "Of what use is education to an Indian with consumption? An Indian child learns to read and write, contracts trachoma, is sent home and goes blind. How does that education benefit the blind Indian?"[33]

With the new century, the Indian Service assigned physicians to most agencies and schools, although it contracted with physicians as specific needs arose. Notwithstanding improvements, many American intellectuals referred to the American Indians as a "vanishing race." By 1920, the population of American Indians reached its nadir at fewer than 250,000. Left unchecked, poor health conditions among the Indians may well have made a reality of the "vanishing race" theory.[34]

## Tuberculosis and Trachoma

Although outbreaks of diseases such as smallpox were infrequent by 1900, tuberculosis and trachoma increased, with tuberculosis galvanizing the attention of the medical world toward the end of the nineteenth century. Medical anthropologist Washington Matthews brought to the attention of the medical establishment the causes and incidence rates of the disease. But it was Inspector William McConnell who led the charge that forced the Indian Service to address the issue. While examining the Indian school at San Carlos (Apache), Arizona Territory, McConnell lamented the fact that government schools were filled at all costs. Students "are superficially examined and others not," McConnell wrote to Secretary Ethan Allen Hitchcock in July 1899. "Tuberculosis frequently develops, and apparently for no other reason than to maintain a full attendance, [students] are kept until the last stage is reached, when to prevent a death occurring at the school, they are carted home, to their tepe (sic), where in some instances even a few days suffices to bring the end. In this manner the disease is disseminated among the pupils in the schools, and the few days they occupy the home tepe may be, and no doubt is, frequently the cause of the other members of the family becoming affected."[35]

Visiting the Blackfeet in Montana, McConnell found that two and often three children shared a single bed—with one pillow. "No child sleeps alone," McConnell informed Hitchcock in June 1901. "Among the children thus packed away are sandwiched in cases of both pulmonary and lymphatic tuberculosis." Out of 15 Shoshone boys sent to Carlisle Indian School, 11 died there or soon after arriving at home. "The word murder is a fearful word," the inspector wrote, "but yet the transfer of pupils and subjecting them to such tearful mortality is little less."[36]

Bureaucracy compounded matters. Once assigned to an agency, physicians were usually at odds with the Indian agent or superintendent who controlled the dispensation of medical supplies and the purse. Drugs ought to be selected by physicians, not the agents, Dr. Breen of Fort Lewis, Colorado, wrote to commissioner William Jones in 1898, and the agent "should not be allowed to interpose his opinion against the opinion of the medical supervisor." Furthermore, the dispensing of medicine required "an intelligent physician" with the support of a medical division. Joseph G. Bullock, physician at Oneida Indian School near Green Bay, Wisconsin, sought to formalize an Indian medical service in 1898, pointing to the deplorable health conditions as justification. Jones disagreed and the movement withered away.[37]

Indian Service regulations reflected little concern for healthcare. In the 1884 departmental regulations, the Indian Service made no mention of medical matters. With charges of school overcrowding and admitting contagious students placed at his feet, Jones was forced to act. In an education circular sent to all Indian agencies and schools, Jones declared war upon "dust, filth, foul odors, and all disease breeding spots." Schools were to be filled to capacity, but "with sound and healthy children. There must, most positively, be *no overcrowding* in the dormitories to the detriment of the children sleeping in them. If you have an insufficient number of healthy children to fill up your school, do not place any more therein."[38]

Jones in 1903 ordered Indian Service physicians to make detailed statistical reports on the conditions of adult Indians, students returned from off-reservation schools, and the local non-Indian population. Physicians noted death rates, conditions of buildings in relation to disease, and other pertinent information that might influence the health and well-being of American Indians. In initiating the first comprehensive health survey, Jones discovered conditions were worse than supposed. Tuberculosis was more pronounced among American Indians than non-Indians, even though most Indians lived in regions of the country that were healthful and believed to be unfavorable for the development of the disease.[39]

With the study in hand, Jones sent another circular letter to all Indian school and agency personnel outlining additional regulations designed to improve Indian health. Students were to be examined by physicians before admittance to Indian schools. Any child with symptoms of tuberculosis was prohibited from enrolling. To prevent the spread of tuberculosis, Jones ordered school superintendents to clean dormitories and ensure that they received adequate sunlight. Physicians were to provide weekly talks to students on personal hygiene and treat all optical ailments.

To implement these regulations, Jones proposed converting a non-reservation school, "favorably situated as to climate and hygienic conditions," into a sanitarium school for tubercular children. In 1905, commissioner Francis Leupp recommended constructing the sanitarium in the Southwest, eventually selecting a site adjacent to Phoenix Indian School in Arizona Territory.[40] Leupp moved deliberately in attacking Indian health challenges, although it was not until 1908 that he exhibited any meaningful interest in the campaign against tuberculosis. From that point onward tuberculosis was foremost on his agenda due to "its fatal nature threaten[ing] to decimate the tribes."[41]

Leupp in 1908 dispatched Elsie E. Newton to prepare an exhibit at the Sixth Annual Tuberculosis Congress in Washington, D.C. Concurrently, the Smithsonian Institute detailed Dr. Ales Hrdlicka to survey tuberculosis among the Indian tribes. The morbidity and mortality rates among the Indians, Hrdlicka reported to the Tuberculosis Congress, "exceed by far those among the whites generally, and their average exceeds the very high rate among the American negroes." The causes were familiar: overcrowded homes and schools, spitting, poverty, undernourishment, and even milk from tubercular cows. Phoenix Indian School demonstrated the seriousness of the matter. Twenty-eight Tohono O'odham students enrolled at the school in 1907 after a physician's examination showed they were in good health. By the following July, five returned home with symptoms of tuberculosis, with two succumbing to the disease.[42]

A year later Leupp ordered a medical survey of Haskell Indian School. As in nearly all Indian schools, Haskell dormitories were overcrowded, poorly lighted, and inadequately ventilated. "The people slept two, three, or more in single beds. Both pulmonary and glandular cases [of tuberculosis] were found occupying beds with supposedly healthy pupils." Students shared towels and drinking cups, and a lack of fresh air in the dormitories was "the rule rather than the exception. No attention was paid to decayed teeth and tooth brushes were not regularly used or their use insisted upon. Spitting on the floor was a common occurrence."[43] Leupp recognized that if such conditions existed at Haskell, one of the top Indian schools in the nation, they likely permeated the entire Indian school system.

Diagnosing the prevalence of tuberculosis at Haskell was the key to focusing Indian Service attention on the health conditions of all schools, with the report serving as the impetus for the campaign against tuberculosis. The Indian Service ordered all infected students to return home and then isolated and monitored all suspected tubercular cases. Leupp ordered dorms to be ventilated and forbade administrators to place more than one student to a bed. The new regulations immediately took effect throughout the Indian Service.

Leupp employed Joseph A. Murphy, a tuberculosis expert, to conduct the investigation at Haskell. Leupp was so impressed with Murphy that he appointed him as the Indian Service's first chief medical supervisor in 1908. He then established a medical division to coordinate the fight against disease. Leupp charged Murphy with finding ways to combat the scourge of tuberculosis and other infectious diseases. Addressing the National Education Association later that year, Murphy asked whether the United States was "guilty of criminal negligence" for not doing more to prevent the spread of tuberculosis. Acknowledging that the Sixth International Congress on Tuberculosis had awakened the public as to the seriousness of the disease, Murphy now reminded Indian Service teachers, matrons, disciplinarians, and superintendents that their duties went further than "the mental welfare of the child." It included "an interest in the[ir] physical welfare also."[44]

Murphy and three assistants spent a year inspecting schools throughout Indian Country. The old policy of sending diseased children home, where they almost always died, was not "ideal." Leupp, prompted by Murphy, saw to the construction of screened porches to house tubercular children at several Indian school hospitals, a policy that his successor Robert G. Valentine continued. Leupp also established tubercular hospital camps at Colville, Washington, and Laguna, New Mexico. Valentine initiated an educational campaign to further "a more intelligent comprehension of disease by the children themselves." The challenges of dealing with disease were so acute that from 1908 on all commissioners prominently highlighted health matters in their *Annual Report*.[45]

Trachoma was also a concern to the Indian Service. In a letter sent to Leupp in 1909, U.S. Surgeon General Walter Wyman explained that the "increasing prevalence of trachoma in the United States (had) attracted widespread attention ... and because of the continuance of this disease and the seriousness of its sequel it must be regarded as a distinct menace to the public health." To deal with trachoma, Leupp moved quickly, seeking funds from Congress, which appropriated $12,000 for treatment and prevention. Due to the rising prevalence of trachoma in the Southwest, Leupp established a trachoma hospital at the Phoenix Indian School and staffed it with a trachoma specialist. By 1911, more than 700 cases of trachoma were treated.[46]

Two trachoma specialists in Phoenix visited Indian schools and agencies in the Southwest while a third was responsible for tribes in the Pacific Northwest. By the end of 1909, the specialists examined nearly 20,000 American Indians for trachoma, with 20 percent afflicted with the disease. To mitigate the outbreak, Congress appropriated $40,000 in 1910, "to relieve distress among the Indians and to provide for their care and for the prevention and treatment of tuberculosis, trachoma, smallpox and other infectious and contagious diseases." This first general appropriation for Indian health enabled the Indian Service to take its first meaningful steps in the fight against tuberculosis and trachoma.[47]

A U.S. Public Health Service survey of Indian Country in 1913 confirmed what some members of Congress refused to believe. The Public Health Service reported tuberculosis rates in Indian Country ranging from 32.7 percent of the Pyramid Lake Paiute to 1.3 percent of New York Indians, with a national Indian trachoma rate of 22.7 percent. American Indians were dreadfully ill with no relief in sight. It was time for Congress to reckon with poor Indian health conditions. A $90,000 appropriation for Indian healthcare in 1913 more than doubled to $200,000 in 1914.[48] With increased appropriations, Commissioner Cato Sells (who replaced Valentine in 1913) pushed forward the campaign to improve Indian healthcare.

To control the spread of disease, especially trachoma and tuberculosis, the Public Health Service recommended the construction of hospital facilities on reservations. The removal of Indian patients to off-reservation facilities was ill-advised, both to prevent the spread of disease to off-reservation communities and to limit climatic changes that often compounded matters. More nurses and specialists were needed to provide home treatment and instruction to those unable to visit agency hospitals or dispensaries.[49] With political support in Congress aided by the Public Health Service, the number of Indian hospitals, which stood at 48 in 1913, increased to 87 by 1920.

Beyond the fight against tuberculosis and trachoma, foremost on Sells' list of goals was reducing infant mortality. Sells continued the "Save the Babies" campaign initiated by Valentine and instituted a corollary measure known as "Swat the Fly."[50] He made the primacy of the "Save the Babies" campaign clear in his address before the Congress on Indian Progress. "It is our duty to protect the Indian's health and to save him from premature death," the commissioner stressed.

> Before we educate him, before we conserve his property, we should save his life. If he is to be perpetuated, we must care for the children. We must stop the tendency of the Indian to diminish in number, and restore a condition that will ensure his increase. Every Indian hospital bed not necessarily occupied with those suffering from disease or injury should be available for the mother in childbirth. It is of first importance that we begin by reestablishing the health and constitution of Indian children. Education and protection of property are highly important, but everything is secondary to the basic condition which makes for the perpetuation of the race.[51]

In another circular letter sent to every Indian Service employee, the commissioner outlined the fundamental purpose of the program. "No race," Sells stressed, "was ever created for utter extinction." The Indian problem could not be solved without Indians and Indians could not be educated unless they were kept healthy. The goal of the Indian Service was to perpetuate "an enduring and sturdy race" and this meant beginning with the "unborn generation." With 60 percent of all Indian infants dying prior to their fifth birthday, Sells asked: "Of what use to this mournful mortality are our splendidly equipped schools?" Sells challenged Indian Service employees to "redouble [their] energy and zeal throughout the service, for it means personal work and tireless patience." With the increased attention focused on infant mortality, Sells remarked in 1917 that "the Indian is no longer a vanishing race."[52] Despite a decreasing infant mortality rate, infant diseases remained high among American Indians, as seen in Table 1.3.

The entrance of the United States into World War One restricted, reduced, and, in some cases, repealed the fight against disease. The war effort devastated the Indian medical service, with 40 percent of all medical positions vacant. The end of the war brought inflation and an overall reduction in Indian health appropriations, hampering long-term advancements in the campaign against disease. If the war alone diverted Indian medical resources it would have been significant. But added to the war-time reductions was the worldwide influenza epidemic of 1918-1919, which struck especially hard in the American Southwest. Out of an Indian population of 304,854, there were 73,651 cases of influenza, with 6,270 Indians (more than 2 percent of the Indian population) dying. The combination of war-time vacancies in the Indian medical service and the devastating influenza epidemic reduced the progress made in the campaign against disease. Every Indian Service trachoma specialist was reassigned to combat the influenza outbreak, leaving trachoma work unattended.

Table 1.3

*Infant Mortality Among American Indians: 1914-1920*

| Year | Births | Deaths | Under Three | Percent Under Three |
|------|--------|--------|-------------|---------------------|
| 1914 | 6,964 | 5,778 | 2,391 | 41 |
| 1915 | 6,542 | 5,632 | 1,897 | 33 |
| 1916 | 6,092 | 4,570 | 1,303 | 28 |
| 1917 | 5,340 | 4,494 | 1,379 | 30 |
| 1918 | 5,571 | 4,682 | 1,541 | 32 |
| 1919 | 6,344 | 9,462* | 1,644 | 17 |
| 1920 | 6,510 | 6,070 | 1,436 | 23 |
| Totals | 42,868 | 40,788 | 11,591 | 28 |

*Increase due to outbreak of influenza in 1918-1919

(Source: *Tuberculosis Among the North American Indians*, 1921)

## Efforts to Transfer the Indian Medical Service into the Public Health Service

Not entirely the result of their own doing (Congress controlled the purse), the Indian medical service, and the Indian Service in general, was vulnerable to criticism, with some critics charging the Service with being "stupid or venal, or both." Otis O. Benson, a former Indian Service physician, declared "open season" on the Indian Service by opining in the American Medical Association that limited pay, inadequate equipment, unclear and convoluted channels of authority, and Indian resistance to medical advice, combined with Congressional parsimony, limited the success of the medical program. Other critics were less kind. "There is," Frederick L. Hoffman of the Prudential Insurance Company wrote in the *Journal of the American Medical Association*, "broadly speaking, no Indian health service, and very little is done to prevent occurrences of disease."[53] Hoffman advocated the immediate transfer of the Indian medical service into the Public Health Service.

An increasingly conservative Congress, mindful of the critics and their charges, and looking for ways to economize government activities and spending, considered a transfer in 1919. In September, the House Committee on Indian Affairs opened hearings on the proposed transfer. Only by integrating the Indian medical service with the Public Health Service, conventional wisdom held, could efficiency be attained and the first steps in the final assimilation of the Indians be accomplished.[54]

While Congress was keen on the idea of consolidation, neither the Indian

Service nor the Public Health Service favored or endorsed such a plan. Surgeon General Robert Blue, while acknowledging such a transfer should eventually occur, opposed consolidation on the grounds that it would be difficult to secure competent physicians to fill the needs of the Indian medical service. Of greater concern was the isolation of most reservations, particularly in the West. Blue did not wish to inherit what he viewed as a political liability and a logistical nightmare. A more immediate consideration for Blue was the medical care of returning World War One veterans. American servicemen were overwhelming the Public Health Service and, as enfranchised citizens, were of "more importance." Congressman Carl Hayden (D-AZ), a member of the Committee on Indian Affairs, emphasized nothing should disturb the Public Health Service in caring for the troops. Clinging to arguments of cultural inferiority, Blue placed culpability for the high incidence of disease in Indian Country on the strange practices and habits of the Indians.[55]

The Indian Service also opposed consolidation. Medical Director Robert E. Lee Newberne, recognizing it "would be pleasing" to be associated with the Public Health Service, argued healthcare was too closely allied with the educational and social goals of the Indian Service to warrant such action. Unless Congress was prepared to turn the whole department over to the Public Health Service, Newberne opined, the move was ill-advised. Commissioner of Indian Affairs Cato Sells concurred, suggesting that any talk of consolidation was a "radical variance" with standard administrative practices. If the Public Health Service were to assume responsibility for Indian health, Sells opined, it would do no better than the Indian medical service unless "additional appropriations were made." The bottom line, the commissioner rationalized, was that the Indians were in a "critical transformation period" of evolving from one "social plain to another" and only the Indian Service was equipped to manage this transformation.[56]

The medical establishment and Indian medical service critics did not waver in their desire to effect the transfer. Hoffman argued the transfer called for "the highest considerations of Indian policy" because there was "no health service worthy of the name" in Indian Country. Hoffman was vociferous in his critique of the Indian medical service, calling it "as deplorable as it was disgraceful" and "the most regrettable apathy on the part of the nation which has assumed responsibility for the medical needs of the Indian population." Reformer John Collier and the American Indian Defense Association, an organization dedicated to the protection of Indian rights, also supported the transfer, eyeing it as the means of improving care. Haven Emerson labeled the Indian medical service "the most disgraceful apology for scientific or humane medical care" in the nation.[57]

The House Committee on Indian Affairs debated the matter on several occasions and, in January of 1921, opined the Indian medical service did "exactly the same activities" as the Public Health Service, except it was nowhere "as efficient as [it] would be if transferred to the Public Health Service." Not only would the transfer improve the delivery of healthcare, the committee asserted, but it would also economize government and provide a more "competent authority" to direct the health services for Indians. Homer Snyder (D-NY), chairman of the

House Committee on Indian Affairs, saw practical reasons to integrate the two medical programs. Foremost among these was economy. That it would hasten assimilation and reduce the need for Indian-only appropriations was a strong underlying rationale. While the Committee favorably reported on the transfer bill, the House as a whole took no action and the effort died.[58] Nonetheless, the Public Health Service began detailing medical officers and supervisors to the Indian medical service in 1926, continuing the practice up to the Indian Transfer Act of 1954.

## New Efforts to Consolidate with the Public Health Service

It was fifteen years before the transfer issue again reached a level of political discussion. Chief Medical Supervisor James Townsend, detailed from the Public Health Service in 1933, faced difficulties in battling tuberculosis and trachoma in Indian Country. Townsend urged Commissioner of Indian Affairs John Collier, who in 1920 supported the transfer, to act. Transferring the Indian medical service into the Public Health Service was the only viable way to improve healthcare for American Indians and Alaska Natives, for whom the Indian Service assumed responsibility in 1931. In a 1936 letter to Collier, Townsend outlined his rationale for the transfer. As the relationship between the several states and the newly renamed Division of Indian Health grew more amicable, and as the allocation of federal funding under New Deal legislation such as the Johnson-O'Malley Act and the Social Security Act increased and provided the states and private sector an incentive to cooperate with the health program, now was the time to chart the course of Indian health policy. A professional career health organization for physicians and nurses such as the Public Health Service would attract and retain more qualified personnel.

Townsend believed the Indian Service could continue its existing relationship, with the Public Health Service exercising supervisory control over the Division of Indian Health, as it had done since 1926. On the other hand, the Indian Service could terminate its relationship with the Public Health Service and operate independently. To Townsend and other similarly-minded medical professionals, however, there was a third, preferable option: merge the two agencies, with the Public Health Service given control over the operation of the Division of Indian Health.[59]

Townsend informed Collier that it was not advisable to continue the then-existing structure of Public Health Service supervisory control. The most telling reason was that detailing Public Health Service officials to the Indian Service and granting them supervisory authority over Indian health personnel degraded the morale of Division of Indian Health employees. As long as the Public Health Service supervised the Indian medical service, "deserving physicians" would be hindered from any advancement to supervisory positions. Furthermore, because Public Health Service medical officers frequently transferred out of Indian hospitals to meet the exigencies of Public Health Service hospitals, stability and an intimate understanding of Indian health needs was impossible. On the other hand, the Indian Service was unable to provide adequate staffing on its own. As long as the Public Health Service administered oversight, Indian Service physicians could not expect to gain such training, leaving the agency in a perpetual state of dependency. This was unwise. To withdraw the support of the Public Health Service could imperil Indian health and foster another government organization that would parallel the Public Health Service. "This policy is not sound," Townsend opined, "and it is extremely doubtful whether the Indian Medical Service could ever in reality be a career service." If the relationship were severed, the Division of Indian Health would continue as a non-career organization unable to compete with the Public Health Service for personnel.[60]

The only option was a complete integration and merger of the Division of Indian Health with the Public Health Service. While the former lacked much, the latter was an established public health service "well equipped through tradition and appropriations for conducting adequate clinical service and a high standard of public health work and research." The Public Health Service could provide staff with a better chance of promotion and with salaries commensurate with their duties. But most importantly, Townsend promised better medical care for American Indians and Alaska Natives. Fewer services would be contracted out, as Indians utilized Public Health Service hospitals where service in Indian hospitals was not available.[61]

Both Townsend and the critics recognized there would be "differences and misunderstandings" within both agencies if a transfer were effected. This was inherent in any government consolidation. Nonetheless, Townsend encouraged Collier to initiate the transfer as "expeditiously as possible." If Collier needed a precedent, one existed. The Indian Service had once been in the War Department, but in 1849 had transferred to the Interior Department.

While Collier supported integration in 1920, he did not share Townsend's sentiments in 1936. The difference between then and now, Collier opined, was that the Indian Service had authority under New Deal legislation to contract services with state agencies. By pooling resources with the states, Collier argued, comprehensive healthcare could be provided for both the Indian and non-Indian population, fulfilling a Congressional desire for both economy and integration.[62] Collier hoped to leverage federal resources for Indian healthcare into a cooperative relationship with state health departments to improve Indian health services.

In a letter to Interior Secretary Harold Ickes, Collier opposed the transfer, urging the secretary to grant the Indian Service authority to employ its own chief and medical directors—outside the administration of the Public Health Service. Ickes concurred with Collier and, in a letter to President Franklin Roosevelt, supported the position that Indian Service, rather than Public Health Service, medical officers administer the Division of Indian Health. Collier found allies in Ickes and Roosevelt and fended off further integrative action. As war clouds appeared on the horizon, further discussion of a transfer vanished.[63]

In February of 1941, Townsend was recalled by the Public Health Service and, in April, was replaced by J. R. McGibony, who had been detailed to the Indian Service in 1937 as a hospital administrator. Neither McGibony nor Congress addressed the transfer issue until after World War Two. In 1947, Fred Foard, new director of the Division of Indian Health, and Congress again considered the propriety of a transfer. By then both Collier and Ickes were out of office and Congress contemplated the termination of all federal services to Indians. The Congressional desire to terminate the Indian medical service did not wane until the transfer into the Public Health Service was complete in 1955.[64]

# Notes

1. Virgil J. Vogel, *American Indian Medicine* (Norman: University of Oklahoma Press, 1970), 13; Henry F. Dobyns, *Their Number Became Thinned* (Knoxville: University of Tennessee Press, 1983), 275-276; Alfred W. Crosby, *The Columbian Exchange* (Westport, CT: Greenwood Publishing Company, 1972), 40; Russell Thornton, *American Indian Holocaust and Survival: A Population History Since 1492* (Norman: University of Oklahoma Press, 1987), 61-90, 497, and 505.

2. Herman J. Viola, *Diplomats in Buckskins: A History of Indian Delegations in Washington City* (Bluffton, North Carolina: Rivilo Press, 1995), 152-167.

3. "An Act making provisions for the civilization of the Indian tribes adjoining the frontier settlements," 3 Stat. 516 (1819). Ruth M. Raup, *The Indian Health Program 1800-1955* (Washington, D.C.: United States Department of Health, Education and Welfare, Public Health Service, 1959), 1.

4. *Tuberculosis among the North American Indians* (Washington, D.C.: Government Printing Office, 1923), 93. *Annual Report of the Commissioner of Indian Affairs*, 1892, (Washington, D.C.: Government Printing Office, 1893) 299 (hereafter *Annual Report*). "The Indian Service Health Activities" (Office of Indian Affairs, Bulletin 11), 1922. Grant Foreman, *Indian Removal* (Norman: University of Oklahoma Press, 1932), 110, 184-185 and 222-223. Foreman notes that out of 1,600 Creeks who left for the Indian Territory on March 20, 1837, 177 died by August 1.

5. "An Act to provide the means of extending the benefits of vaccination, as a preventive of smallpox, to the Indian tribes, and thereby, as far as possible, to save them from the destructive ravages of that disease," 4 Stat. 514 (1832).

6. Elbert Herring to Lewis Cass, January 31, 1833, in "Letter from the Secretary of War, transmitting a report of the Commissioner of Indian Affairs in relation to the execution of the act extending the benefit of Vaccination to the Indian Tribes, &c," February 2, 1833, *House Document 82*, 22nd Congress, 2nd session. Many of the vaccine points arrived out-of-date, requiring the agents to purchase new points. "Small Pox among the Indians, Letter from the Secretary of War on the Subject of the Small Pox among the Indians," *House Document 51*, 25th Congress, 3rd session. Commissioner of Indian Affairs T. Hartley Crawford wrote to Secretary J. R. Poinsett on December 14, 1838, that smallpox had yet to be arrested on the Upper Missouri River due, in his estimation, to

apathy on the part of the Indians. There were 10,145 vaccinations distributed as follows: Sioux 3,000; Potawatomie and Miami 86; Indians of Illinois 513; Sioux 665; Osage 2,177; Shawnee and Kickapoo 1,645; Chippewa and Ottawa 2,070. *House Document 82*, 22nd Congress, 2nd session, 4. Cass sent a circular letter to all Indian agents in Illinois and Michigan requiring them to explain the vaccination process to the Indians, a feat that required "some time and perseverance."

7. Most treaties asserted federal protection of tribes in exchange for land or a pledge by tribes to not engage in political intercourse with other foreign states. This has generally been interpreted to mean that the United States would provide the means to preserve the health of the Indians. This fiduciary responsibility is supported by federal court rulings and legislation and is the basis of the federal Indian trust responsibility.

8. "Articles of a Treaty made and concluded at Fort Armstrong, Rock Island, Illinois, between the United States of America and the Winnebago Nation of Indians, September 15, 1832," 7 Stat. 370, at 372.

9. *Ratified Treaties 1854-1855*, RG 75, T-494, National Archives and Research Administration, Roll 5.

10. "Treaty between the United States of America and the Nez Perce Indians concluded at Camp Stevens in the Walla-Walla Valley, June 11, 1855," 12 Stat. 957. *Ratified Treaties, 1856-1863*, RG 75, T-494, roll 6.

11. "Treaty between the United States of America and the Cheyenne and Arapaho Tribes of Indians concluded October 28, 1867," 15 Stat. 593.

12. J. G. Townsend, "Indian Health-Past, Present and Future," in Oliver LaFarge, Ed. *The Changing Indian*, (Norman: University of Oklahoma Press, 1942), 30.

13. *Tuberculosis among the North American Indians*, Report of a Committee of the National Tuberculosis Association (Washington, D.C.: Government Printing Office, 1923), 93.

14. "Condition of the Indian Tribes: Report of the Joint Special Committee appointed under Joint Resolution of March 3, 1865," 39th Congress, 2nd Session, *Senate Report 156*, (Washington D.C.: Government Printing Office, 1867), 3-4.

15. *Annual Report*, 1877, 94. *Annual Report*, 1879, 9.

16. *Annual Report*, 1878, 79.

17. *Annual Report*, 1879, 9.

18. *Annual Report*. 1890, xxi.

19. *Annual Report*. 1888, xxxv.

20. *Tuberculosis among the North American Indians*, 95.

21. Prior to this time a number of temporary hospitals had been established. "The Indian Service Health Activities," 2.

22. *Annual Report*, 1884, 81.

23. *Annual Report*, 1889, 14. *Annual Report*, 1890, xxii.

24. *Annual Report*, 1892, 63.

25. *Annual Report*, 1894, 290.

26. *Annual Report*, 1893, 344.

27. *Annual Report*, 1899, 249.

28. Robert A. Trennert, "White Man's Medicine vs. Hopi Tradition: The Smallpox Epidemic of 1899," *Journal of Arizona History* (33:4, Winter 1992), 349-366.

29. McConnell to Secretary of Interior, February 20, 1899, Office of the Secretary of

Interior, Official Letters of W. J. McConnell, RG 75.

30. *Annual Report*, 1905, 404.

31. *Tuberculosis among the North American Indians*, 8.

32. *Tuberculosis among the North American Indians*, 10.

33. Warren K. Moorehead, *The American Indians in the United States: 1850-1914* (Freeport, NY: Books for Liberty Press, 1969 reprint edition of the 1914 original), 265.

34. Thornton, *American Indian Holocaust*, 101, notes that "some scholars have argued that because of vaccinations late 19th century American Indians felt the effects of smallpox less than adjacent populations of non-Indians." Thornton adds that latter nineteenth-century outbreaks were "for the most part" localized outbreaks.

35. Washington Matthews, "Consumption Among the Indians," *Transactions of the American Climatological Association*, 1886, 234-241. Matthews, "Further Contribution to the Study of Consumption Among the Indians," ibid., 136-155. McConnell to Secretary Hitchcock, July 29, 1899. Office of Indian Affairs, Official Letters of W. J. McConnell, U.S. Indian Inspector, RG 48.

36. McConnell to Hitchcock, June 17, 1901, Office of the Secretary of the Interior, Indian Division, Indian Inspection Reports, Blackfeet, RG 48. McConnell to Hitchcock, July 5, 1901, Office of the Secretary of the Interior, Appointments Division, Indian Inspectors, W. J. McConnell, RG 48.

37. Report of William Jones to Secretary Bliss, *Annual Report*, 1898, 341. *Annual Report*, "Report of the Superintendent of Indian Schools," 1898, 340-341.

38. *Regulation for the Indian Department*, (Washington, D.C.: Government Printing Office, 1884), 97-99. *Annual Report*, 1894, 89-92. Education Circular no. 102, September 21, 1903. Circular no. 85, dated November 6, 1902, (RG 75, M1121, Office of Indian Affairs, Circulars, roll 9) directed off-reservation schools to admit only "sound and healthy children." A physician's certificate was to accompany each student before they could be admitted to school. Emphasis in the original.

39. *Annual Report*, 1904, 33-38. Hrdlicka, "Tuberculosis among Certain Indian Tribes in the United States," Bureau of American Ethnology, Bulletin 42 (Washington, D.C.: Government Printing Office, 1909), 4.

40. Francis E. Leupp, "Outlines of an Indian Policy," *Outlook* (79, April 15, 1905), 946-950. *Annual Report*, 1905, 1-15.

41. Francis Paul Prucha, *The Great Father: The United States Government and the American Indians*, Volume II (Lincoln: University of Nebraska Press, 1984), 847.

42. Hrdlicka visited the Menominee, Oglala Sioux, Quinault, Hoopa and Mojave, in addition to Phoenix Indian School. "Fighting the White Plague," *Annual Report*, 1908, 24. Hrdlicka, "Tuberculosis among Certain Indian Tribes of the United States," 8, 17, 25-26, 33-36. Hrdlicka provides a rather extensive bibliography on tuberculosis among the Indians (37-43).

43. Hrdlicka, "Tuberculosis among the North American Indians," 97.

44. Joseph F. Murphy, "The Prevention of Tuberculosis in the Indian Schools," *Journal of Proceedings and Addresses of the Forty-Seventh Annual Meeting*, (Winona, MN: National Education Association, Secretary's Office, 1909), 919-924. Murphy lamented the tendency of the schools to "handle the mass rather the individual," a practice that frequently neglected Indian welfare. Improved selection and inspection of dairy products, more fresh

air in dormitories, and proper ventilation and disinfecting of the schools were essential.

45. Murphy, *Manual on Tuberculosis: Its Causes, Prevention and Treatment*, (Washington, D.C.: Government Printing Office, 1910). Valentine, in the 1909 *Annual Report* (5-6), outlined the following "line of attack." Better nourishment; improved sanitary conditions; complete sterilization of dishes; revised methods of sweeping and dusting; fumigation of all schools and books; establishment of a traveling health exhibit; a course on physical development and healthcare; distribution of a pamphlet on tuberculosis prevention and cure; establishment of tuberculosis camps; and more sanitary homes for Indians with proper ventilation.

46. "Trachoma in Certain Indian Schools," *Senate Report no. 1025*, 60th Congress, second session, 1909, 2. "An Act for the Investigation, Treatment, and Prevention of Trachoma among the Indians," February 20, 1909, 35 stat. 642 (1909).

47. 36 Stat. 271. Not everyone was satisfied with the appropriations. Moorehead, *The American Indian in the United States*, 267, noted "there is no earthly excuse why instead of three or four, there should not be fifteen or twenty doctors on every reservation. There is no reason why our rich, powerful Government does not appropriate two to three million dollars a year to put an end to the miseries we ourselves have introduced."

48. "Contagious and Infectious Diseases among the Indians," *Senate Document no. 1038*, 62nd Congress, third session, (Washington, D.C.: Government Printing Office, 1913), 81. For fiscal year 1915 Congress appropriated $100,000 for the construction of six hospitals—one each among the Blackfeet, Turtle Mountain Chippewa, Mescalero Apache and Pima and one near Tucson, Arizona, and Carson, Nevada. An additional $10,000 was set aside to equip the old Fort Spokane military reservation with an Indian hospital. Plans were made to build hospitals on the Red Lake and Fond du Lac reservations in Minnesota, and within the Choctaw Nation, Oklahoma (to be built using Choctaw-Chickasaw tribal funds). "Letter from the Secretary of the Interior (Franklin Lane) to the House Committee on Indian Affairs," *House Document 1254*, 63rd Congress, 2nd session, 1-2. The appropriation was provided for in the 1915 Indian Appropriation Act, 38 Stat. 582.

49. "Contagious and Infectious Diseases among the Indians," 82-84. For a list of Indian hospitals operating in 1912, see "Report of the Joint Commission on Indian Tuberculosis Sanitarium and Yakima Indian Reservation Project," *House Document 505*, 63rd Congress, 2nd session, exhibit c, 19-20.

50. Circular no. 707, November 9, 1912 (supplemented January 6, 1914) and Circular no. 1263, February 15, 1917, RG 75, M1121, Office of Indian Affairs, Circulars, rolls 10-11.

51. *Annual Report*, 1916, 4.

52. *Annual Report*, 1916, 7. *Annual Report*, 1917, 19. Hrdlicka, in "The Vanishing Indian," *Science* (46:1185, September 14, 1917), 266-267, observed that the "genuine Indian is rapidly passing away," and thus was vanishing. The Indians, however, were beginning to increase in number, as shown by the 1920 census.

53. Elinor D. Gregg, *The Indian and the Nurse* (Norman: University of Oklahoma Press, 1965), 92. Otis O. Benson, M.D., "Conditions in the Indian Medical Service," *Journal of the American Medical Association* (81:16, October 20, 1923), 1381-1382. Frederick L. Hoffman, "Conditions in the Indian Medical Service," *Journal of the American Medical Association*, (75:7, August 14, 1920), 493-494.

54. "Indians of the United States: Hearings before the Committee on Indian Affairs on the Condition of Various Tribes of Indians," 66th Congress, 1st session (Washington, D.C.: Government Printing Office, 1919), 46-66.

55. "Indians of the United States: Hearings before the Committee on Indian Affairs on the Condition of Various Tribes of Indians," 46 and 53.

56. "Indians of the United States: Hearings before the Committee on Indian Affairs on the Condition of Various Tribes of Indians," 57. "Reorganizing the Indian Service," *House Report no. 1189*, 66th Congress, 3rd session, (Washington, D.C.: Government Printing Office, 1919), 3.

57. Hoffman, 493-494. Hoffman criticized the lack of pharmacists, inadequate dental care, no eye specialists and inadequate pay. The government had a treaty obligation—or at a minimum a "human obligation," to provide adequate healthcare. "Conditions in the Indian Medical Service," *Journal of the American Medical Association*, 81:10 (September 8, 1923), 848-849. Haven Emerson, "Morbidity of the American Indians," *Science* 68:1626 (1926), 229-231.

58. "Reorganizing the Indian Service: Report of the Committee on Indian Affairs," *House Report no. 1278*, 68th Congress, 1st Session, February 1, 1921 (Washington, D.C.: Government Printing Office, 1921). *House Report no. 1228*, January 25, 1921.

59. "A Statement Relative to the Past, Present and Future Medical Facilities Provided the Indians in the United States and the Natives of Alaska by the United States Government," *United States Code and Administrative News* (Washington, D.C.: Government Printing Office, 1954), 2932-2933.

60. "A Statement Relative to the Past, Present and Future Medical Facilities Provided the Indians in the United States and the Natives of Alaska by the United States Government," *United States Code and Administrative News* (Washington, D.C.: Government Printing Office, 1954), 2932-2933.

61. "A Statement Relative to the Past, Present and Future Medical Facilities Provided the Indians in the United States and the Natives of Alaska by the United States Government."

62. "Indian Conditions and Affairs: Hearings before the Subcommittee on General Bills of the Committee on Indian Affairs, House of Representatives," 74th Congress, 1st session, *House bill no. 7781*, (April 2, 1935), 743-746.

63. *House Report no. 870*, 83rd Congress, 1st session, in *United States Code and Administrative News* (Washington, D.C.: Government Printing Office, 1954), 2928.

64. *Indians at Work* (8:7, March 1941), 9. Townsend served as Director of Indian Health for eight years. For McGibony's career statistics see "New Director Appointed for Indian Medical Service," *Indians at Work* (8:10, June 1941), 9-10. McGibony graduated from the University of Georgia Medical School in 1927. "McGibony Named Director of Health of Indian Service," *Journal of the American Medical Association* (117:2, July 12, 1941), 974. With Collier's resignation in 1945 and Ickes' in 1946, the Indian Service lost its direction. Collier's successor, William Brophy, was absent on sick leave for much of his three-year tenure. Brophy's successor, John R. Nichols, served just one year before he, too, resigned. Consequently, between 1945 and 1950 control of the Indian Service passed to the Congress by default. In 1946, Congress began termination hearings.

# CHAPTER TWO

## Overcoming Generations of Neglect

In July 1953, a veteran cardiologist and internal medicine specialist named James "Ray" Shaw became director of the newly renamed Branch of Indian Health. At the time Shaw was a twenty-year Public Health Service Commissioned Corps Officer who had served as medical advisor on loan to the Indian Service and as Director of the Public Health Service's Division of Hospitals. As chief of the Indian medical service, Shaw concerned himself with integrating Indian health services with those of state and local governments. His foremost goal was to improve American Indian and Alaska Native health status, no small task for a people plagued by a "backlog of disease and disability accumulated through generations of neglect."[1]

To meet this goal, Shaw and Surgeon General Leonard A. Scheele aggressively advocated a transfer of the Indian health program into the Public Health Service where prospects for increased funding for hospital construction and services were available. Modernized and expanded medical facilities were essential if American Indians were to be given a fair chance to compete in the American economy. American Indians demanded an expanded public health program and access to a wider array of services. Shaw tired of Public Health Service officials being subordinate to Indian Service bureaucrats. If progress in the campaign against disease among the Indians was to be made, former director Fred Foard (1952-1954) and Shaw agreed, was it too much to expect that the Public Health Service staff delivering such care administer the health program?[2]

### Fostering the Transfer of Indian Health Services

Nearly every state and national medical organization favored the consolidation of the Branch of Indian Health with the Public Health Service, noting the latter had provided a variety of services for the former since the 1920s. In 1945, the Senate Committee on Indian Affairs, in a discussion on repealing the Indian Reorganization Act, which Commissioner of Indian Affairs John Collier had championed as the means of restoring the many positive attributes of Indian tribes, asked whether it would be advantageous for the Indian health program to be "part of a relief and welfare function appertaining to local government?" By 1953, Congress answered this question by calling for the termination of all federal programs for American Indians and creating the Department of Health, Education and Welfare.[3]

The cessation of World War II created a wave of conservatism and nationalism in the United States, adding momentum to the proposed transfer. Under President Harry Truman's Fair Deal, the executive branch considered ways to integrate, consolidate, and eliminate duplicative government programs. In 1948, Truman charged a federal commission with identifying ways to reduce government waste. Known as the Commission on the Organization of the Executive Branch of the Government and chaired by former President Herbert Hoover, the commission concluded state and local health authorities had to assume a greater responsibility for public health functions in Indian Country.[4]

The commission recommended Indian Service hospitals and physicians charge fees for services rendered to Indian patients. Furthermore, it encouraged greater use of contract physicians and utilization of off-reservation hospitals operated by the federal government, but only until state and local health authorities assumed responsibility for such care. More directly, the commission recommended Indian Service hospitals be converted into community hospitals as quickly as possible, an idea Interior Secretary Oscar Chapman supported as a means of reducing expenditures and improving services. Such a path would hasten the "gradual liquidation of [Indian Service] hospitals and the absorption of Indian patients into other Federal or non-Federal systems."[5]

Beginning in 1951, the Indian Service adopted the policy of not operating any hospital or clinic when care was available from state and local health facilities or where federal contracts for medical services under the authority of the Johnson-O'Malley Act could be consummated. Commissioner of Indian Affairs Dillon Myer enforced a policy of operating facilities only when Indians could not receive care elsewhere or could not receive care without being segregated. In effecting this policy, Myer closed the Fort Berthold Indian Hospital in August of 1951, and proposed closing seven more Indian hospitals in 1952. A year later, he negotiated a contract with the State of South Dakota providing for the transfer of public health and preventive services in Indian Country to that state.[6]

Acting on the advice of the Hoover Commission and the critical need for hospital services in rural America, both Houses of Congress considered bills calling for the construction of joint-use facilities. In 1949, Congressman Harold Patten (D-AZ) introduced HR 3635 authorizing non-Indians to use Indian Service hospitals. While supporting the concept of integrating Indian services, Chapman recommended several modifications, including protecting Indian priority to services at such facilities. When Congress enacted Public Law 291 in 1952, it incorporated Chapman's basic concerns and granted statutory authority to the secretary to transfer any Indian hospital to state or local agencies. It also gave the secretary authority, if the health needs of the Indians could be better served, to enter into contracts with any federal, state, or territorial government or political subdivision thereof for health facilities.[7]

Indians were given service priority over non-Indians in any hospital transferred to outside authorities. The admittance of non-Indian patients, while authorized, was permissible only where there were an insufficient number of local hospital beds or health facilities available. Moreover, access was permissible only if Indians were not utilizing such services. With the Indian Service seeking to economize and Congress granting legislative authority to close Indian hospitals, as well as the advent of the federal relocation policy that forced thousands of Indians from reservations to urban centers, Myer and his successor Glenn Emmons closed eight Indian hospitals between 1951 and 1955.[8]

Mindful of its ultimate desire to withdraw services, the Indian Service established a new office of public health services within the Branch of Indian Health. A trained public health physician was appointed to direct the activities of this office, which was designed to administer and develop programs aimed at terminating the federal government's Indian-only healthcare responsibilities. Among its duties, the new public health officer developed a comprehensive medical-dental program that incorporated provisions focused on effective tuberculosis control, which by 1956 consumed 40 percent of the Indian health budget. Shaw encouraged Congress to consider funding and authorizing environmental sanitation services as one means of combating tuberculosis.[9]

The fundamental goal of the public health program was to improve services to American Indians and Alaska Natives and then find ways to transfer those services (and responsibilities) to state and local agencies. Paralleling this goal was the aim of developing direct services from local agencies. In areas where such services were unavailable, the Indian Service agreed to provide them but only until state or local agencies assumed this responsibility. In some states, public health services were already provided under Johnson-O'Malley contracts, particularly in Wisconsin, Minnesota, and California. With nearly half of the Indians living in areas where local health services were either underdeveloped or nonexistent, the Indian Service had few options but to continue providing such care.[10]

By the 1950s, Congress was increasingly of the mind to radically restructure the federal-Indian relationship. When it adopted House Concurrent Resolution 108, in August of 1953, Congress called for termination of federal supervision for Indians "at the earliest possible time" and the abolition of all government facilities "whose primary purpose was to serve any Indian tribe or individual." With the passage of Public Law 83-280 that same month, Congress conferred jurisdiction on several states for criminal and civil offenses involving Indians in Indian Country. Although not directly related to healthcare, Public Law 280 and House Concurrent Resolution 108 established a Congressional intent of terminating federal responsibility for Indians, a proposition apparent in the divestiture of some Indian health responsibilities to state and local governments.[11]

The goal of transferring the Branch of Indian Health to the Public Health

Service was but one step toward the Congressional objective of divesting the Indian Service of all responsibility for American Indians and Alaska Natives. The Hoover Commission, which concerned itself with identifying the means of assimilating medical services into state and local health agencies, was an important impetus for change. But it was not the only agency, public or private, to recommend consolidation. The American Medical Association long favored consolidation and officials within the Public Health Service threatened the withdrawal of assistance unless they were given full control of the Indian medical service.[12]

World War II had an important effect in shaping the Indian policy of the mid-twentieth century. Thousands of American Indians served in the war, which transformed the United States into an economic and military powerhouse. But it also mistakenly convinced the federal government that American Indians desired and were prepared to have federal services terminated. As a result, the Indian Service prepared a number of reports on Indian progress prompting Congress to begin termination and the consolidation of services.

Congress enacted dozens of laws repealing and/or terminating federal laws related to American Indians in the early 1950s. In March of 1952, Congressman Walter Judd (R-MN) introduced HR 6908, which proposed transferring Indian health responsibilities and services to the Public Health Service. The following January, Senator Edward Thye (R-MN) introduced Senate Bill 132, which also called for the transfer of health services. These bills were the first consolidation proposals since 1919, when the House Committee on Indian Affairs held hearings on such a transfer.[13]

## The Indian Health Transfer Act

When the Senate concluded its fifteen-year, 23,000 page investigation of Indian affairs in 1943, the Committee on Indian Affairs voiced its support for transferring Indian hospitals to the Public Health Service. With Congress preoccupied with the war, the first bill calling for the transfer was not introduced until March 1947. Interior Secretary Julius Krug opposed the bill on the grounds the challenges of Indian administration were so closely related that it was imprudent to separate health services from other Indian services. The Bureau of the Budget and the Federal Security Administration also opposed the bill and it was never reported out of committee.[14]

In 1949, William P. Shepard, of the Metropolitan Life Insurance Company and former president of the National Tuberculosis Association and then-president of the American Public Health Association, began a sustained effort to bring about the transfer. Assisted by James E. Perkins, Managing Director of the National Tuberculosis Association, and Noble J. Swearington, Shepard obtained endorsements from most major health organizations in the country. Combined, these organizations applied sustained pressure on Congress to effect the transfer.

The American Medical Association, the American Public Health Association, the Association of State and Territorial Health Officers, the Governor's Interstate Council on Indian Affairs, the National Tuberculosis Association, and numerous state agencies all rallied behind the proposal. A number of Indian tribes, including the Minnesota Chippewa, and the National Congress of American Indians and the Association on American Indian Affairs, also supported the efforts of Shepard. In 1953, the House of Representatives approved Resolution 303, which recommended the transfer.[15]

Support for the move was premised on the belief that it would alleviate the chronic shortages in the physician and nursing corps of the Indian Service. In supporting the transfer, the Senate subcommittee pointed out that in 1953, there were sixty Indian hospitals staffed by just sixty-three Indian Service physicians. To fill the need, the Public Health Service detailed eighty physicians to the Branch of Indian Health. It was apparent the Indian Service had not overcome its long-standing shortage of personnel and likely would not without policy changes. On the other hand, the Public Health Service was a career organization that could offer what the Indian Service could not: professional growth, fewer and shorter details to isolated health centers, better benefits, and increased pay. The former would also be able to recruit physicians and nurses more effectively than the latter, simply because of its career status and its accredited health centers and hospitals. The Public Health Service also encouraged and provided for postgraduate health research opportunities and study.[16]

With such a transfer, the Public Health Service would assume direct medical supervision of the Indian health program, thereby eliminating the inevitable conflicts that arose when agency superintendents exercised administrative control over health matters. On the Navajo Nation, for instance, funds secured by the Branch of Indian Health to help fight tuberculosis were spent by the agency superintendent for a warehouse and community center instead. Moreover, transfer would enable the Public Health Service to function as a nationwide unit in accordance with professional evaluations of health needs and services and provide the Indian health program with leadership that was in tune with the challenges facing Indian Service physicians.[17]

As a professional and career organization, the Public Health Service was more likely to expand university relationships that would aid the campaign against poor health in Indian Country. Research into, and development of, preventive medicines would be more effectively hatched in the Public Health Service since it was single-mindedly focused on health issues. On the other hand, the Indian Service had never been able to focus on health issues, as it was concerned with Indian resources, land, education, and other trust responsibilities. The bottom line for Congress was economy and the elimination of service duplication, although there was a belief the Public Health Service would bring Indian healthcare up to an acceptable level.[18]

By turning responsibility for healthcare over to existing federal, state, and local agencies, the Congressional goal of terminating Indian-only services could begin. Since the Public Health Service administered grants-in-aid for public health work, it understood the capacity of state and local health agencies to provide services for American Indians and Alaska Natives. It was also in a position to know which state health programs were available and to what extent Indians were receiving services available to them as American citizens. As part of the new Department of Health, Education and Welfare, the Public Health Service also had direct access to other federal agencies that provided care under grants for maternal and child health, public assistance, and other health-related services.[19]

Support was not unanimous, as the departments of Interior and Health, Education and Welfare opposed it. While the House debated the bill in 1953, the Interior Department voiced its opposition. "The various service programs for Indians are so closely related," Assistant Secretary Orme Lewis wrote Congressman A. L. Miller (R-NE), "that it is deemed inadvisable to separate the administration of the health services from the administration of other services to Indians." The following year, Interior dropped its opposition to the transfer and threw its weight behind the measure after it was convinced the Public Health Service could attain health objectives more readily than the Indian Service. In a letter to Senator Hugh Butler (R-NE), chairman of the Committee on Interior and Insular Affairs, Lewis wrote of the department's changed view. "Such a transfer would place the program in a department where decisions having to do with health and welfare of people could be readily and expeditiously made without the time-consuming process of negotiation of such matters between separate departments with divergent primary responsibilities."[20]

The Department of Health, Education and Welfare continued to oppose the transfer. Secretary Oveta Culp Hobby in a letter to Butler argued there had been good progress in transferring Indian responsibilities to state and local governments. The transfer, Hobby opined, would "increase the difficulties of pursuing the policy of integrating the Indians." Hobby feared a new administrative structure would be created in the Public Health Service to deal with Indians as "separate and distinct," leading to confusion in an Indian policy advocating incorporation of the Indians into American society. "The transfer of responsibility in itself would not constitute the solution to the health problems of the Indians," Hobby argued. "These problems are difficult and deep seated, involving the geographic location, economic status, cultural and educational levels, and lack of social and political integration of this special segment of the Nation's population." The Bureau of the Budget also opposed the transfer, believing the move to be inconsistent with the intent of Congress to "integrate medical care for Indians with local health services."[21]

Numerous tribal councils and leaders opposed consolidation, fearing the liquidation of all federal services provided to Indians under treaty or legislative obligations. Francis Pipestem, Chairman of the Otoe Tribal Council, exhibited opposition representative of many tribal leaders when he opposed the transfer on the grounds the law did not "define the Federal responsibility for providing services to the Indians" and did not "authorize the Public Health Service [to] enter into agreements with the various tribes." Indian opposition, Congressman Judd noted, was justified as "so often in the past, whenever any change was made in the existing pattern of care for them, they lost something."[22]

Despite objections, the House Committee on Interior and Insular Affairs made clear its desire to transfer the Indian health program as part of the overall termination of federal responsibility for Indians. The Public Health Service carried the Branch of Indian Health for many years, the Committee concluded. National policy now "called for turning over this responsibility to State or local agencies wherever feasible—all aiming at erasing the line of distinction between services for Indians and the non-Indian population." Health was to be the first step in the complete liquidation of the Indian Service. State health agencies and national health groups emphasized the desirability of a transfer for many years. Now was the time, Senator Thye argued, as it would "improve the health services for the Indian people" and coordinate public health programs that would "further the long-range objective of the integration of the Indian people."[23]

The Oklahoma Congressional delegation remained an obstacle for the transfer. Oklahoma tribes received a "very high percentage" of all funds appropriated for Indian healthcare at the time, largely because the state congressional delegation exerted considerable political strength in the Interior and Insular affairs committee and the Indian Affairs committee before it became a subcommittee of the former. With strong opposition from the Oklahoma delegation, the bill could not be reported out of committee and called before the House for a vote. Judd, however, remained vigilant in his efforts to see the bill enacted. When he caught the delegation missing a committee meeting after a late night party, Judd mustered the bill out of committee and before the House for a vote.[24]

Congress approved the Indian Health Transfer Act on August 5, 1954, and with President Dwight Eisenhower's signature the bill became law, taking effect on July 1, 1955. Public Law 83-568 authorized the transfer of "all functions, responsibilities, authorities, and duties . . . relating to the maintenance and operation of hospital and health facilities for Indians, and the conservation of the health of Indians . . . [to] the Surgeon General of the United States Public Health Service." Indian Commissioner Glenn Emmons called the transfer "the biggest reduction of program responsibilities in the history of the [Indian] Bureau." On July 1, 1955, 56 hospitals, 13 school infirmaries, and 970 buildings valued at nearly $40,000,000, as well as 3,500 health employees shifted from the Indian Service to the Public Health Service. To mitigate Indian fears over the closure of additional Indian hospitals, Congress prohibited the Public Health Service from closing any Indian health facility prior to July 1, 1956, unless the consent of the governing council of the affected tribe was secured. Any existing contractual arrangements between the Indian Service and state and local health agencies remained in effect.[25]

With the passage of the Indian Health Transfer Act, Public Law 291, which authorized the Secretary of the Interior to enter into contracts providing for the transfer of specific Indian health facilities to state or local governments, was repealed. Section two of the transfer act granted this authority to the Secretary of Health, Education and Welfare but added a provision that Public Law 291 did not have: The Public Health Service could reassume management and operation of any facility that did not provide adequate care to the Indians.

## Settling into the Public Health Service

The transfer of the Branch of Indian Health was not expected to produce an immediate fiscal economy. In fact, Public Health Service officials, including Shaw, warned Congress that the transfer would temporarily increase the cost of the program. Nonetheless, a new era in Indian healthcare was set to commence, one expected to bring increased appropriations, better services, more qualified personnel, and an improved level of health among American Indians and Alaska Natives.[26]

With the transfer, the Branch of Indian Health was renamed the Division of Indian Health and placed within the Bureau of Medical Services. The division included an Office of the Division Chief and six branches: Hospital and Medical Services; Nursing Services; Sanitation Services; Field Health Services; Dental Services; and Program Analysis. The Hospital and Medical Services Branch provided medical care through Public Health Service Indian hospitals and contract facilities. The Field Health Services Branch developed and oversaw the public health program and administered non-hospital field facilities. The nursing, dental, and sanitation service branches were responsible for programs in their respective fields. Program Analysis reviewed and evaluated health statistics and data for program operations. All management and fiscal services were centered in the Bureau of Medical Services.[27]

The area office structure of the Division of Indian Health more closely resembled that of the Indian Service than the regional Public Health Service area offices. The Public Health Service made this administrative decision since its regional offices were far removed from centers of Indian population, whereas the offices of the Indian Service were better aligned with the Indian constituency served by the program. The close interrelationship between the health and other programs for American Indians also required the Division of Indian Health to have access to Indian Service area offices. Consequently, there were six area and three subarea offices established.[28]

With the expiration of Indian Service jurisdiction on June 30, 1955, Secretary of Health, Education and Welfare Marion B. Folsom issued regulations defining Indian eligibility for health services. The new regulations paralleled the Indian Service practice of local discretion in determining eligibility. Services were to be "made available, as medically indicated, to persons of Indian descent belonging to the Indian community served by the local facilities and program, and non-Indian wives of such persons." An individual was deemed eligible for services if the community in which he lived regarded him as Indian. Evidence of "Indianness" included tribal membership or enrollment, living on tax-exempt land, ownership of restricted property, active participation in tribal affairs, or "other relevant factors" that the Indian Service recognized as constituting membership. Doubtful cases were left to the discretion of the medical officer in charge of the facility. Individuals "clearly able to pay the cost of hospital care" were expected to do so, with some services being conditioned upon payment. No fees would be charged for preventive services such as immunizations, health exams for school children, and prenatal clinical visits.[29]

In an effort to obtain outside advice on the operation of the program, Scheele created an Advisory Committee on Indian Health in 1956. The nine member committee, which included three American Indians, evaluated the effectiveness of the Indian health program in light of cultural and welfare considerations. A second committee, the Interconstituent Committee on Services to Indians, was established that same year in an effort to coordinate the health program with related federal, state, and local programs serving Indians and Alaska Natives. This committee concerned itself with the issue of eligibility for services and increasing Indian utilization of other health services available to them, both of which were important since the Public Health Service initially took the position that no Indian had a "legal entitlement to medical services."[30]

## Health Services for American Indians and Alaska Natives

As head of the Division of Indian Health, Shaw and the Public Health Service worked to increase the Indian health budget to better manage health challenges. Shaw found an ally in Congress during the 1956 Indian health appropriation hearings. Believing the end of Indian-only services was at hand, Congress was willing to appropriate funds if the Public Health Service quantified the time needed to prepare the Indians for assimilation. The House Appropriations Committee explained American Indians had been provided health services for over a hundred years but were "still the victim of an appalling amount of sickness." Staff housing was lacking or inadequate and the workload of medical professionals tested their "patience and endurance." This all pointed to "a gross lack of resources equal to the present load of sickness and accumulated neglect." The challenge, the committee agreed, could not be approached with timidity. The committee requested the full extent of the need, the time frame to cure the need, and the cost required to bring Indian health to an acceptable level.[31]

The committee asked Folsom for a comprehensive evaluation of Indian health and the resources required to improve health conditions. Congress was willing to make resources available but predicated any appropriation on the creation of baseline data. Time was of the essence, for if American Indians were to be emancipated from federal supervision and services, they first had to be free of disease. Aided by the Indian Service and scholars from five universities, Folsom submitted the requisite reports to Congress in April of 1957. The final report was uncanny in its similarities to past health studies: "Indians of the United States today have health problems resembling in many respects those of the general population of the nation a generation ago." Diseases largely controlled among the nation at-large still caused widespread illness and death among American Indians. Table 2.1 illustrates the ten most reported communicable diseases among American Indians and Alaska Natives between 1952 and 1954.[32]

Table 2.1
*Ten Most Reported Communicable Diseases: 1952-1954*
(Per 100,000 Population)

| Disease | American Indians | Alaska Natives |
|---|---|---|
| Influenza and Pneumonia | 2,906 | 2,957 |
| Dysentery | 857 | N/A |
| Measles | 842 | 4,850 |
| Tuberculosis | 643 | 2,094 |
| Gonorrhea | 467 | 1,267 |
| Syphilis | 385 | 116 |
| Trachoma | 279 | 557 |
| Chicken pox | 249 | 1,345 |
| Mumps | 213 | 1,579 |
| Whooping Cough | 128 | N/A |

(Source: *Public Health Service Survey*, Washington, D.C.: GPO 1957 & *Alaska Health Survey*, University of Pittsburgh, 1954)

The causes of the egregious health conditions were many and varied. Inadequate health services, substandard and overcrowded housing, and a lack of adequate sanitation facilities were among the chief causes. The health concerns with the greatest urgency were tuberculosis, pneumonia and other respiratory diseases, diarrhea and enteric diseases, accidents, eye and ear diseases, dental disease, and mental illness.[33]

To bring the level of health to an acceptable standard the Public Health Service promoted the need for a comprehensive preventive health program. Closely allied with this was the necessity of correcting the gross environmental sanitation deficiencies in Indian homes and communities, which, due to the level of poverty in Indian Country, could only be accomplished through a federally supported construction program. Fred Foard argued this point in 1949, connecting typhoid, diphtheria, diarrhea, and other diseases with poor sanitation. A sanitation program was the cornerstone of any preventive health program.[34]

The Public Health Service identified the sanitation deficiencies in Indian Country and then categorized them into five broad areas. The lack of domestic water, necessitating the transportation of water from communal sources located great distances away, was a prime cause of disease. The continued use of contaminated water sources for domestic purposes was an additional cause of disease, followed by inadequate vector control resulting from improper waste and refuse disposal, unsafe excreta disposal causing parasitic infections, and a general lack of basic sanitation practices within the home. Overcrowded and poorly repaired houses, many of which still had earthen floors, hampered mitigation efforts. In 1950, Indian families were four times as crowded as non-Indian families (2.2 people per room versus 0.6). Reservations were also dispersed in isolated areas. The Tohono O'odham in Arizona, for example, lived in 73 villages, half of which were inaccessible by graded roads. Except for the agency town of Sells and a few surrounding villages, none of the villages on the 2.8 million-acre reservation had electricity, and domestic water was transported as far as ten miles.

To raise Indian health conditions to an acceptable level required additional health facilities, field units, and a sanitation facilities construction project. Folsom estimated five to ten years' time to raise the health status of the Indians to a minimal level. Thereafter, the federal health program could be progressively scaled back as the effects of the preventive health and sanitation services and facilities lessened the impact of communicable diseases, enabling state and local governments, as well as the Indians themselves, to assume responsibility for health services.

The Public Health Service was careful to couch the preventive program within the context of the overall well-being of the Indians. In his report to Congress, Folsom stressed the challenge was more than just health. "To achieve good health," the Surgeon General wrote, "Indians need more than measures aimed directly at disease prevention and control. They need better general education, vocational training, housing, food, roads, and means of transportation." In addition to these physical needs, there were deep social and cultural issues to consider. "They need more understanding and acceptance by the rest of the population, particularly their own non-Indian neighbors." If any one component of the delicate puzzle were ignored, the challenge would be prolonged. The annual cost of operating such a program would be in the neighborhood of $60 to $65 million, not including $45 million spread over a ten-year period to improve hospitals, clinics, and housing. An additional $29 million would be needed to construct sanitation facilities.

The study convinced Congress that its fiduciary obligation included ensuring that American Indians and Alaska Natives enjoyed a minimal level of healthcare and appropriating resources to mitigate the challenge. With additional resources, the Public Health Service hired more and better-qualified staff and provided a wider array of services. Shaw focused his energies on constructing additional hospitals and satellite facilities or contracting for such services. To improve the overall quality of healthcare, it was essential to have a wider array of facilities upon which to ground preventive health services in Indian Country and ensure they became a part of the broader community health services.

# The Indian Health Facilities Act

Just two months after Folsom delivered his report to the House appropriation committee, Senator Lee Metcalf (D-MT) and Representative Leroy Anderson (D-MT) each introduced a health facilities bill. Forthwith, the Public Health Service amended the bills, with one reintroduced by Anderson. The modified bill authorized the Surgeon General, after consultation with tribal nations, to provide financial assistance to public or other nonprofit organizations for the construction of community hospitals if they provided services to Indians. In other words, the Public Health Service would provide local governments or nonprofit groups planning to construct hospitals with the capital equal to the proportion of the Indian population in the area. The Bureau of the Budget, which had opposed the transfer act, enthusiastically supported this bill, viewing it as "ultimately furnish[ing] health services to Indians in the same manner as they are provided to the rest of the population."[38]

With Foard and Metcalf leading the way, Congress enacted into law the Indian Health Facilities Act in 1957. Known as Public Law 85-151, the act granted the Surgeon General statutory authority to use Indian health funds to construct joint-use community hospitals whenever he "determine[d], after consultation with Indians, that the provision of financial assistance to one or more public or other non-profit agencies or organizations for the construction of a community hospital constitute[d] a method of making needed hospital facilities available for such Indians which is more desirable and effective than direct Federal construction."[39]

The law had a dual purpose. Because of the age, condition, obsolescence, and caliber of construction of many Indian health facilities inherited by the Public Health Service, the Surgeon General, if he were to properly discharge his responsibilities, would have had to immediately replace a dozen or more outdated and ill-repaired Indian hospitals. This would have been a political challenge of considerable magnitude given that Congress was no longer interested in funding Indian-only services. A parallel purpose was providing adjacent non-Indian communities lacking financial resources with the means of opening a hospital. Such joint-use facilities would aid Indians and non-Indians and hasten the ultimate objective of integrating the Indians.[40]

Shaw enthusiastically supported the bill. Committed to integration of the Indians, Shaw recognized the remote location of most Indian reservations and the small tribal populations would mean "an extremely small hospital" if services were segregated. Two-thirds of the Indian hospitals had fewer than forty beds, with a third having fewer than thirty. "For hospitals of this size," Shaw argued, "it is not possible to provide staffs and ancillary services sufficient to meet the array of complicated medical problems inherent in the Indian health situation."[41]

Table 2.2

*Priority List of Proposed Construction and Modernization of Hospitals, 1958*

| | | *Number of Additional Beds Needed in:* | | |
|---|---|---|---|---|
| *Service Unit* | *Rank* | *Federal* | *Community* | *Undetermined* |
| Turtle Mountain | 1 | 36 | | |
| Navajo | 2 | 113 | | |
| San Carlos | 3 | 36 | | |
| Standing Rock | 4 | 27 | | |
| Fort Peck | 5 | | 25 | |
| Red Lake | 6 | | | 21 |
| White Earth | 7 | | 16 | |
| Mescalero | 8 | | | 13 |
| Jicarilla | 9 | | | 12 |
| Fond Du Lac | 10 | | 8 | |
| Mole Lake | 11 | | 4 | |
| Nett Lake | 12 | | 3 | |
| Grand Portage | 13 | | 2 | |
| Elko-Ruby Valley | 14 | | 4 | |
| Hoopa Valley | 15 | | 15 | |
| Colorado River | 16 | | 30 | |
| Fort McDermott | 17 | | 2 | |
| Wind River | 18 | | 15 | |
| Lac de Flambeau | 19 | | 4 | |
| Fort Berthold | 20 | | 10 | |
| Pima | 21 | 28 | | |
| Fort Totten | 22 | | 5 | |
| Papago | 23 | | | 22 |
| Mt. Edgecumbe | 24 | | 13 | |
| Pine Ridge | 25 | | 8 | |
| Anchorage | 26 | | 33 | |
| Flathead | 27 | | 5 | |
| Navajo | 28 | 25 | | |
| TOTAL | 28 | 265 | 202 | 68 |

(Source: Division of Indian Health, Washington, D.C., 1958)

The Indian Health Facilities Act did not authorize any new expenditure of funds but simply allowed Indian facility monies to be used for the construction of joint-use hospitals. By granting discretionary authority to the Surgeon General to undertake cooperative projects with non-Indian communities, the campaign against disease intensified. Financial assistance was limited to the reasonable cost of the community facility that was attributed to Indian health needs, as determined by the

Surgeon General. Community hospitals remained eligible for federal funding under the Hill-Burton Program, which made federal grants available for community health facilities. While constructed with federal funds, such hospitals were not under federal supervision, maintenance, administration, or control, although signed agreements guaranteed they were open to American Indians.[42]

To carry out his statutory charge of conserving the health of the Indians, the Surgeon General ordered Shaw to evaluate all health facilities available to American Indians and Alaska Natives and determine which tribes could be better served by community facilities rather than direct federal services. Shaw classified Indian hospitals into three categories: those acceptable and meeting state criteria for standards; those potentially acceptable and failing state criteria but having construction funds available to improve the facilities; and those not acceptable and not meeting state standards and having no funding available for repairs. Using such criteria, Shaw categorized twenty-four acceptable, thirteen potentially acceptable, and seventeen not acceptable Indian hospitals (see Table 2.2). The Public Health Service was prevented from closing or reducing the capacity of any hospital and no program related to the reduction of tuberculosis and infant mortality could be curtailed until the Indian rates were comparable with non-Indian rates.[43]

The purpose of the study was to determine an "orderly and timely development" of health facilities construction, something the Indian Service had never done. In so doing, Shaw established a priority list based on bed needs unmet and adjusted by several factors, including tribes considered closest to having federal supervision withdrawn and proximity to private and/or parochial health facilities. In the first seven years of Public Health Service administration, fourteen community hospitals and seven new or replacement Public Health Service Indian hospitals were constructed and four hospitals were modernized. The Gallup Indian Hospital was the first designed to be a referral and consultation center for the greater Southwest.[44]

## The Indian Sanitation Facilities Construction Act

While the health survey stimulated a building program, it also pointed to a number of continuing health challenges, most notably sanitation services. It was a long-known fact in Indian Country that sanitation facilities were lacking. In 1955, there were just thirteen sanitary engineers and sanitarians in the Indian health program assisted by thirty-one Indian sanitarian aides. No other resources were available to mitigate environmental deficiencies.[45]

Throughout the 1950s, sanitary engineers and Indian sanitarian aides conducted reservation-wide sanitation surveys. More than 80 percent of American Indian and Alaska Native families hauled or otherwise imported domestic water supplies, with over 70 percent of this water coming from contaminated or potentially contaminated sources. Less than 20 percent of Indian homes were equipped with adequate waste disposal, with 12 percent having no facilities at all.

Not surprisingly, post-neonatal infant mortality remained five times the non-Indian rate. [46]

While sanitation was essential for improving Indian health, the Surgeon General lacked authority to construct and maintain sanitation facilities in Indian Country. He was further hampered in that if he could construct such facilities (and he was legally proscribed from doing so) they would have been built on Indian land under the jurisdiction of the Indian Service. Fragmented authority vested the Public Health Service with responsibility to conserve the health of the Indians without granting it authority to construct sewage and water supply facilities. To complicate matters, the Interior Department possessed the authority to construct sanitation facilities but was powerless to transfer such projects to state, local, or tribal entities. [47]

Officials of the Public Health Service, Department of Health, Education and Welfare, Indian Service, Department of the Interior, and the Office of Management and Budget held a series of meetings to untangle the jurisdictional web. Out of these meetings grew a concerted effort to secure the legislative authority for the Surgeon General to construct and maintain sanitation facilities. Included was a proviso authorizing the Surgeon General to acquire non-Public Health Service land for use in such facilities. In January of 1956, Folsom convened a meeting with select members of Congress to solicit bipartisan support for Indian sanitation facilities legislation. From this dialogue came the introduction of several bills in the 85th Congress for specific tribes. One of these bills became law in 1957, and authorized the Surgeon General to construct sanitation facilities for Elko Indian Colony in Nevada. [48]

The Elko legislation did not address the matter of authorizing the Surgeon General to construct and maintain sanitation facilities throughout Indian Country. Without such authorization, Congress would have had to enact legislation on a project-by-project basis. In April of 1958, acting Secretary of Health, Education and Welfare Elliot Richardson requested Congress draft a bill granting the Surgeon General universal authority to construct such facilities throughout Indian Country. Although the bill died at the end of the 85th Congress, it was reintroduced along with eight similar bills in 1959. Secretary of Health, Education and Welfare Arthur Fleming exhorted Congress to provide the Surgeon General with broad authority to construct sanitation facilities. "Few families and few communities," the secretary reminded Congressman Oren Harris (D-AR), "are able to . . . provide essential sanitation facilities from their own resources." [49]

On July 31, 1959, the Indian Sanitation Facilities Construction Act became law, providing the Surgeon General statutory authority to construct sanitation projects to mitigate "the serious environmental problems" in Indian Country. Public Law 86-121 amended the Indian Health Transfer Act by authorizing the Surgeon General to "construct, improve, extend, or otherwise provide and maintain, by contract or otherwise, essential sanitation facilities, drainage facilities, and sewage and waste disposal facilities . . . for Indian homes, communities, and lands." The Surgeon General was also authorized to acquire land or rights-of-way for constructing sanitation facilities and upon the completion of the facility transfer it "to any State or Territory or subdivision or public authority thereof, or to any Indian tribe, group, band or community." Any domestic improvements transferred to the occupant of the Indian home so served.[50]

The passage of the law could not in its own right relieve the environmental deficiencies among the Indians. "Sanitation improvements at reservation areas depend first upon acceptance by the Indians of modern concepts of the interrelationship between disease and insanitary living conditions," Fleming informed Harris, "and, second, upon provision and use of basic sanitation facilities—safe water supplies, safe sewage disposal and refuse disposal facilities." These tasks would not be easily accomplished among some tribes. A 1954 study in Arizona found assistance difficult to render because of deep-seated Indian "resistance to change." The same study concluded resistance occurred because of entrenched social attitudes and "habitual patterns of living" that were contrary to effective, modern preventive health measures. While individuals might accept change, community acceptance was more difficult, and the latter was foundational for preventive programs to be successful.[51]

## Signs of Progress

The operational improvements of the Division of Indian Health were significant during its first years in the Public Health Service. While there were still challenges, initial signs pointed toward progress. Additional medical staff, including specialists from nearly every field of medicine, and improved and modernized health facilities made their mark. In the first years of Public Health Service responsibility, the full-time medical staff of the Indian health service grew 45 percent, passing the 5,000 mark by 1959. Physicians more than doubled to 300 and included pediatricians, surgeons, and maternal and childhood specialists. The number of dentists tripled to 100, as did dental assistants and technicians. Sanitary engineers and sanitarians expanded from fourteen to sixty-eight, and sanitarian aides more than doubled to sixty-eight. Graduate nurses increased from 783 to 890, with practical nurses increasing from 289 to 486. Pharmacists, medical social workers, community workers, medical record librarians, dietitians, and nutritionists all increased four- or five-fold. The urgency and the need were so real that *espirit de corps* was at its peak. For the first time, it appeared the Division of Indian Health might provide comprehensive care to American Indians and Alaska Natives.[52]

In an effort to make healthcare more relevant, the Public Health Service expanded training opportunities for American Indians and Alaska Natives. Nurses trained at the School of Practical Nursing in Albuquerque, New Mexico, while advanced training was available at Shiprock, New Mexico, and Rapid City, South Dakota. Dental technicians trained at four facilities in the West and sanitarian aides received training at Sandia Pueblo, New Mexico. As the end of the decade approached, over one-half of the employees of the Indian health service were

American Indian or Alaska Native, although most were in support staff roles such as aides.

The expansion of services, increasing appropriations, growing numbers of medical specialists, and legislatively sanctioned construction projects meant little if Indian health conditions did not improve. In order to determine the effectiveness of the program, health conditions must be measured in terms of overall improvement. When viewed in this light the Public Health Service made important advances in some areas, tuberculosis and infant mortality in particular. Overall, Indian health conditions remained at least a generation behind the national standard, with Alaska Native health conditions lagging by two generations. Diseases controlled among non-Indians were still the cause of disproportionate numbers of American Indian and Alaska Native deaths.

Table 2.3
*Tuberculosis Incidence Rates: 1954-1959*
(Per 100,000 Population)

| Year | American Indian | Alaska Native | U.S. General Population |
|------|-----------------|---------------|-------------------------|
| 1954 | 571.5 | 2,452.4 | 62.4 |
| 1955 | 563.2 | 2,325.7 | 60.1 |
| 1956 | 474.3 | 2,283.8 | 54.1 |
| 1957 | 426.9 | 1,649.7 | 51.0 |
| 1958 | 421.8 | 978.7 | 47.5 |
| 1959 | 338.2 | 1,048.0 | 42.6 |

(Source: *Indian Health Highlights*, 1964)

The most dramatic reduction in Indian Country was the incidence rate from the old Indian nemesis tuberculosis, which declined 49 percent among American Indians (571.5 to 292.3 per 100,000) and 78 percent among Alaska Natives (2,452.4 to 547.5 per 100,000) after the introduction of antibiotics and improved health education. Although it had been the leading cause of death among American Indians and Alaska Natives in 1949, the tuberculosis mortality rate declined so sharply that by 1960 it dropped to the ninth leading cause of death.[53] Table 2.3 shows the declining incidence rate of tuberculosis.

Corresponding with the decreasing tuberculosis rate was a declining infant mortality rate, which was aided by more hospital deliveries. Between 1954 and 1962, the mortality rate for Indian infants declined 36 percent, yet remained 150 percent higher than the non-Indian rate. Among Alaska Natives the infant death rate was double the Indian rate and three times the overall national rate. For post-neonatal infants the rate was even higher. The Indian rate of 26 deaths per 1,000 live babies was nearly 4 times the overall rate of 7 deaths. The leading causes of infant mortality remained respiratory, digestive, infective, and parasitic diseases.[54]

Table 2.4

*Top Five Causes of Death among American Indians and Alaska Natives:*
*1954-1960*
(Per 100,000 Population)

| Mortality Rates among American Indians/Alaska Natives | | | | U.S. All Groups | |
|---|---|---|---|---|---|
| Disease | *1954-56* | *1956-58* | *1958-60* | *1959* | *1960* |
| Accidents | | | | | |
| U.S. | 154.0 | 154.1 | 151.1 | 52.2 | 52.3 |
| Alaska | 175.3 | 183.0 | 181.5 | 115.2 | 110.5 |
| Heart Disease | | | | | |
| U.S. | 137.6 | 139.3 | 142.7 | 363.4 | 369.0 |
| Alaska | 91.8 | 95.4 | 77.1 | 111.5 | 118.1 |
| Influenza/Pneumonia | | | | | |
| U.S. | 87.9 | 93.8 | 82.8 | 31.2 | 37.3 |
| Alaska | 138.7 | 130.1 | 117.3 | 39.8 | 44.2 |
| Malignant Neoplasms | | | | | |
| U.S. | 63.5 | 63.7 | 67.1 | 147.4 | 149.2 |
| Alaska | 45.0 | 58.1 | 57.0 | 57.1 | 52.2 |
| Infant Disease* | | | | | |
| U.S. | 60.8 | 57.0 | 50.2 | 26.2 | 25.8 |
| Alaska | N/A | N/A | 74.0 | 42.9 | 40.5 |

*Per 1,000 Live Births

(Source: *Indian Health Highlights*, 1964)

Owing to some improvement in sanitation matters, progress was also made in reducing gastroenteric diseases. Although the death rate from such diseases diminished among American Indians, it actually doubled among Alaska Natives. With non-Indians six times less likely than American Indians and Alaska Natives to experience such health challenges, it was apparent that gastroenteric diseases remained a major contributor to ill-health among the Indians. Biliary disease was significantly higher among American Indians than non-Indians as well.[55]

By 1959, the leading causes of death were new to Indian Country. Heart disease, accidents, influenza, pneumonia, gastroenteric diseases, malignant neoplasms, cirrhosis of the liver, vascular lesions of the central nervous system, as well as chronic diseases such as tuberculosis, were double or more the non-Indian rates. American Indians and Alaska Natives were less likely than non-Indians to be afflicted with malignant neoplasms, heart disease, and vascular lesions, but that was largely because they did not live as long and did not face many of the chronic geriatric diseases. Nonetheless, rates for these diseases were increasing. Table 2.4 compares the mortality rates of the five leading causes of death among American Indians and Alaska Natives with those of non-Indians.

The reduction in morbidity and mortality (particularly due to declines in the incidence rate of tuberculosis) is reflected in the increased average life span among American Indians. Between 1954 and 1962 the average age at death for Indians rose from thirty-eight to forty-three, although among Alaska Natives it remained at thirty years of age. With more services and better care, life expectancy among American Indians also increased, rising from fifty-one to sixty-two, still far short of non-Indian life expectancy, which was seventy years of age.[56]

While there were instances of health improvement, Indian health indices remained far behind those of non-Indians. Tuberculosis, gastroenteric, and infant mortality rates all declined, although morbidity rates for these diseases remained high. The geographical isolation, social and linguistic barriers, cultural differences, environmental and sanitary hazards, lack of economic resources, and the proclivity of American Indians and Alaska Natives to accept Western medicine still affected the overall health of the people and complicated the implementation of a comprehensive community health program. Added to these challenges were transportation difficulties, both for Indian patients and medical personnel, and the continued overlay of an imposed healthcare system that did not always consider the cultural views and needs of its clients.[57]

Consequently, while there was progress made in the formative years of Public Health Service responsibility, additional progress was dependent upon the increasing utilization of, and appropriations for, sanitation facilities and improved preventive health measures. While *espirit de corps* was high, it yet remained to be seen if the Public Health Service would do a better job of melding traditional Indian medicine and practices with Western ways.

# Notes

1. Shaw succeeded Fred Foard, who retired from the Public Health Service in October 1952 to become director of the North Carolina State Department of Health. "Medical News," *Journal of the American Medical Association* (150:16) December 20, 1952, 1614. Shaw assumed command of the Branch of Indian Health on July 31, 1953, and was assisted by Dr. Frank French and Dr. Joseph Dean. Between October 1952 and July 1953 Burnet M. Davis was acting director of the medical service. "Government Services," *Journal of the American Medical Association* (152:14) August 1, 1953, 1357. *Annual Report of the Secretary of Health, Education and Welfare*, 1960, 132.

2. Scheele outlined his immediate task as controlling the preventable communicable

diseases that accounted for the low Indian average age of death (36 vs. 61 for non-Indians). "Washington News," *Journal of the American Medical Association* (158:11), July 16, 1955, 14. Fred T. Foard, "The Federal Government and American Indians' Health," *Journal of the American Medical Association* (142:5), February 4, 1950, 328.

3. "The Indians' Health and Public Health," *American Journal of Public Health* (44:11), November 1954, 1461-1463. The *Journal* saw obvious advantages in placing the health program under the "immediate and sole direction" of Public Health Service professionals. Advantages included obtaining new facilities, equipment and technology; unshared control of funds by medical officers who understood better than the Indian Service bureaucrats the needs of a public health program; easier access to all the special skills and the broad competencies of the Public Health Service; and staffing benefits. Hazards could include the Public Health Service competing with itself for medical funds, both in terms of allocation and authorizations. "Aspects of Indian Policy," Senate Committee on Indian Affairs, Senate Committee Print, 79th Congress, 1st session (Washington, D.C.: Government Printing Office, 1945), 4, 16.

4. Donald Fixico, *Termination and Relocation: Federal Indian Policy, 1945-1960* (Albuquerque: University of New Mexico Press, 1986), 49. The Hoover Commission recommended a new Department of Natural Resources be created for all remaining Indian programs.

5. Authority already existed in a 1938 law that provided for the collection of fees from those Indians able to pay. 52 stat. 311. "Providing for Medical Services to Non-Indians in Indian Hospitals," *House Report no. 641* 82nd Congress, 1st session, June 25, 1951, 2-3. Chapman argued such a law would help recruit physicians because they would provide care to a "greater variety of patients" and would be able to increase their pay through private practice on the side (while still being contractually bound to provide care for Indians). An initial bill passed the House on June 20, 1949, but the Senate failed to take action. *Commission on the Organization of the Executive Branch of Government: Functions and Activities of the National Government in the Field of Welfare* (Washington, D.C.: Government Printing Office, 1949), 66. The Hoover Commission suggested Public Health Service physicians be detailed to the Indian Service for a minimum of 3 and preferably 4 or 5 years so they would better understand the needs of the Indian community they served.

6. *Annual Report of the Secretary of the Interior*, 1952, 395. Myer argued final decisions regarding the closing of any health facility would not be made without tribal consultation. Nine community or sectarian hospitals provided care at Fort Berthold, with a small agency health staff maintained for residual needs. The Ft. Berthold tribal council, State health council, the State hospital, medical and pharmaceutical associations and the State Commission on Indian Affairs all supported the plan. *Annual Report of the Secretary of the Interior*, 1953, 34. New contracts were also signed expanding state and county services to Indians.

7. "Providing for Medical Services to Non-Indians in Indian Hospitals and for Other Purposes," *House Report no. 797* 81st Congress, 1st session, June 14, 1949. The revised bill (HR 4815) allowed physicians to contract for services but without becoming federal employees, prioritized Indian access to services, and provided procedures for the disposition of funds from non-Indian patients. "Providing for Medical Services for Non-Indians in Indian Hospitals," *Senate Report no. 1095* 81st Congress, 1st session, September 20, 1949.

66 stat. 34.

8. The closing of hospitals was not without anxiety. The fact remained that when hospitals closed Indians lost their traditional services and had to apply to county or state health departments for medical attention. Many Indians feared discrimination and the bureaucracy involved and threatened to go it alone. Fixico, 46. Public Law 291 (HR 1043) was reported (2229), passed the Senate (2747), examined and signed (2869 and 2873), sent to the president (p. 3091) and approved (p. 3756) in the *Congressional Record* (98), 1952.

9. "Urgent Deficiency Appropriation Bill, 1956," *Hearing before the Committee on Appropriations, United States Senate on HR 9063* 84th Congress, 2d session, March 16, 1956, 480.

10. *Annual Report of the Secretary of the Interior*, 1953, 36.

11. "Concurrent Resolutions: Indians," 67 stat. B132 (1953). "An Act to confer jurisdiction on the States of California, Minnesota, Nebraska, Oregon and Wisconsin, with respect to criminal offenses and civil causes of action committed or arising on Indian Reservations within such states, and for other purposes," 67 stat. 588.

12. W. F. Braasch, B. J. Branton and A. J. Chesley, "Survey of Medical Care Among the Upper Midwest Indians," *Journal of the American Medical Association* (139:4, 1949), 221, asked whether it was wise to have an agency in one government department directed by officials in another or whether the PHS should carry on a general practice of medicine (which the Indian situation demanded). Braasch and his colleagues argued in opposition to both. In regards to the latter, they noted the mission of the Public Health Service was not the "general practice of medicine" but preventive medicine. In the final analysis, Braasch and his colleagues argued for transfer of the health program and a separate budget within the Public Health Service and the transfer of preventive health measures to the state boards of health.

13. *Congressional Record* (98), 1952, 1900. Representative Harold A. Patten (D-AZ) also introduced legislation (HR 7232) to effect the transfer. The Meriam Report of 1928 raised the issue of whether or not the federal government should grant authority for state and local governments to provide services for American Indians. Lewis Meriam, the principal author of the study, argued the sooner state and local governments were brought to the point of rendering services and the Indians to the point of accepting the services from local governments the better. Lewis Meriam, *The Problem of Indian Administration*, (Baltimore: Johns Hopkins Press, 1928), 221.

14. "Survey of Conditions among the Indians of the United States," *Senate Report no. 310: Analysis of the Statement of the Commissioner of Indian Affairs in Justification of Appropriations for 1944, and the Liquidation of the Indian Bureau* 78th Congress, 1st session, June 11, 1948, 9 and 22. "Transfer the Maintenance and Operation of Hospitals and Health Facilities for Indians to the PHS," *Senate Report no. 1530* 83rd Congress, 2d session, June 8, 1954, 9. Subcommittee hearings were held on March 28, 1948. The Bureau of the Budget, which surveyed the Indian health program in 1948, found a need for a new approach to Indian health problems but did not favor the transfer (16).

15. James R. Shaw, "Indian Health in Historical Perspective," unpublished paper courtesy of the author, University of Arizona, Tucson, October 18, 1982, 12. The American Medical Association Board of Trustees, for example, approved a resolution that encouraged Congress to effect the transfer. On April 20, 1953, George Lull, Secretary and General Manager of the American Medical Association, wrote a letter to Congressman William

Henry Harrison (R-WY), Chairman of the Subcommittee on Interior and Insular Affairs, and encouraged him to enact the necessary legislation. "Committee on Legislation," *Journal of the American Medical Association* (152:2), May 9, 1953, 169; (149:3), May 17, 1952, 283; (151:9), February 28, 1953; and (155:8), June 19, 1954, 753. *Transfer of Indian Hospitals and Health Facilities to Public Health Service, Hearings Before a Subcommittee of the Committee on Interior and Insular Affairs United States Senate on HR 303* 83rd Congress, 2nd session, 1954.

16. "Organizational News," *Journal of the American Medical Association* (149:3), May 17, 1952, 283. "Transfer the Maintenance and Operation of Hospitals and Health Facilities for Indians to the Public Health Service," *House Report no. 870* 83rd Congress, 1st session, July 17, 1953, 3-4.

17. John Todd, Interview with Dr. James R. Shaw, Unpublished Document in the Commissioned Corps Centennial Archives, History of Medicine Division, Library of Medicine, Bethesda, Maryland, 1988.

18. *Senate Report no. 1530*, 8. Shortly after the transfer, the Public Health Service announced it had contracted with the Phipps Institute of the University of Pennsylvania for a three-year health project designed to reduce tuberculosis among the Jicarilla Apache, Consolidated Utes, United Pueblo Tribes, and the Mescalero Apache. "Government Services: Public Health Service," *Journal of the American Medical Association* (160:7), February 18, 1956, 576.

19. *Senate Report no. 1530*, 8. Both the Consolidated Ute Tribe and the Southern Ute Tribe contracted with Blue Cross-Blue Shield for their healthcare needs in 1955. "Urgent Deficiency Appropriation Bill 1956," 464. Raup, *The Indian Health Program 1800-1955*, 26.

20. Orme Lewis to A. L. Miller, May 5, 1953, in *House Report no. 870*. Lewis to Hugh Butler, May 27, 1954, *Senate Report no. 1530*, 10.

21. Oveta Culp Hobby to Hugh Butler, May 28, 1954, *Senate Report no. 1530*, 17. "Hearings on the Proposed Transfer of Indian Hospitals and Health Facilities to the Public Health Service," *Hearings before the Committee on Interior and Insular Affairs United States Senate* 83rd Congress, 2d session, May 28 & 29, 1954, 9.

22. *Hearings before the Committee on Interior and Insular Affairs United States Senate*, 92, 130-131.

23. *House Report no. 870*, 14. The Committee recommended that the educational responsibilities of the Indian Service be turned over to other agencies serving non-Indians as soon as practicable programs could be worked out. *Congressional Record*, (100), 8959.

24. Oklahoma's delegation included five Democrats (Ed Edmondson, Carl Albert, Tom Steed, John Jarman, and Victor Wickersham) and one Republican (Page Belcher). Todd, 7.

25. The Bureau of the Budget requested $125,000 so the Public Health Service could begin the initial steps of transfer before July 1. Letter of Percival F. Brundage, acting Director of the Bureau of the Budget, to the president, March 21, 1955, in "Proposed Provision-Department of Health, Education and Welfare, Communication for the President of the United States," *Senate Document 16*, 84th Congress, 1st session, March 23, 1955. "Transferring the Maintenance and Operation of Hospitals and Health Services for Indians to the Public Health Service," *House Report no. 2430* 83rd Congress, 2d session, July 21,

1954, for the Conference Report with amendments. "An Act to transfer the maintenance and operation of hospital and health facilities for Indians to the Public Health Service, and for other purposes," 68 stat 674. *Annual Report of the Secretary of the Interior*, 1955, 231. *Annual Report of the Secretary of Health, Education and Welfare*, 1955, 122.

26. "Labor-Health, Education and Welfare Appropriations for 1959," *Hearings before the Subcommittee of the Committee on Appropriations United States Senate* 85th Congress, 2d session, April 1, 1958. Shaw argued that more Indians were using the services and that more money was needed to operate the program.

27. *Health Services for American Indians*, 98.

28. Area offices included Portland, Oregon; Aberdeen, South Dakota; Oklahoma City, Oklahoma; Albuquerque, New Mexico; and Phoenix, Arizona. Alaska was set up as an independent area office. Sub-area offices were established at Billings, Montana; Bemidji, Minnesota; and Window Rock, Arizona. Both offices operated independently as far as medical and other program supervision was concerned. Area office staff included a medical officer, an assistant medical officer, two graduate nurses, a sanitary engineer, a dental officer, a social worker, and several other sundry employees. *Health Services for American Indians*, 98-99.

29. *United States Code of Federal Regulations*, Section 36.12 and Section 36.13, 1956.

30. The Committee's American Indian members included N. B. Johnson, Chief Justice of the Oklahoma Supreme Court; Anna Wauneka, Chair of the Navajo Nation's health committee; and Frank Ducheneaux, Chairman of the Cheyenne River Sioux. Non-Indian members included Robert Atwood (Alaska); Dr. Robert Neff Barr (Minnesota); Former director of the Indian Medical Service, Dr. Fred Foard (North Carolina); Dr. Alexander H. Leighton (New York); Dr. James Perkins (New York); and Dr. Raymond F. Peterson (Montana). "Indian Health Advisory Committee," *Journal of the American Medical Association* (161:6), June 9, 1956, 547. Assistant Indian Commissioner William Zimmerman, Jr., argued if the Public Health Service continued to hold the view that health services were "an act of grace" it was "headed for trouble." William Zimmerman, Jr., "The Role of the Bureau of Indian Affairs," *The Annals of the American Academy of Political and Social Sciences*, May 1957, 37-38.

31. *House Report no. 228* 84th Congress, 1st session, 12-13. *Health Services for American Indians*, vii.

32. *Health Services for American Indians*, 1. Thomas Parron, *Alaska's Health: A Survey*, (The Graduate School of Public Health, University of Pittsburgh, 1954), III-1.

33. *Health Services for American Indians*, 1.

34. *Health Services for American Indians*, 175. "Interior Department Appropriation Bill for 1950," *Hearings before the Subcommittee of the Committee on Appropriations House of Representatives* 81st Congress, 1st session, part 1, January 26, 1949, 633.

35. *Health Services for American Indians*, 21. Bertram S. Krauss, *Indian Health in Arizona: A Study of Health Conditions among Central and Southern Arizona Tribes* (Tucson: Bureau of Ethnic Research, University of Arizona, 1954), 24. Living in small one- or two-room adobe houses, the cool winters and lack of heat resulted in a high incidence of respiratory illnesses among the Papago. While the neighboring Pima had to haul water, it was not as great a distance as the Papago. And the Pima were considerably better off, many homes having electricity. Many San Carlos Apache still lived in flimsy wooden houses,

tents, or wickiups.

36. *Health Services for American Indians*, 175. A number of Congressmen inquired of Shaw whether the time could be shortened if Congress appropriated larger amounts of money. Shaw replied it was possible but not probable. "Department of Labor and Health, Education and Welfare Appropriations, 1958," *Hearings before the Subcommittee of the Committee on Appropriations House of Representatives* 85th Congress, 1st session, February 18, 1957, 675-688.

37. *Health Services for American Indians*, 3.

38. Metcalf introduced S. 2021 and Anderson introduced HR 2380. "Constructing Indian Hospitals," *House Report no. 574* 85th Congress, 1st session, June 17, 1957, 2. "Construction of Indian Hospitals," *Hearings before the Committee on Interstate and Foreign Commerce House of Representatives on HR 204 and HR 2380* 85th Congress, 1st session, April 9, 1957. Congress had built several joint hospitals prior to this. For example, it enacted emergency legislation to construct a joint use hospital in Bernalillo County, New Mexico, as authorized by the act of October 31, 1949 (63 stat. 1049). "Indian Hospitalization Payments to Bernalillo County, New Mexico," *House Report no. 1052* 85th Congress, 1st session, August 13, 1957. "Indian Hospitalization Payments to Bernalillo County, New Mexico," *Senate Report no. 992* 85th Congress 1st session, August 17, 1957. "Authorizing Funds Available for Construction of Indian Health Facilities to be used to Assist in the Construction of Community Hospitals which will Service Indians and Non-Indians," *Senate Report no. 769* 85th Congress, 1st session, July 30, 1957, 6.

39. "Construction of Indian Hospitals," 11-14. G. D. Carlyle Thompson, Executive Officer and Secretary of the Montana State Board of Health and the Chairman of the Indian Health Council of the Association of State and Territorial Health Officers, and Robert Barr, Executive Officer and Secretary of the Minnesota State Board of Health and a member of the Surgeon General's advisory committee on Indian Health, also urged Congress to enact the bill. "An Act to authorize funds available for construction of Indian health facilities to be used to assist in the construction of community hospitals which will serve Indians and non-Indians," 71 stat 370. James R. Shaw, "Historical Development of Indian Health Services," unpublished history of the Indian Health Services, University of Arizona, October 18, 1982.

40. Alan Sorkin, *American Indians and Federal Aid* (Brookings Institute, 1971), 61-62. Twelve Indian hospitals had been built before 1925 and just eleven were accredited at the time. "Authorizing Funds Available for Construction of Indian Health Facilities to be Used to Assist in the Construction of Community Hospitals which will Serve Indians and Non-Indians," 3. "Washington News: Grants for Indian and Non-Indian Hospitals" *Journal of the American Medical Association* (163:16), April 20, 1957, 25.

41. *Plan for Medical Facilities Needed for Indian Health Services* (Washington, D.C.: Public Health Service, Division of Indian Health, 1958), 19.

42. *Senate Report no. 769*, 2. M. B. Folsom to Lister Hill, Chairman of the Senate Committee on Labor and Public Welfare, "Indian Health Facilities-Funds," *United States Code and Administrative News*, vol. II (Washington, D.C.: Government Printing Office, 1957), 1548. The proportionate sharing of overhead construction and basic operating and equipment costs (i.e., X-ray facilities, operating rooms, heating facilities, etc.) tended to reduce the per-bed construction costs for both Indian and non-Indian communities involved. By enabling the Division of Indian Health to participate in joint health ventures, additional

health facilities and hospitals were established in or near small Indian and non-Indian communities, both of which were unable to support a facility individually. Folsom correctly viewed the law as an "alternative for carrying out the Public Health Service's responsibility for the conservation of Indian health."

43. *Plan for Medical Facilities Needed for Indian Health Services*, 6-7. "Declaring the Sense of Congress on the Closing of Indian Hospitals," 86th Congress, 2d session, January 19, 1960, 1-2. If the Public Health Service sought to close a hospital, ninety days notice had to be given and no facility was to be closed if it created a shortage of facilities or intensified the shortage in any given area.

44. Table 2.2 shows the priority rank established by the Division of Indian Health and the number of beds needed and whether such beds could be provided via federal Indian Health Service hospitals, Community hospitals or undetermined hospitals. The Navajo service unit was listed twice to illustrate the high priority for modernizing existing hospitals (rank #2) and the lower priority for residual needs (rank #28). New Public Health Service facilities were constructed in Shiprock, New Mexico (75 beds); Eagle Butte, South Dakota (30 beds); Sells, Arizona (50 beds); Gallup, New Mexico (200 beds); Keams Canyon, Arizona (38 beds); Kotzebue, Alaska (53 beds); and San Carlos, Arizona (36 beds). Remodeled hospitals were in Pine Ridge, South Dakota; Rosebud, South Dakota; Browning, Montana; and Whiteriver, Arizona. New hospitals were planned for Crow Agency, Montana; Point Barrow, Alaska (12 beds); Fort Yates, North Dakota (27 beds); Phoenix, Arizona (200 beds); and Lawton, Oklahoma (80 beds). "Review of the Indian Health Program," *Hearing before the Subcommittee on Indian Affairs of the Committee on Interior and Insular Affairs House of Representatives* 88th Congress, 1st session, May 23, 1963, 53. *Annual Report of the Secretary of Health, Education and Welfare*, 1961, 198.

45. *Celebrating Thirty Years of Progress: The Indian Health Service and the Sanitation Facilities Construction Program* (Washington, D.C.: Indian Health Service, 1989), 8. By 1957, there were eighty sanitarian aides. Shaw asked for additional funds to expand training because their Indian peers "enthusiastically" accepted the aides. *Department of Labor and Health, Education and Welfare Appropriation for 1958, Hearings before the Subcommittee of the Committee on Appropriations House of Representatives*, 669.

46. *Indian Health Highlights* 12. "Amending the Act of August 5, 1954," *Senate Report no. 1876* 85th Congress, 2d session, July 22, 1958, 2. Acting Health, Education and Welfare secretary Elliot Richardson supported the sanitation facilities construction legislation, as it would "provide an improved legislative base for the correction of gross deficiencies in basic sanitation facilities and improvements for Indians."

47. "Indian Sanitation Facilities," *Senate Report no. 589* 86th Congress, 1st session, June 29, 1959, 4.

48. *Sanitation Facilities Construction: Project Administration Management*, Part I (Washington, D.C.: Indian Health Service, Division of Environmental Health, 1986), I-3. "Elko Indian Sanitation Facilities," *Hearing before the Subcommittee on Health and Science of the Committee on Interstate and Foreign Commerce House of Representatives* 85th Congress, 1st session, April 10, 1957, 2. The project was funded under 71 stat. 353.

49. "Indian Sanitation Facilities," 2. These bills were HR 849, HR 966, HR 1338, HR 1768, HR 1979, HR 2349, HR 2546 and HR 3188. Arthur Fleming to Oren Harris, Chairman of the Committee on Interstate and Foreign Commerce, "Indian Sanitation

Facilities," 4. "Amending the Act of August 5, 1954," *Senate Report no. 244* 86th Congress 1st session, May 11, 1959.

50. "An Act to amend the act of August 5, 1954, and for other purposes," 73 stat. 267. Albert H. Stevenson, "Sanitary Facilities Construction Program for Indians and Alaska Natives," *Public Health Reports* (76:4) April 1961, 317-322.

51. Fleming to Harris, "Indian Sanitation Facilities." *Indian Health in Arizona*, 18 and 24. In the first three fiscal years subsequent to the enactment of Public Law 121, 168 construction projects were authorized, 72 of which were completed

52. *Indian Health Highlights*, xvi.

53. *Indian Health Highlights*, xi. Arthur Fleming, "Indian Health," *Public Health Reports* (74:6, 1959), placed the tuberculosis rate drop at 40 percent between 1953 and 1957. The decrease among Alaska Natives was 63 percent. With the decreasing tuberculosis rate, the 330-bed tuberculosis sanitarium in Tacoma, Washington, was closed in 1960.

54. *Indian Health Highlights*, xvi. "Infant Death Rate of American Indians Dropped 30% Since 1954" in *Journal of the American Medical Association* (180:11), March 17, 1962, 44.

55. Maurice Sievers and James Marquis reported that biliary or gallstones occurred more frequently among American Indians than non-Indians possibly due to the Indians' greater propensity for diabetes, obesity and early childbearing. Maurice L. Sievers and James R. Marquis, "The Southwestern American Indian's Burden: Biliary Disease," *Journal of the American Medical Association* (182:5), November 3, 1962, 570-572.

56. *The Indian Health Program of the United States Public Health Service* (Washington, D.C.: Division of Indian Health, 1963), 16.

57. Fleming, "Indian Health," 521-522. Fleming notes that one Public Health Service dentist traveled 10,000 miles a year treating his patients on the Navajo Reservation. In Alaska, some medical personnel drove dog sleds or flew their own airplanes.

# CHAPTER THREE

## Beginnings of a Community Health Program

In August of 1962 Shaw retired as director of the Division of Indian Health and became Associate Coordinator of Research and Professor of Microbiology at the University of Arizona in Tucson. An orthopedic surgeon named Carruth J. Wagner succeeded him. Wagner came from the Public Health Service Office of Health Mobilization and worked to establish community health. In 1965, the American Academy of General Practice presented Wagner with the Meritorious Service Award for his efforts in fostering cooperation between private and governmental medicine on behalf of American Indians and Alaska Natives.[1]

As chief of the Division of Indian Health, Wagner worked to implement partnerships in healthcare delivery. He strengthened the management, operation, and delivery of the Indian health service by emphasizing improved administrative management and training of healthcare managers and other health paraprofessionals, and by directing attention on program planning, budgeting, and evaluation. He also established a formal liaison with the American Medical Association.[2] Wagner was promoted in the fall of 1965 to the position of Director of the Bureau of Medical Services, which included oversight responsibility for the Indian health program.[3]

Following the lead of Shaw, Wagner promoted the construction of Indian hospitals and clinics. Despite the fact that, by 1965, the Public Health Service constructed seven new hospitals, nine health centers, twenty-nine field health stations, and fifteen community hospitals, Indian Country continued to face shortages of healthcare services. In addition, several antiquated facilities were closed and, where Public Health Service facilities were not available, the Division of Indian Health utilized 200 private or community hospitals and over 400 contract physicians, dentists, and other specialists. Nearly 20 percent of the Indian health historical budget was spent on contract services in 1963 and continued to consume a comparable percent of the budget throughout the 1960s.[4]

Notwithstanding such services, the backlog of disease in Indian Country meant the Division of Indian Health remained crisis-oriented. As long as Indian health services remained crisis driven, the Division of Indian Health was "unable to significantly alter the overall low health conditions of the Indian people." For most of the history of organized Indian healthcare, hospitals had been the polestar of all medical activities. Due to cultural barriers and the Indians' lack of financial means, adequate preventive or public healthcare was difficult to establish in Indian Country, with the result that the focus of the program centered on treating the ill rather than preventing the illness. Wagner told the House subcommittee on Indian Affairs "the burden of disease is heavy, and much of it is associated with the hazards and rigors of the environment" in which American Indians lived. These factors were compounded by cultural and linguistic factors and geographical and social isolation.[5]

Wagner was cognizant that a crisis-oriented approach to healthcare was still the norm in Indian Country. Inadequate facilities were partly to blame. "This inadequacy is a product of age [and] obsolescence resulting from the transition to modern health practices, lack of facilities and deferred maintenance." In the field, the shortage of hospitals was critical. At the Indian hospital in Anchorage, Alaska, there was a waiting list of 5,000 patients for reconstructive ear surgery. Despite an increased budget and an ambitious building program, the Division of Indian Health provided limited services for American Indians and Alaska Natives and many of these services were provided in field clinics and health centers housed in obsolete, substandard buildings, such as school basements and trading posts. Many health facilities remained without adequate "water, toilet facilities and heat."[6]

Table 3.1

*Indian Health Facilities Historical Budget, 1956-1963*

| Year | Total | Hospitals & Clinics | Personnel Housing | Community Hospitals | Other |
|---|---|---|---|---|---|
| 1956 | $5,535,000 | $2,850,000 | $1,650,000 | -- | $1,035,000 |
| 1957 | $8,762,000 | $6,762,000 | $1,000,000 | -- | $1,000,000 |
| 1958 | $3,130,000 | -- | -- | -- | $3,130,000 |
| 1959 | $6,010,000 | $1,985,000 | $714,000 | $1,750,000 | $1,560,000 |
| 1960 | $4,787,000 | $1,808,000 | $2,500,000 | -- | $479,000 |
| 1961 | $9,714,000 | $1,540,000 | $4,000,000 | $500,000 | $3,674,000 |
| 1962 | $8,285,000 | $1,160,000 | $2,500,000 | $325,000 | $4,300,000 |
| 1963 | $9,335,000 | $3,440,700 | $425,000 | $100,000 | $5,369,000 |

(Source: *Indian Health Program*, 1963)

Antiquated hospitals, clinics, and field stations posed a challenge in providing adequate health services. Despite substandard facilities, the Public Health Service managed to accomplish more in its first ten years than the Indian medical service did as part of the Indian Service. The Public Health Service was respected in the medical world, secured increased appropriations from Congress, and worked harmoniously with its constituents, something the Indian medical service failed to do.

Notable structural improvements were realized in several health facilities. By mid-decade, for example, construction commenced on a new twelve-bed hospital in Barrow, Alaska, an eighty-bed facility in Lawton, Oklahoma, and a twenty-seven-bed structure in Fort Yates, North Dakota. Feasibility studies were completed on the proposed construction of the 200-bed Phoenix Indian Medical Center and a 125-bed facility in Tuba City, Arizona. New health clinics and field stations were constructed. The need for adequate facilities remained urgent, although it was reduced as the Public Health Service dedicated additional resources to improving or replacing existing facilities. The health facilities budget increased from $5,535,000 in 1955 to $9,335,000 in 1963. Table 3.1 shows the breakdown for the health facilities budget.[7]

## Improving Medical Infrastructure

Moving the Indian health program into the Public Health Service was a milestone event in the history of Indian healthcare. But difficulties remained. For instance, the Indian Service (now Bureau of Indian Affairs) and the Public Health Service infrequently communicated. While the latter was responsible for building hospitals, the former was responsible for the road network to make the hospitals accessible. The Bureau of Indian Affairs (BIA) was responsible for education, while the health of the students was the responsibility of the Public Health Service. George Pierre, Chief of the Confederated Tribes of Colville, urged the two government agencies to more closely cooperate in order to ensure that "the national policy for Indian development and welfare is effective and consistent."[8]

The need for medical facilities was only one of the demands competing for available resources. Because of the geographical location of most American Indian and Alaska Native communities, health facilities were (and many still are) located in isolated or sparsely populated areas. In many of these areas, housing facilities for employees were nonexistent. The lack of facilities was a prime factor in the program's inability to recruit and retain skilled professionals, who were indispensable to the health objectives of the Division.

At the time of the transfer in 1955, many of the housing units available for medical staff were "substandard, often mere shacks." Most housing units did not meet minimum federal standards of decency for commissioned corps officers. As temporary stopgaps, the Division of Indian Health acquired 326 used, prefabricated housing units in 1956 and added an additional 600 by 1965. An acute shortage of housing remained a stumbling block in the recruitment of physicians and other medical personnel.[9]

While the Public Health Service emphasized the construction of additional health facilities, its primary objective was to knit a closer relationship between

American Indian and Alaska Native communities and local health committees. Such joint undertakings were essential to the promotion of Indian health. Wagner informed a Senate appropriations committee in 1964 that to remedy this challenge the Division of Indian Health was incorporating American Indian and Alaska Native health aides into the program to make it more acceptable to its constituents while still "attacking poverty." Wagner added that a national epidemiology center was needed to implement a cooperative program of community health. Such a center would be "oriented to diseases and illness that are prevalent among the Indians but not commonly found among the general population." Compiling such data and then analyzing it could lead to a more effective preventive health program.[10]

A systematic method of record-keeping was also necessary to advancing Indian healthcare. The near lack of record-keeping frequently gave the program a public relations black eye. More often than not, poor or nonexistent record-keeping made Indian healthcare appear even more egregious than it really was. Often times the lack of medical records resulted from the great time demands placed on physicians, especially those in the isolated areas. In many Indian health facilities there were simply too few personnel and too great a patient load to maintain complete records. The American Medical Association urged Wagner to establish closer ties with state health associations to improve record-keeping or transfer as much of the program as was feasible to the private sector.[11]

It was imperative to have accurate record-keeping. But while the need was real, the tools to acquire the information were unavailable and few Indian communities were prepared for such joint ventures. Although successfully tested in several tribal communities, joint ventures slowly materialized. But while a national epidemiological center did not come to fruition, medical record librarians increased. In 1962, Shaw established the goal of placing a medical librarian in every hospital exceeding fifty beds. This was accomplished by mid-decade, with most small facilities staffed with clerical personnel trained in medical record-keeping. Records analysis and program development, however, remained elusive.

Corresponding with the increased focus on epidemiological research was a cooperative relationship between the Division of Indian Health and medical, scientific, and educational research groups. Medical needs were great but the available resources to mitigate these needs were limited. In an attempt to offset this continuing challenge, Wagner solicited private sector support for the campaign on disease in Indian Country. His goal was to influence specific areas of research in accordance with American Indian and Alaska Native health needs.[12]

A corollary measure designed to make Wagner's goal of community health a reality was to improve the management of the Indian health program. Wagner emphasized the need for medical officers to improve their hospital management skills. By learning to better manage the local community health facility, Wagner believed that the management infrastructure of the Division of Indian Health would improve. Medical officers trained in hospital management might be more effective in administering the day-to-day planning and fiscal husbandry of the local medical facility, making it more efficient with the use of limited resources. Public health educators were encouraged to earn graduate degrees and, by 1966, one-quarter of health educators had Master's of Public Health degrees.[13]

The Division of Indian Health also underwent internal change. In 1963, a seventh area office was created in Billings, Montana, and three field offices were added. The area offices continued to administer the health programs, but to better facilitate the medical program in Indian Country, each of the areas was subdivided into service units. Most reservations constituted a single service unit, although larger reservations were partitioned into multiple service units. The Navajo Reservation, for example, was divided into eight service units. Smaller reservations were combined into a single service unit.[14]

The service unit was the basic health service delivery organization for the Indian health service, acting much like a county or city health department. The service constituency looked to the health facilities within its service unit as the healthcare provider. Some preventive, mostly curative, services were available at most service units and most had at least one hospital and health center, as well as ancillary field clinics. Within the service units, hospitals remained the hub of all activities, providing both inpatient and outpatient services. Ancillary care via health centers and clinics was scheduled weekly or monthly. It was not uncommon for patients to travel ninety miles to a clinic, "only to find 200 to 300 people in line ahead of them, and leave at the end of the day without seeing a doctor." Some Navajo lived fifty miles from the nearest road, which might be eighty miles from the nearest hospital. At Wanblee, South Dakota, (ninety miles from the Indian hospital in Pine Ridge) one physician and two nurses visited the community weekly where fifty waiting patients often greeted them. The Havasupai in Arizona saw a physician twice a month and had limited nursing services. And a physician and nurse visited the Goshute Indian Community in Utah just once a month, with the nearest Indian hospital 275 miles away. One physician from each service unit was designated field health officer, spending part of his time in public and preventive health activities, most of which was outside the hospital setting. The preventive health activities conducted by field health officers included making home visits, conducting classes on diabetes, tuberculosis, pre- and postnatal care, and immunization clinics.[15]

## Increasing Indian Involvement

Wagner advanced the goal of expanding training programs for auxiliary health workers, both to encourage Indian participation in health services and to enable professional staff, such as physicians, dentists, and nurses, to make more efficient use of their time. This simple but important change greatly facilitated health services. Wagner recognized the only way to reach out to Indian communities was to enable them to take ownership of their health services. He also believed that if the Division of Indian Health were to overcome its shortage and high turnover rates of professional staff, it had to find ways to reduce physician patient loads. It was not uncommon for physicians to see 50 to 100 patients a day. On average there was just one physician for every 900 American Indians and Alaska Natives, with the ratio for dentists 1:2,900. The turnover rate of physicians remained high (83 percent by 1966), and even physicians and dentists serving under the doctor-dentist draft law, which allowed them to serve two years of military service in the Public Health Service, rarely stayed more than the minimum commitment.[16]

To realize the goal of training personnel for auxiliary health workers, the Division of Indian Health had to reach out to American Indian and Alaska Native communities and train local personnel. The historic lack of cultural connectedness plagued the health program, leading to the criticism that the Indian health service did not do enough to involve its constituents in their own healthcare. Although training courses and in-service institutes provided instruction and training in the areas of sanitation, dental, nutrition, nursing, health hygiene, and food service, they were in support roles. In 1964, Wagner initiated a demonstration program of training village health aides in Kotzebue, Alaska, as a means of providing community health services in remote villages and communities. The intent was to attack health issues in a more culturally sensitive manner and relieve healthcare professionals of the many mundane activities that burdened their time.[17]

The village health program promoted active community health awareness by raising the level of health sophistication among the people. It also provided training to health resource personnel on a paraprofessional level and delivered first aid treatment in remote areas. In this respect they were much like modern first-responders. The idea of training village health aides as liaisons between Alaska Native communities and medical personnel was not a foreign concept. In 1947 some Alaska Native villages employed similar aides. Until 1964, however, the responsibilities of the village aides grew informally and usually came as a result of necessity. That spring, the Indian health service initiated two formal five day training sessions, held in Kotzebue, to prepare aides for most aspects of general community health.[18]

An ancillary purpose of training village aides was to spread the effectiveness of the trained medical staff. Geographic inaccessibility of villages and frequent inclement weather kept most professional health personnel at major population centers and hospital facilities. Consequently, rural or village-oriented Alaska Natives requiring medical attention typically received such care on a delayed basis. By utilizing village health aides, who maintained contact with the Public Health Service Indian hospital in Kotzebue via short-wave radio, patients in outlying areas received treatment for everything from minor trauma to otitis media. In a very real sense village health aides were the primary medical care providers in rural Alaska Native villages.

The use of village aides in isolated Alaska Native villages was not the only place such aides were trained or employed. In the continental United States the Navajo Nation represented the most isolated and dispersed tribal nation, being spread over 18,000,000 acres in Arizona, New Mexico, and Utah. When the Public Health Service assumed responsibility for healthcare, it contracted with Cornell University Medical College to establish the Navajo-Cornell Field Health Research Project at Many Farms, Arizona, a community of 2,000 Navajo. The Many Farms Project sought to identify cultural concerns in the delivery of services to the Navajo. Having done that, the program worked to develop practical ways of delivering health services in a culturally meaningful way. Pivotal to the project was the training and employment of Navajos as medical aides, one of the first uses of paraprofessional healthcare workers in the civilian sector in the United States.[19]

Eight Navajo were selected as medical aides and placed in two classes, each consisting of two women and two men. The first class was held in 1956 with the second three years later. Candidates were selected on the basis of interest and willingness, with all but one having experienced an extended period of hospitalization for tuberculosis, an intangible characteristic that Cornell saw as integral to the position since it would allow the aides to empathize with patients while at the same time helping them comprehend the goals of Western medical care. The goal of the Division of Indian Health was that the aides would assist those Navajo who did not comprehend the germ theory accept modern medicine. Many American Indians, including the Navajo, viewed illness as a reflection of disharmony between the spiritual, physical, and emotional forces and, therefore, outside the realm of Western medicine.[20]

In training Navajo aides, Cornell University sought to convey a basic understanding of health and disease in carrying out specific nursing procedures (while under the direction of a public health nurse). The trainees were to collect demographic and health data (and keep accurate records) and complete simple medical instructions and procedures. They were trained to give basic emergency care until a patient could be transported to either a hospital or the care of a physician. The ability to communicate in Navajo and understand Navajo culture was fundamentally more important than formal education.[21]

To carryout the program of medical aides, trainees received instruction in personal health, community hygiene, and basic principles of epidemiology, immunology, sanitation, nutrition, dental care, and family life. Additional training was provided in general medical record-keeping. After the completion of a six month trial basis, during which the trainees were dispatched to three different areas on the reservation, the aides were hired as permanent Public Health Service employees. The use of aides increased by four-fold the territory that could be covered on the Navajo Nation by the public health nurses.

The use of medical aides among the Navajo (central to the holistic concept of the Many Farms Project) helped introduce a system of primary care that was both sensitive to the needs of the people and involved them in community health. When the initial phase of the project ended in July 1962, the Public Health Service hailed it as a success both in terms of community expectations and satisfaction of healthcare delivered. Despite the success, the latter component had a limited impact on disease prevention. Critics charged the Public Health Service with once again attacking Indian health problems without dealing with environmental, social, and economic factors. Despite such criticism, a fundamental paradigm shift was in the making, one that encouraged cultural understanding.[22]

The success of the Indian health service was to a large degree dependent on reaching out to the American Indian and Alaska Native communities and involving them in the delivery of health services. Too often the medical profession treated the recipients of their services as objects, not participants. A Western biochemical approach to medicine "constitute[d] an assault upon a culture where people define themselves in terms of their relationship to others, where they view illness as a sign of being out of harmony with the universe." Colville Chief George Pierre simply argued the Indian health service had to do more in adjusting its professional attitudes and practices to "make them more suitable and acceptable to my people."[23]

## Challenges Remain

The need to extend preventive services was great. While the training of aides was a step in the right direction, conditions demanded a full assault on the leading causes of disease: poverty and the lack of sanitation facilities in Indian homes and communities. At its annual meeting held in Phoenix, Arizona, in 1964, the American Medical Association applauded the Division of Indian Health for its recent efforts to improve sanitary conditions and water problems in Indian Country. But in a 1964 speech to the National Congress of American Indians, President Lyndon B. Johnson declared that poverty continued to be a fact of life for most American Indians and Alaska Natives. Most Indians, the president noted, were "desperately poor." Commissioner of Indian Affairs Philleo Nash affirmed Johnson's remark when he noted: "Our major effort in recent years has been to remedy past neglect."[24]

The Johnson Administration implemented the war on poverty envisioned by President John F. Kennedy. While designed to end poverty throughout the country, several Great Society programs extended assistance to American Indians to eliminate poor health and improve educational opportunities. Using Economic Opportunity Act funds, many tribes constructed tribal governmental buildings and stimulated (for a short time anyway) tribal economic advancement (some tribes developed tribal housing authorities). When Wagner assumed the directorship of the Division of Indian Health, poverty remained widespread among American Indian and Alaska Native communities. In 1962, the average reservation family had a combined annual income of $1,500, 50 percent lower than the $3,000 national poverty line. Reservation unemployment rates were nearly eight times the national average, with the underemployment rates even higher. When Nash noted that nine out of ten American Indian families lived in substandard housing it was no surprise to those involved in Indian affairs. Inadequate housing meant substandard health conditions. Low economic status resulted in poor nutrition, which further reduced resistance to infectious or contagious diseases.[25]

Secretary of Health, Education and Welfare John W. Gardner acknowledged that the scarcity of safe water for domestic use, combined with the lack of sanitary waste disposal facilities, was not only common among American Indian and Alaska Native communities, but was also responsible for the high rates of infectious diseases, particularly among infants. A child's first year of life was fraught with danger due to a variety of socioeconomic and environmental factors, as shown in Table 3.2.[26]

Table 3.2

*Comparison of Death and Birth Rates, American Indian and U.S. General Population, 1964*

| Population Group | Birth rate per 1,000 live births | Death Rate | Average age of death |
|---|---|---|---|
| American Indians | 42.2 | 41.8 | 42 |
| Alaska Natives | 48.6 | 66.8 | 30 |
| U.S. General Population | 23.7 | 25.3 | 62.3 |

(Source: *Healthier Indian Mothers and Babies*, 1964)

Wagner estimated three-quarters of American Indians and Alaska Natives lacked or had unsatisfactory water and waste facilities. Health complications related to the lack of sanitation facilities included gastroenteritis, which ranked at the top of all reported notifiable diseases in Indian communities. The incidence rates of amoebic and bacillary dysentery were more than 50 percent higher than the non-Indian rates, with approximately 35 percent of all American Indian and Alaska Native patients discharged from Indian hospitals treated for infectious diseases. The primary factor was insanitary conditions and overcrowded housing. Other health challenges related to insanitary conditions included infant mortality, which was nearly 70 percent higher than the non-Indian rate. For infants under the age one the mortality rate was four times (among Alaska Natives it was six times) that of the comparable non-Indian rate. Table 3.3 compares the American Indian and national distribution rate of deaths by age. The high American Indian death rate was attributed to insanitary facilities in the home. Twenty percent of all reported Indian deaths in 1965 were infants under the age of one year; for non-Indians, the rate was about 6 percent.[27]

Wagner reported to a House Subcommittee on Indian Affairs in 1963 that more than 80 percent of all reservation Indians hauled water from sources more than one mile from their homes. Of this number, nearly eight out of ten hauled water from contaminated streams, irrigation ditches, stock ponds and unprotected wells and springs. In some instances, they were required to purchase water for domestic purposes at a cost of $1 to $3 per barrel. The lack of disposal facilities for human and household waste contributed to health concerns. In addition to diseases such as diarrhea and dysentery, which were directly related to poor sanitation, vector and rodent infestations and contaminated food supplies resulted from poor sanitation facilities.[28]

Table 3.3

*Percent Distribution of Death by Age*

| Indian Rate | Age Group | Non-Indian Rate |
|---|---|---|
| 14 percent | < 1 | 4 percent |
| 4 percent | 1-4 | 1 percent |
| 10 percent | 5-24 | 3 percent |
| 17 percent | 25-44 | 6 percent |
| 21 percent | 45-64 | 25 percent |
| 33 percent | 65 + | 61 percent |

(Source: Interior Appropriation Hearings, 1969)

Under the provisions of the Indian Sanitation Facilities Construction Act, the Division of Indian Health continued to construct water treatment, storage, and distribution systems, as well as waste collection, treatment, and disposal systems. The Indian health service constructed household appurtenances, such as sanitary pit privies or flush commodes, kitchen sinks, and sundry plumbing accessories, as well as drainage facilities for controlling insect and rodent problems, and subsurface waste disposal. In the first six years of construction, 436 sanitation projects were undertaken, 367 of which were completed. The fact remained, however, that less than 30 percent of the known sanitation need was met. Of the 400,000 American Indians and Alaska Natives, just 24,000 had basic sanitation services.

But while the Office of Environmental Health, established under the authority of the Indian Sanitation Facilities Construction Act, improved or constructed sanitation facilities in existing homes prior to 1965, after mid-decade it coordinated the construction of sanitation facilities with the construction of new Indian homes provided under the Public Housing Administration, Bureau of Indian Affairs, Office of Economic Opportunity, and tribal housing authorities. Wagner informed a Senate appropriation hearing that he hoped the agency would work with the Bureau of Indian Affairs and the Public Housing Administration to construct 3,200 Indian homes, a proposition the director knew would be difficult to fulfill. After 1965 the Indian health service and the Bureau of Indian Affairs jointly planned housing and sanitation construction. Using joint ventures, tribal housing authorities, the Public Housing Administration, and the Bureau of Indian Affairs constructed houses, while the Indian health service constructed sanitation facilities.[29]

## Expanding Services

By the mid-1960s, the number of admissions in Indian hospitals increased 64 percent since 1955. To eligible American Indians and Alaska Natives, the Public Health Service provided services through 49 Indian hospitals, 46 health centers, and approximately 300 health clinics and field stations. But despite the advantages of being in the Public Health Service, the Division of Indian Health still experienced difficulties in maintaining adequate medical staffing for its hospitals and health facilities. While the number of staff increased substantially, the program was still in need of health professionals, as seen in Table 3.4. The Indian health service still had a significantly higher physician to patient ratio than the nation as a whole (Minnesota Indians had a ratio of 1:1,485 with a non-Indian ratio of 1:714, while Oklahoma Indians had a ratio of 1:2,390 with a non-Indian ratio of 1:1,005).[30]

Where Public Health Service facilities were unavailable or where specialized care was absent, contracts with over 200 private or community hospitals, representing nearly 400 physicians, dentists, and specialists, and eighteen state and local health departments provided services. But here, too, there were difficulties in providing services. American Indians often felt they were "treated with contempt and rudeness" and feared that the Indian health service would fail to pay for their care at non-Indian hospitals. Some local communities and, even states, failed to recognize American Indians as citizens "entitled to the same rights and privileges as any other citizen."[31]

But if contract care was difficult to obtain, pharmaceutical services were non-existent. In 1951, the Public Health Service assigned Dr. Allen Brands to the Division of Commissioned Officers where he was responsible for assigning commissioned corps officers to hospitals and clinics under the Bureau of Medical Services. Brands was also responsible for loans to Bureau of Indian Affairs hospitals. Of the sixty-three Indian hospitals and scores of clinics then in operation, Brands found no pharmacists. Astounded at this deficiency, Brands made an investigatory trip to several Indian hospitals in Oklahoma, where he hoped to convince Bureau of Indian Affairs officials and area medical officers of the need for pharmacists. What he found during his travels was startling: Some prescription drugs were in excess of twenty years old. In all of the facilities he examined, nurses and physicians carried heavy patient loads, which were exacerbated by their responsibilities to order, package, stock, and dispense drugs. When the Public Health Service assigned Brands to the Bureau in 1953, to serve as pharmacist in the central office of the Branch of Indian Health, there were just two pharmacists in the whole of the Indian Service—and both were located at the Indian hospital in Mt. Edgecumbe, Alaska.[32]

Brands established an ambitious goal of placing at least one pharmacist in every large Indian hospital where he could store, package, label, and dispense all medicines for that facility. For smaller hospitals and clinics, Brands utilized area offices, where a single person served as an area pharmacy officer. These persons then provided indirect pharmacy services, in effect acting as a central purchasing, packaging, and labeling center. Prescriptions were filled at the central location and given to outpatients by nurses and doctors who no longer had to count and repackage drugs. Area pharmacists also visited smaller facilities to periodically inspect drugs, with surplus or outdated supplies returned to the area pharmacy for redistribution or disposal.[33]

Table 3.4

*Comparison of Health Professionals, 1955 and 1962*

| Category | 1955 | 1962 |
|---|---|---|
| Service Population* | 370,000 | 380,000 |
| Physicians | 125 | 279 |
| Dentists | 40 | 101 |
| Graduate Nurses | 783 | 916 |
| Sanitary Engineers/sanitarians | 14 | 59 |
| * approximation | | |

(Source: *Review of the Indian Health Program*, 1963)

The redistribution of drugs was a critical aspect of the pharmacy program. With high professional turnover rates, it was not uncommon for drugs to be ordered by a physician who subsequently left the hospital or clinic before the medicine arrived. Replacement physicians, not familiar with the prescription, often disposed of it. Brands lamented that some physicians took advantage of Indian patients by testing new drugs on them first "so they would know about them when they left the service for private practice."[34]

Brands initiated other changes enabling pharmacists to contribute to the well-being of American Indians and Alaska Natives. In 1962, pharmacists filled prescriptions from patient medical records rather than from prescription forms. This not only saved time but it also improved safety, as physicians no longer were required to write prescriptions on separate forms and record them in the patient's medical record. Filling prescriptions from a patient's medical record allowed pharmacists to prevent the dispensing of incompatible drugs or prescribing drugs that caused allergic reactions or performed similar functions as previously dispensed drugs.

Like many other functions of the Indian health service, new pharmacies were established with great difficulty, both in terms of personnel and physical facilities. Filling the Division's need for pharmacists was as challenging as finding physicians and other medical specialists. Finding places to house them was difficult. At the health facility in Rapid City, South Dakota, for example, the pharmacy was located in an old school building. In Shawnee, Oklahoma, it was housed in the old laundry building. The pharmacy at Red Lake (Chippewa), Minnesota, was housed on the back porch of an old building across the street from the hospital. In some facilities, pharmacies were located in the general waiting area of the hospital. In these facilities, patients often objected to the manner in which drugs were dispensed. In Whiteriver, Arizona, the Apache complained about lack of privacy. At their request the Division of Indian Health established private offices for pharmacists to dispense drugs, as well as to instruct and counsel patients in the proper use of prescriptions.[35]

Since many patients could not read, write, or speak English, the Indian health service developed creative ways of dispensing drugs. One of the more creative was to place pictorial labels on prescription bottles. Designed by George Dick of the Fort Defiance (Navajo) Indian Hospital in Arizona, pictorial labels were introduced among the Navajo in 1962 because of the high non-English speaking population. Pictures on bottles designated the patient by circling the image of the appropriate family member (baby, boy, woman, etc), the time of day (by position of the sun or moon) the medicine was to be taken, and the proper dosage.

To further reduce physician caseloads, Brands proposed authorizing pharmacists to provide non-prescription drugs for American Indian and Alaska Native patients without first having to visit a physician. In off-reservation towns and cities, people went to the local community pharmacy to obtain prescriptions for minor illnesses. So, Brands argued, "Why couldn't the Indians be treated the same way?" Some hospitals, such as the Indian hospital in Cherokee, North Carolina, reported up to 90 percent of the patient load could be directed to the pharmacist if the Indian health service concurred with the recommendation of Brands. Allowing pharmacists to prescribe drugs would allow physicians to spend more time with those truly in need of care. For two years the concept was debated before Wagner rejected it, arguing that the Public Health Service was a physicians' organization. If a patient was ill enough to seek treatment, he was ill enough to see a physician. A few months later, Wagner was promoted to the Director of the Bureau of Medical Services and Erwin S. Rabeau assumed the Directorship of the Division of Indian Health. In 1967, Rabeau authorized pharmacists to provide drugs to patients without a medical prescription.[36]

## Health Status

The operational improvements, the increasing number of services, the administrative changes, and the addition of new programs meant little if there was no substantive change in American Indian and Alaska Native health. While conditions improved, the average age of death for American Indians remained forty-two years (for Arizona Indians it was just thirty-one and in neighboring New Mexico it was thirty-three). The national average was 50 percent higher at sixty-two years of age. The low Indian averages reflected high infant mortality rates in Arizona and New Mexico. Tuberculosis, which was the number one cause of death among American Indians and Alaska Natives in 1956, dropped 64 percent by 1966.

Infant mortality rate likewise declined over 41 percent. Yet, the fact remained childhood diseases, including tuberculosis rates, remained higher among American Indians and Alaska Natives than the general population, as seen in Table 3.5.[37]

Table 3.5

*Age-Specific Death Rates from Tuberculosis, 1961-1963*

| Age Group | Indian (1961-1963) | All Races (1962) |
|---|---|---|
| under 5 | 6.5 | .8 |
| 5-14 | 2.8 | .5 |
| 15-19 | 5.1 | .2 |
| 20-24 | 9.0 | .5 |
| all ages | 56.6 | 5.1 |

(Source: *Childhood Tuberculosis*, 1967)

While the one-time leading causes of death were declining, new health concerns were arising, partially due to the increasing life-expectancy among American Indians and Alaska Natives and partially because of dietary changes. Diabetes, for instance, was prevalent in the Southwest and devastated the Pima and Tohono O'odham (Papago). By the mid-1960s, the Pima had the highest rate of diabetes mellitus ever recorded among any population group. A 1963 survey reported 31.3 percent of Pima aged thirty and over had diabetes and a 1965 study indicated 49 percent of the Pima over the age of thirty had diabetes. Malignant neoplasms (cancer), homicide, suicide, and accidental deaths all increased sharply in the first decade of Public Health Service responsibility for Indian healthcare. In the Southwest, biliary disease (gallbladder), portal cirrhosis, enteric infections, glaucoma, and other diseases were widespread. Alcoholism and mental illness also increased. And even though the infant mortality rate decreased, it remained one of the leading causes of death in Indian Country, with nearly one-quarter of American Indian and Alaska Native deaths infants. Table 3.6 highlights the changing health status of American Indians and Alaska Natives between 1955 and 1966.[38]

Believing trachoma to be an issue of the past, research on the disease came to a halt by 1960, with most researchers and funding turning to other issues. The lack of adequate sanitation facilities and hygiene education, however, led to episodic increases in the disease, striking especially hard in the Southwest. Among the Pueblos, Pima, Tohono O'odham, Apache, and Navajo the disease returned to its prewar rates. When the Third National Conference on American Indian Health convened in New York City, in November of 1964, it focused most of its efforts on the issue of trachoma. Trachoma rates increased from 1,000 per 100,000 in 1963, to nearly 2,300 per 100,000 in 1964. Two years later, after a trachoma abatement program was begun, the rate remained 1,600 per 100,000. The Indian health service believed the high rates in the Southwest resulted from poor sanitation conditions in Indian boarding schools, the hot, dry, and windy climate, and the overcrowding and inadequate water supplies prevalent in many Indian homes. In the Pima village of Blackwater, a "significant reservoir of [trachoma was present] in preschool children."[39]

Table 3.6

*Changes in Causes of Death: 1955-1966*
(per 100,000 Population)

| Cause of Death | 1955 | 1966 | Difference |
|---|---|---|---|
| Accidents | 714 | 1,003 | + .40 |
| Diabetes | 64 | 115 | + .80 |
| Gastrointestinal | 165 | 107 | - .35 |
| Homicide | 77 | 102* | + .32 |
| Infant Mortality** | 63 | 37 | - .41 |
| Malignant Neoplasms | 296 | 386 | + .30 |
| Maternal Deaths | 16 | 7# | - .56 |
| Suicide | 39 | 64 | + .64 |
| Tuberculosis | 253 | 91 | - .64 |

(* 1965 rate)
(** Per 1,000 Live Births)
(# 1967 Rate)

(Source: *Trends in Indian Health*, 1989)

The inescapable conclusion was that treatment alone could not eradicate trachoma. Overcoming the challenge required treatment plus environmental changes. Sources of safe water and a relevant health education program that people could understand was essential. To ensure the implementation of such a program, the Association on American Indian Affairs urged the Indian health service to plan and execute a trachoma program "with the advice and active participation of representatives of the tribal councils." In 1966, Wagner initiated a five year trachoma prevention program, with three teams of specialists working out of the Public Health Service hospitals in Phoenix and Keams Canyon, Arizona, and Gallup, New Mexico. In fiscal year 1967, specialists screened 40,931 individuals for trachoma, with 4,883 (11 percent) infected. Over 70 percent of the new cases were children under the age of 19.[40]

The prevalence of measles was a concern for children, even though the development of an effective measles vaccine and its availability to American Indians and Alaska Natives in 1963 was a landmark accomplishment. The immunization program, much like vaccination programs for polio, diphtheria, whooping cough, and similar diseases, targeted school-aged children, largely leaving adults unprotected. Due to the absence of vaccinations for non-school-aged children, the American Indian and Alaska Native incidence rate of measles remained six times the non-Indian rate, with whooping cough ten times more prevalent. Any further progress in the campaign against such childhood diseases was "dependent upon increased emphasis on home-centered, physician-directed, community health programs." Despite the lack of community health programs, a measles immunization program reduced the number of measles cases by 67 percent by 1967. Table 3.7 shows the infant mortality rate (all cases) for American Indians and Alaska Natives. [41]

Table 3.7

*American Indian and Alaska Native Infant Mortality Rates, 1960-1966*
(Per 1,000 live births)

| Year | American Indians | Alaska Natives | All Natives | U.S. All Races |
|------|------------------|----------------|-------------|----------------|
| 1960 | 47.6 | 73.6 | 50.3 | 26.0 |
| 1961 | 42.3 | 64.0 | 44.4 | 25.3 |
| 1962 | 41.8 | 66.8 | 44.2 | 25.3 |
| 1963 | 42.9 | 50.7 | 43.6 | 25.2 |
| 1964 | 35.9 | 54.8 | 37.6 | 24.8 |
| 1965 | 36.4 | 65.4 | 39.0 | 24.7 |
| 1966 | 37.7 | 51.4 | 39.0 | 23.7 |

(Source: *Evaluation of Public Health Service Program*)

Other diseases robbing children of good health included otitis media and related forms of inner ear infection, which often resulted in hearing loss. Nearly 80 percent of Alaska Native children suffered from otitis media, and an estimated one-quarter of all Inuit in Alaska suffered from hearing impediments. Hunger and malnutrition also remained prevalent in Indian Country.[42] But children were not alone in facing health challenges. While cultural loss and identity crises were not new, the loss or disintegration of culture, high levels of poverty, low educational achievement, and haunting childhood experiences manifested themselves in an alarming rate of mental illness among adults. Distraught by poverty and loss of cultural security, many American Indians and Alaska Natives were emotionally imbalanced, unable to take advantage of opportunities to stop the cycle, exacerbating the spiral. Suicide, alcoholism, glue sniffing, delinquency, and broken homes were simply symptoms of a larger, underlying challenge. Some statistics suggested that as many as one in four American Indians were affected by mental illness.[43]

The fact was the Division of Indian Health remained crisis-oriented. While there was movement toward preventive services, the backlog of disease and ill-health made the task difficult to accomplish, tarnishing the *espirit de corps* so popular during the initial years of Public Health Service auspices. The priorities and policies of the Division of Indian Health seemed to favor the temporary relief of the few over the expense of life and health for the many. Adequate healthcare, basic sanitation services, and culturally appropriate treatment remained elusive.

# Notes

1. "Awards, Honors," *Journal of the American Medical Association* (192:7) May 17, 1965, 46. The award had been given only five times, with Wagner the first recipient since 1952. Wagner initiated numerous private Indian health-university medical research projects including, but not limited to, Cornell University, the Phipps Institute, the American Medical Association, the University of Arizona, the University of Utah and several state departments of public health.

2. "Council on Medical Service," *Journal of the American Medical Service* (186:4) November 26, 1963, 391.

3. "Medical News," *Journal of the American Medical Association* (195:5) January 31, 1966, 42. Todd, "Interview with Carruth J. Wagner." Wagner continued to impact Indian health care policy during his tenure with the Bureau of Medical Services. He retired in 1968 with thirty years of Public Health Service to his credit.

4. "Review of the Indian Health Program," 14. Contract care totaled $5,032,652 in 1955 and increased to $10,700,000 by 1963.

5. Edgar S. Cahn and David W. Hearne, Eds. *Our Brother's Keeper: The Indian in White America* (New York: New American Library, 1969), 56. "Review of the Indian Health Program," 3.

6. *Justifications of Appropriation Estimates for Committee on Appropriations*, fiscal year 1966, United States Department of Health, Education and Welfare, CIHF-41. National Commission on Community Health Services, "Health Is a Community Affair," in *Making Health Resources Available to All Beneficiaries* (Washington, D.C.: United States Department of Health, Education and Welfare, Public Health Service, Division of Indian Health, January 9, 1967), 9.

7. *Indian Health Program*, 1963.

8. George Pierre, *American Indian Crisis* (San Antonio, TX: The Naylor Company, 1971), 87. Cahn, *Our Brother's Keeper*, 62, was more succinct: "The two agencies rarely coordinate efforts." A 1968 House Appropriations Committee reported that the Division of Indian Health and the Bureau of Indian Affairs rarely communicated. As an example, they reported on a particular Indian boarding school that had a mild strep throat epidemic among its students. The students were treated by the nearby Indian health clinic but the Indian Bureau was never informed. An Indian health official claimed there was virtually no communication between the two governmental agencies. "Department of the Interior and Related Agencies Appropriations for 1969," *Hearings before the Subcommittee of the Committee on Appropriations House of Representatives* 90th Congress, 2nd session, Part III, 502-503.

9. *Justifications of Appropriation Estimates for Committee on Appropriations*, fiscal year 1966, CIHF-61. For fiscal year 1966, $1,405,000 was available to construct personnel housing; only $891,000 was utilized.

10. *Annual Report of the Department of Health, Education and Welfare*, 1963, 151.

"Interior Department and Related Agencies Appropriation Bill, 1965," *Senate Report no. 971* 88th Congress, 2d session, April 4, 1964, 1272. Wagner noted the successful Indian training program for nursing assistants and practical nurses, which was held at the Rapid City Tuberculosis Hospital. In 1964, twenty Indian women graduated from the program.

11. "Council on Medical Service."

12. For example, Cornell University and its Many Farms Projects among the Navajo; the Phipps Institute and its continuing work on tuberculosis among American Indians; various schools of public health also joined up with particular Indian tribes to conduct studies particular to area or tribal needs.

13. Wallace W. Jonz, "Staffing Health Education Programs for American Indians," *Public Health Reports* (81:7) July 1966, 627-630. In 1966 there were thirty-nine health education specialists (ten of whom had M.P.H. degrees) and six community health education aides (all of whom worked on the Navajo Reservation). In order to work in the area offices or at headquarters, health education specialists needed a minimum of five years experience and a M.P.H. degree.

14. The area offices included: Anchorage, Alaska; Portland, Oregon; Billings, Montana; Aberdeen, South Dakota; Phoenix, Arizona; Albuquerque, New Mexico; and Oklahoma City, Oklahoma. Field Offices were in Bemidji, Minnesota; Window Rock, Arizona; and Mt. Edgecumbe, Alaska. The Fort McDowell Yavapai-Apache, Salt River Pima-Maricopa, Ak-Chin and Gila River Pima-Maricopa Indian Communities, for example, were all under the Gila River (Sacaton) service unit.

15. Cahn, *Our Brother's Keeper*, 59 and 63. Cahn quoted a February 19, 1969, *New York Times* report that noted twenty Navajo infants were dead on arrival at medical stations on the western side of the reservation because of travel delays in reaching the nearest clinic. "Healthier Indian Mothers and Babies," *Public Health Reports* (79:6), June 1964, 468. *The Indian Health Program of the United States Public Health Service* (Department of Health, Education and Welfare, Public Health Service, 1963), 5.

16. *Annual Report of the Department of Health, Education and Welfare*, 1963, 151. George Blue Spruce, "American Indians as Dental Patients," *Public Health Reports* (76:12) December 1961, 1059-1062. In 1963, there was just one Indian physician and no Indian dentists in the health program. Testimony of Wagner in "Review of the Indian Health Program," 38-39. "Department of the Interior and Related Agencies Appropriations for Fiscal Year 1967," *Hearings before a Subcommittee of the Committee on Appropriations United States Senate* 89th Congress, 2d session, March 8, 1966, part 2, 1440. Medical Director Erwin Rabeau complained that for years the retention rate of two year enlistments was zero.

17. Pierre, *American Indian Crisis*, 88; Cahn, *Our Brother's Keeper*, 66-67. An Indian health psychiatrist went so far as to acknowledge that the Division of Indian Health didn't "believe it is important to involve the people we are serving in the provision of the service." Some health professionals failed to see that the Indian community might have something to contribute to the improvement of health conditions.

18. Thomas J. Harrison, "Training for Village Health Aides in the Kotzebue Area of Alaska," *Public Health Reports* (80:7) July 1965, 565, 571.

19. Kurt W. Deuschle, "Training and Use of Medical Auxiliaries in a Navajo Community," *Public Health Reports* (78:6), June 1963, 461. William Brodt, "Implications

for Training Curriculums from a Task Inventory Survey of Indian Community Health Representatives," *Public Health Reports* (90:6) December 1975, 553.

20. In 1963 President John F. Kennedy presented Navajo Councilwoman Annie D. Wauneka the Presidential Medal of Freedom for her work in helping the Navajo accept modern medicine. The daughter of Navajo Chief Henry Chee Dodge, Wauneka was among the first women to win the award. She had also been presented with the Hughes Memorial Award by the Arizona Press Women's Association in 1958; the Indian Achievement Medal in 1959; and was honored by the Arizona Public Health Association in 1959, as an "outstanding worker in public health." "Presidential Medal of Freedom Awarded to Annie D. Wauneka," *Public Health Reports* (78:10) October 1963, 838.

21. Deuschle, 464.

22. J. Adair and K. W. Deuschle, *The People's Health: Medicine and Anthropology in a Navajo Community* (New York: Appleton-Century-Crofts, 1970). Walsh McDermott, Kurt W. Deuschle, and Clifford R. Barnett, "Health Care Experiment at Many Farms," *Science* (175:1) January 7, 1972, 29. "Making Health Resources Available to All Beneficiaries," 9.

23. Cahn, *Our Brother's Keeper*, 65. Cahn opined that as the educational system was seeking acculturation, so, too, "Indian health care has the effect of a form of cultural war. Indians often must reject their traditions to secure the white man's medicine." Cahn suggested that American Indians resisted such choices through alcoholism and suicide or "thinly disguised efforts at self-destruction." Pierre, *American Indian Crisis*, 87, urged physicians to confer with Native Americans and seek to "benefit from their counsel."

24. "Council on Medical Service," *Journal of the American Medical Association* (190:4) October 26, 1964, 355. "Remarks to Members of the National Congress of American Indians," January 20, 1964, *Public Papers of the Presidents of the United States: Lyndon Baines Johnson, Containing the Public Messages, Speeches and Statements of the President 1963-1964*, Vol. 1 (Washington, D.C.: Government Printing Office, 1965), 149-152.

25. Carl W. Taylor, Jr., and Armin L. Saeger, Jr., "Maternal Health and Socioeconomic Status of Non Reservation Indians," *Public Health Reports* (83:6), June 1968, 465-473. Taylor and Saeger examined socioeconomic conditions in eastern Oklahoma and found that non-reservation Indians were healthier than reservation Indians. The more "socially Indian" one was the more rural, less educated, and more impoverished one was.

26. *Annual Report of the Department of Health, Education and Welfare*, 1966, 153. Infant mortality rates dropped significantly by the mid-sixties largely due to more babies being born in hospitals, but there was no equivalent decline in the infant death rate once infants left the hospital and returned home. Infants between one month of age and one year of age faced the greatest danger. "Healthier Indian Mothers and Babies," 468.

27. William Lasersohn, "Acute Diarrheal Disease in a Zuni Village," *Public Health Reports* (80:5), May 1965 457-461. Lasersohn reported that diarrhea reached "epidemic proportions" every summer largely due to poor sanitation and overcrowding. Frank R. Lemon, "Health Problems of the Navajos in Monument Valley, Utah," *Public Health Reports* (75:11) November 1960, 1055-1061. A. Rubenstein, J. Boyle, C. L. Odoroff, and S. J. Kunitz, "Effects of Improved Sanitary Facilities on Infant Diarrhea in a Hopi Village," *Public Health Reports* (84:12) December 1969, 1093-1097. *Justifications of Appropriation Estimates for Committee on Appropriations*, fiscal year 1966, CIHF 78-79.

28. "Department of the Interior and Related Agencies Appropriations for 1965," *Hearings before a Subcommittee of the Committee on Appropriations House of Representatives* 88th Congress, 1st session, February 19, 1963, 1504.

29. *Justifications of Appropriation Estimates for Committee on Appropriations*, fiscal year 1967, CIHF-259. 50 Stat., 888. Providing every American family with a "decent, safe and sanitary dwelling" was the main impetus behind the United States Housing Act of 1937. Despite the passage of the law, it was not until 1961 that the public housing program, through an administrative function, initiated a low-rent Indian housing program. In a White House ceremony on September 19, 1961, President Kennedy authorized Indian tribes to legally establish, under Indian law, tribal housing authorities that could be empowered to plan, develop, and operate low-income public housing projects. The extension of the 1937 Public Housing Act to Indian communities in 1961 was the first significant housing construction effort for Indian communities. "A First for Indian Citizens," *15th Annual Report of the Housing and Home Finance Agency, 1961* (Washington, D.C.: Government Printing Office, 1961), 208. *Report on Indian Housing*, United States Senate Select Committee on Indian Affairs (Washington, D.C.: Government Printing Office, 1979), 23. "Interior Department and Related Agencies Appropriation Bill, 1965," 1302-1303.

30. "Council on Medical Service," 355.

31. Carruth J. Wagner and Erwin S. Rabeau, "Indian Poverty and Indian Health," Health, Education and Welfare Indicators (Washington, D.C.: Department of Health, Education and Welfare, March 1964), xxx. *Making Health Resources Available to All Beneficiaries*, 5-6.

32. "Urgent Deficiency Appropriations Bill, 1956," 462.

33. Allen Brands, *History of Pharmacy in the Indian Health Service* Unpublished manuscript in the Commissioned Corps Centennial Archives, History of Medicine Division, National Library of Medicine, Bethesda, Maryland, 1981, 14.

34. Brands, *History of Pharmacy*, 15.

35. Brands, *History of Pharmacy*, 24-25.

36. Brands, *History of Pharmacy*, 36.

37. "Review of the Indian Health Program," 38. The life expectancy for an Indian baby in 1961 was sixty-two years versus seventy years for a non-Indian baby. While no figures were given for Alaska, Wagner acknowledged that it was much lower than among American Indians. Helen M. Wallace, "Childhood Tuberculosis with Reference to the American Indian," *Public Health Reports* (82:1) January 1967, 30-34. Wallace argued better data collection, follow-up, diagnosis, prevention, and evaluation of data was necessary to further reduce childhood tuberculosis.

38. Maurice L. Sievers, "Disease Patterns Among Southwestern Indians," *Public Health Reports* (81:12) December 1966, 1078-1079. M. Miller, T. A. Burch, P. H. Bennett and A. G. Steinberg, "Prevalence of Diabetes Mellitus in American Indians: Results of Glucose Tolerance Tests in the Pima Indians of Arizona," *Diabetes* (14) July 1965, 439-440. Because of the high rate of diabetes and gallbladder disease among the Pima, The National Institute of Arthritis and Metabolic Disease proposed to build and staff a twenty-five-bed research unit within the proposed Phoenix Indian Medical Center. The unit later became the first research unit to be incorporated into a PHS Indian hospital. "Metabolic Research Unit for Phoenix Medical Center," *Public Health Reports* (82:4) April 1967, 338. A portable

clinic and epidemiological station were built in Sacaton to research the role of diet and other environmental factors on diabetes. "Washington News," *Journal of the American Medical Association* (197:4) July 25, 1966, 21. Sievers, "Disease Patterns Among Southwestern Indians," 1075-1083. Sievers was head of the Phoenix Indian hospital's department of medicine and based his findings on eight years of studying Southwestern Indians (1957-1964). James E. Brown and Chris Christiansen, "Biliary Tract Disease among the Navajo," *Journal of the American Medical Association* (202:11) December 11, 1967, 1050-1052. Frank G. Hesse, "Incidence of Cholecystitis and Other Diseases among the Pima Indians of Southern Arizona," *Journal of the American Medical Association* (170:15) August 8, 1959, 1789-1790. Wagner told the House Subcommittee on Indian Affairs that the Indian health service had no mental health program, meaning "no plans to identify the causes of mental illness." While Wagner was planning to bring consultants in to make recommendations on a "service-unit by service unit basis," he had no resources with which to start any preventive mental health program. "Review of the Indian Health Program," 33. A number of general hospitals provided outpatient psychiatric services in the early sixties (Crow, Shiprock, Ft. DeFiance, Tahlequah). In 1968, Rabeau told Special Senate Indian Education committee that the Indian health service was gradually shifting from concentrating on clinical services to planning and implementing a comprehensive program in which mental health concepts were to be integrated into the daily operation of the hospital staff and community. "Indian Education," *Hearings before the Special Subcommittee on Indian Education of the Committee on Labor and Public Welfare United States Senate* 90 Congress, 1st and 2d session, May 24, 1968, part 5, 2194.

39. *Appropriation Hearings for the Department of the Interior for Fiscal Year 1979*, H181-41, Part 4, 234. John C. Cobb and Chandler R. Dawson, "Trachoma among Southwestern Indians," *Journal of the American Medical Association* November 1961 (175:5), 406. Stanley O. Foster, "Trachoma in an American Indian Village," *Public Health Reports* (80:9) September 1965, 829-832. Foster visited the Blackwater (Pima) Community and found an average of 5.3 persons per home, approximately one-third of which had bathrooms and only 10 percent of which had satisfactory fly control. Of 404 persons examined, 10.9 percent had active infection and 32.4 percent had inactive disease. Sixty-six out of 109 adults had inactive trachoma. An active home treatment program was begun after the survey and within twelve months the prevalence rate among first graders fell from 71 percent to 19 percent

40. Agnes Fahy and Carl Muschenheim, "Third National Conference on American Indian Health," *Journal of the American Medical Association* (194:10) December 6, 1965, 1096. Sulfanilamide treatment had largely been replaced with tetracycline. *Annual Statistical Review* (Department of Health, Education and Welfare, Public Health Service, Indian Health Service, 1969), 38. Fahy and Muschenheim, (1095-1096) surveyed 900 San Carlos Apache near Bylas and found 35 percent of those under the age of four; 61 percent of those between the ages of five and eighteen; and 43 percent of those over the age of nineteen infected with active trachoma. Every person over the age of 15 had either an active or a healed case of trachoma.

41. "Department of the Interior and Related Agencies Appropriations for Fiscal Year 1970," *Hearings before a Subcommittee of the Committee on Appropriations United States Senate* 91st Congress, 1st session, March 20, 1969, 1396. *Justifications of Appropriation Estimates for Committee on Appropriations*, Fiscal Year 1968, IHA-26. *Annual Statistical*

*Review*, 39.
    42. Cahn, *Our Brother's Keeper*, 58.
    43. Fahy and Muschenheim, 1093.

# CHAPTER FOUR

## On the Threshold of a New Era?

In December 1965 President Johnson appointed surgeon Erwin "E. S." Rabeau as the third director of the Division of Indian Health. Rabeau worked his way up the Public Health Service as a Commissioned Corps Officer on loan to the BIA. In 1957, he was assigned as the Clinical Director of the Anchorage Indian hospital, where he subsequently became the Deputy Area Director. Three years later he was assigned to the Bemidji (Minnesota) sub-area office where he served as the Chief Medical Officer and Deputy Area Director. Two years later he became Director of the Aberdeen Area Office. In 1963, Rabeau moved to Washington, D.C., and became Deputy Director of the Division of Indian Health, remaining there until he was appointed director.

Rabeau advocated American Indian participation in the healthcare process and the expansion of community medicine. For his leadership efforts, the Inter-Tribal Council of the Five Civilized Tribes of Oklahoma recognized him for his "enlightened policies on Indian health and for the progress made in improving the health of American Indians and Alaska Natives." Rabeau stepped down as director in 1969 and moved to Tucson, Arizona, where he became the director of the newly established Indian Health Service Office of Program Development. He remained director of research until 1981, when he retired from the Public Health Service to become deputy director—then director—of the Alaska State Health Department, where he remained until his death in 1984.[1]

### Reorganization of the Indian Health Program

In the latter 1960s, the Indian health service and the Department of Health, Education and Welfare underwent two reorganizations. To implement the changes initiated by such Great Society legislation as Medicare, the Elementary and Secondary Education Act, and sundry civil rights acts, secretary John Gardiner in

1966 reorganized the entire executive department, including the Division of Indian Health. While the Bureau of Medical Services was renamed the Bureau of Health Services, the Public Health Service remained unchanged, with the Surgeon General retaining a direct line of communication with the secretary. Two years later, the department again reorganized, this time for political reasons. The Public Health Service became an agency under the Assistant Secretary for Health and Scientific Affairs. While the Surgeon General was given expanded duties, he was demoted in terms of line communication with the secretary. While the Public Health Service was demoted, the Division of Indian Health was elevated. Within the newly reorganized Public Health Service, three new agencies replaced five old ones. The new agencies included the Health Services and Mental Health Administration, the Consumer Protection and Environmental Health Services, and the National Institutes of Health. Elevated to the Bureau level, the Division of Indian Health was placed in the Health Services and Mental Health Administration and renamed the Indian Health Service.[2]

The regional administrative structure was also modified when the Window Rock (Navajo) subarea office became the eighth area office of the Indian Health Service in 1967. Although area offices existed to provide support for local service units, serving more or less as the intermediary between local service units and the IHS headquarters, they tended to reduce local initiative, as bureaucratic red tape prevented enterprising service units from improving health services. The result was isolation and a feeling of impotence, with "capable people . . . mov[ing] from a sense of futility to lethargy." While intensifying its preventive efforts by using service units as the basic comprehensive health program and third-party sponsors for referral medical care in contract health facilities, the Indian Health Service remained crisis-oriented. By 1969, there were ninety service units within the Indian Health Service.[3]

Rabeau accelerated the program of employing trained administrators in administrative and management positions within the health program. Historically, the Indian Health Service filled administrative positions with physicians, who may have had little or no administrative expertise. By bringing trained administrators on board to run hospitals and clinics, the Indian Health Service sought to improve its management capacity and at the same time prevent its already limited supply of physicians from growing thinner. A corollary initiative encouraged physicians to earn Master's of Public Health (MPH) degrees.

Until the 1960s, physicians in medical and administrative positions dominated the Indian Health Service and the medical world. In the 1960s, hospital administrators still directed most medical facilities in the United States, with physicians remaining outside the hospital system. Within the Indian Health Service, however, most administrators were physicians, meaning they were within the hospital system. Rabeau recognized the importance of changing this management scheme and made it a practice to appoint, not without controversy, non-physicians to administrative positions. In the process, career civil service employees were afforded opportunities to move into management roles, while also reducing the high turnover rate in administrative leadership when physicians serving their 2-year military duty in the Public Health Service were given the positions.[4]

The question over who was more qualified to fill service unit and area office administrative positions at times grew heated. To many physicians, the physician-administrator was more acceptable than non-physician-administrators, as the former understood medical jargon, shared the same professional heritage, and understood clinical medicine. But at the same time, there were physicians who mistrusted physicians-turned-administrators, viewing them as incompetent medical professionals. Non-physician administrators were not left unscathed either. Some physicians felt trained administrators over emphasized the most efficient medical procedures, even to the extent that they lost sight of patient needs. These physicians believed the quality of healthcare was subjected to the "bald numbers of services dispensed." Ignored was the fact that unless medical services made an impact on the recipient, thereby improving his health in some way, the patient simply returned again and again as treatment failed. The growing number of patients in IHS facilities did not necessarily indicate better care as much as it reflected "evidence of the system's inability to provide meaningful treatment."[5]

Although there was disagreement over who should serve as administrative officers, it was agreed that the management structure of the Indian Health Service needed to improve. The need for consistent and effective management was evident. "I have about 400 pounds of paper in my office at present called program plans," service unit director Robert Kane wrote in 1972. "I also recently disposed of another 100 pounds of paper which represents past attempts at program plans. Each year, and sometimes twice a year, we are asked to produce a program plan. Each time, the guidelines, prototypes, and emphasis are changed," usually by bureaucrats in Washington, D.C. "[E]ach year," Kane continued, "we are asked to prepare a construction document which is to request and justify needed medical facilities. Each year the rules regarding the preparation of this document are changed. It is purely accidental if plans for any two years are alike even though we . . . try to keep (them) consistent." The effect of planning efforts was insignificant.[6]

To its credit, the Indian Health Service recognized its need for administrative changes, not only for determining resource allocation schedules that might improve the delivery system and, indirectly, health conditions, but also as a means of reinforcing the management infrastructure of the program. The emphasis of encouraging professionals, particularly physicians and dentists, to earned MPH degrees was one way to improve program management. Nonetheless, as the number of physicians earning MPH degrees increased, the number of practicing physicians decreased, exacerbating the already meager supply of doctors. To balance these losses, the Indian Health Service encouraged young physicians to join the health program by offering a two-year general practice residency at its hospital in Gallup, New Mexico.[7]

# Recurring Staffing Concerns

While moderately higher appropriations allowed the Indian Health Service to increase its personnel by nearly 50 percent by 1967, there continued to be a shortage of professional and support staff. Nearly 70 percent of the physicians and dentists were in the health program in lieu of military service and serving two-year commitments, meaning high turnover rates and lack of continuity. Furthermore, while the Public Health Service salary schedule was better than the Bureau of Indian Affairs, it was still less than what one might receive in private practice. The average private practice physician earned $36,000 in 1968 ($24,500 for dentists) while an Indian Health Service physician earned $13,400 (with $24,000 the maximum salary). With a modest salary schedule, it was increasingly difficult to attract the wide array of medical specialists needed, requiring the program to contract with private physicians for most specialty services. As costs escalated, contract care services were limited.[8] Overall, IHS appropriations increased, as shown in Table 4.1.

Table 4.1

*Annual Appropriations for the Indian Health Service: 1958-1967*

| Year | Appropriation | Year | Appropriation |
|------|---------------|------|---------------|
| 1958 | $40,100,000   | 1963 | $56,836,000   |
| 1959 | $42,327,000   | 1964 | $58,960,750   |
| 1960 | $45,700,000   | 1965 | $62,940,000   |
| 1961 | $50,271,000   | 1966 | $67,548,000   |
| 1962 | $53,010,000   | 1967 | $73,671,000   |

(Source: 1968 Appropriation Hearings)

Physicians and other professional staff also left the agency because of social and professional isolation, limited advancement opportunities, and lack of professional recognition. More importantly, a growing schism between "white careerist" physicians, who maintained status quo and were resistant to change, and the "two-year men," who fulfilled their military obligation but were more enthusiastic and willing to bend the health program to fit Indian needs, emerged. Careerists lost their sense of commitment and the *esprit de corps* so prevalent when the Public Health Service first assumed responsibility for the program. This was due in part to the growing politicization of the agency and loss of a common goal. Some physicians were concerned "the plight of the Peace Corps" had "befallen the Indian Health Service." The result was that some physicians were "more interested in what they can get from [the Indian Health Service] than what they can contribute."[9]

Challenges remained in the nursing corps as well. While nursing salaries were comparable to private practice nurses, the fact remained that it was difficult to attract good nurses, especially in isolated locations. Indian hospitals remained understaffed due to high turnover or a simple inability to fill vacancies. Shortages were likely until "more Indian RNs [were] brought into the service." Table 4.2 shows comparative changes in physician, dentist, pharmacist, and public health nursing patient loads between 1955 and 1966, both for the IHS and the general population.[10]

The high patient-to-health professional ratio meant more than high demands on physicians, nurses, pharmacists, and dentists. It decreased utilization of such services, since many American Indians were "conditioned to expect time and attention from their healers." When a Navajo visited a medicine man, for example, a treatment could last hours or perhaps days. Yet, with a shortage of personnel and high patient loads, most medical professionals could expect to spend no more than 5 to 7 minutes with each patient, which was approximately one-third to one-half of the time allotted by private practice physicians. Increasing the patient load also infringed on the quality of care given.[11]

Table 4.2

*Patients Served by Healthcare Professionals, Select Years: 1955-1966*

| Profession | Indian Health Service | | U.S. General | |
|---|---|---|---|---|
| | *1955* | *1962* | *1956* | *1962* |
| Physician | 2,200 | 1,460 | 1,220 | 840* |
| Dentist | 7,000 | 4,600 | 3,670 | 1,800 |
| Public Health Nurse | 4,000 | 3,500 | 3,300 | 2,500 |
| Pharmacist | 51,400 | 6,460 | 5,000 | 1,500 |

*excludes physicians in fulltime teaching or research

(Source: *American Indians and Federal Aid*, 1968)

## American Indian Participation in Health Services

One means by which to overcome the shortage of health professionals and foster self-determination was to train American Indians and Alaska Natives for the medical professions. In 1969 nearly 60 percent of IHS personnel were American Indian; yet, less than 1 percent of all physicians and dentists was American Indian. More than 1,000 American Indians and Alaska Natives had entered the health field, but most were in low level, non-policy impacting positions.[12]

The goal of involving American Indians and Alaska Natives in the conservation of their own health slowly materialized. For most of Shaw's tenure, the Indian Health Service focused on securing the physical and professional resources necessary to elevate health conditions. Wagner, although interested in jointly planning a health program with American Indian and Alaska Native communities, focused much of his attention on program management. It was during Rabeau's tenure that the idea of client participation in their own healthcare appeared on the threshold of reality.

From the beginning, Rabeau pledged his support for American Indian and Alaska Native participation in the planning, directing, and evaluation of the Indian Health Service. "We consider the Federal Indian health program to be your program, carried out in accordance with your wishes and your requests," Rabeau told tribal leaders. "The Indian Health Service is the instrument for providing services which are planned, conducted and evaluated in cooperation with you as individuals and as organized tribal and community groups."[13]

Indian involvement was essential, especially as the nature of health challenges evolved. Some administrators, such as Sanitation Director Irving Schlafman, believed Indian involvement was not only wise, but also fiscally sound because the agency was rapidly pricing itself out of business. "We are convinced," Schlafman argued, "that proper involvement of responsible tribal representatives can do much to optimize our precious resources and to cause infinitely greater numbers of other resources ... to impact upon unmet health needs."[14]

American Indian and Alaska Native participation was fundamental to improving health conditions. "Getting the Indian communities more knowledgeable and more involved in their healthcare," Stanley Stitt, retired Portland Area Office Director, remarked, "was essential if diseases and illnesses that were controlled among non-Indians were to be controlled among Native Americans." Furthermore, many health administrators believed Indian communities had a right to voice their opinion regarding healthcare needs. "The survival of any society," one administrator opined, "is dependent upon the human necessity for self-identity and self-determination. Individual Indians and tribal groups have now recognized this need and are insisting upon being heard, if only to survive as a cultural group."[15]

Ultimately, the success of the Indian Health Service depended on tribal involvement and ownership. Decisions regarding policy, direction, and assistance required joint undertakings. Tribal health and advisory boards desired to assist area office directors in promoting local leadership and policy. Active involvement was crucial at the grass roots level. Phoenix Area Health Educator Henry J. Keneally, Jr., saw the success of the program dependent not so much on the excellence of professional staff or the number and size of modern health facilities as it depended on its "ability to work with Indian beneficiaries."[16]

The idea of involving American Indians and Alaska Natives in the decision-making process was difficult for traditional Public Health Service administrators. "The successful partnership," Charles McCammon, Director of the Phoenix Area Office, wrote in 1970, "demands time and effort and willingness to work at a pace acceptable to the individuals concerned, as well as within the restrictions of the [federal] system." Careerists encouraged Indian involvement at the lower levels of the Indian Health Service but too often rejected putting American Indians in administrative positions where they would compete with them.[17]

Rabeau recognized the policy of Indian participation would result in challenges to career Public Health Service employees and to Indians as well. "Some of our professionals were concerned that lay [tribal] individuals or groups would be in a position to override professional decisions," the director explained, and "some of the beneficiaries understandably took the position that [tribal participation] was some more of the double talk meant for image only and not for action."[18]

The concept of Indian involvement was revolutionary when viewed in light of the termination mind-set of Congress in the 1950s. Yet, in the latter 1960s, a time when termination waned and the concept of self-determination waxed, it reflected a change in the overall viewpoint of the federal government. For nearly one hundred years, federal bureaucrats controlled reservations. Once American Indians were sequestered on reservations the federal government ignored their involvement and tribal consultation.

In the nineteenth century, the Bureau of Indian Affairs introduced the agency system as a new form of management in Indian Country. Superintendents exercised plenary authority and, as the local arm of the Indian Service, they surrounded themselves with non-Indian employees and a select group of agency Indians. With this staff, superintendents enforced policy decisions with little or no input from the tribal governments. In effect, the Indian Service progressively undermined local autonomy. Medical services were administered in such a manner as to de-emphasize community control and participation. No matter how diligently it worked toward the goal of preventive care, the Indian Service struggled without the involvement of the tribal community.

The passage of the Indian Reorganization Act of 1934 marked a shift in federal Indian policy. For the first time, the federal government sought to repair some of the damage it had caused in undermining community and tribal institutions by encouraging tribal organization. After decades of being organized to depend on the superintendent and his staff, many tribes struggled with making decisions. Even with the Indian Reorganization Act, tribal councils did not change the existing structure of authority. In fact, some councils simply became extensions of the Bureau of Indian Affairs. Decision making remained in the hands of an external institution, rather than in an internal, community organization. Dependency was institutionalized through the bureaucratic reach of the federal government. Bureaucratic control inhibited the growth of local decision-making institutions.

It was not surprising, then, that when Rabeau spoke of a partnership in healthcare many American Indians remained skeptical. Was partnership simply an extension of the old practice of consultation, which did not require consent? Or was it a sincere attempt to involve American Indians in their own healthcare? With decades of bureaucratic control, some professional employees failed to see the efficacy of Indian involvement. Some physicians even failed to see how non-professionals could participate in program decision making, while older, long-term bureaucrats habitually made decisions for tribal communities and saw little need to give up such authority, especially since they believed they had the resources and knowledge the tribes lacked. The question many American Indians and Alaska Natives asked was: "How far would the Indian Health Service go in gaining community involvement?"

Rabeau promoted American Indian and Alaska Native involvement in the health program at three levels. Individual involvement was in some respects the most important initial step in improving well-being, at least until health status improved and tribes assumed control over their own programs. At the time of the transfer act, the old Division of Indian Health was charged with conserving and improving the health status of American Indians and Alaska Natives. Yet, as the Bureau of Indian Affairs had seen—and the Public Health Service was aware—this could not be done by simply treating illness as it occurred. If American Indian health status was to improve, a preventive health program was the cornerstone upon which success would be built.

A decision to establish a preventive health program implicitly committed the Public Health Service to increasing American Indian and Alaska Native involvement. Community involvement in a preventive health program underscored the desire of American Indians and Alaska Natives to improve their health status. For such a program to be successful, tribes or tribal health boards had to be vested with decision-making authority. Such boards could then work with the Indian Health Service on directing programs. On a more practical level, American Indians and Alaska Natives would have to internalize improved health, demand improved sanitation conditions, and be empowered to explore ways to enhance their lives. They would then have to blend Western medicine with traditional beliefs on healing. Because of a century of bureaucratic rule, they would also need know-how, technological assistance, and the resources to successfully implement such a program. Without this personal involvement, it would be difficult to improve health conditions.

To increase community understanding of medical resources and ways individuals could initiate better preventive care, the Indian Health Service considered the establishment of a community health program. Confronted with the chronic shortage of professional staff, a rural and essentially isolated constituency, with cultural and linguistic barriers, the Indian Health Service developed the concept of community health aides. In the mid-1960s the Indian Health Service initiated another demonstration community health aide program. Funded by the Office of Economic Opportunity and established on the Pine Ridge Oglala Sioux Reservation in South Dakota, the aides were provided thirteen weeks of formal instruction in nursing, child care, home management, and sanitation, and then sent out as community health workers. While critics reproved the program because aides too often focused on the specific task of their visit to individual homes (rather than using their visit to introduce additional health education concepts), taken as a whole, the program was a success in that it "brought about earlier diagnosis and commencement of treatment, thereby lessening the impact of illness." As importantly, it pushed the portal of entry for health services to the doorsteps of individual homes.

The response to the community health aide program was positive and served as the model for the permanent establishment of Community Health Representatives, or CHRs, in 1968.[19] The CHR program, administered through contracts between the Indian Health Service and the tribal communities ($1.3 million in fiscal year 1969), employed trained health aides who served as extensions for physicians, nurses, sanitarians, and other healthcare professionals. Selected and employed by the tribe, and representing their tribal community, CHRs were liaisons between the Indian Health Service and Indian tribes and tribal organizations. They interpreted local needs, attitudes, and practices related to healthcare for the Indian Health Service, which in turn directed the agency's resources on those particular issues.[20]

Community Health Representatives assumed important roles in their communities. The advice of the health professionals, for instance, could be conveyed through CHRs in a way that bridged the communication gaps between the Indian and non-Indian world. The challenge, however, was that tribal communities and the Indian Health Service, while agreeing on the purpose of the program, differed in priorities. Tribal communities viewed the program as helping the Indian Health Service "understand the culture and wishes of the tribe" while IHS administrators saw CHRs as "helping the Indians understand PHS programs and philosophy."[21]

What made the CHR program unique was for the first time in the history of federal-Indian healthcare, a medical worker lived in the Indian community and was selected, employed by, and responsible to the tribe. Theoretically, the program was free of interference from the Indian Health Service, as health professionals cooperated with the representatives but did not control them. At the service unit level, some health personnel interactions resulted in de facto control of the program while in others efforts to remain distinct resulted in ignoring the CHRs. In some tribal communities, the CHRs were quickly accepted but "threatened (local) political leaders to the extent that they sought either to dominate the CHRs or to isolate them."[22]

Supporters lauded the program for its importance in fostering community health. CHRs utilized their community's culture and adapted principles of healthcare and prevention. They accessed outside resources to assist their communities in dealing with specific health issues. As importantly, each tribe independently developed programs unique to their needs.[23]

In Alaska, geographical factors necessitated a different approach. The isolation of, and inclement weather in, Alaska Native villages prevented healthcare professionals from providing immediate services to scattered Native communities. To mitigate this challenge, the Indian Health Service provided advanced training for Alaska village aides allowing them to provide additional interim health services. By utilizing short-wave radios, aides treated patients under the supervision of health professionals at hospitals in Kotzebue, Nome, and Anchorage. The use of Village Chemotherapy Aides was also utilized, aiding in the reduction of tuberculosis incidence rates. By 1969, 185 Alaska Natives were employed as village health aides, while an additional 185 CHRs were employed in the continental United States.[24]

The CHR and Alaska village aide programs were not the only means of encouraging American Indian and Alaska Native involvement. The Indian Health Service initiated other programs to supplement services provided by professionally trained staff, as well as increased the involvement of American Indians in the delivery of healthcare. The School of Practical Nursing, located in Albuquerque, New Mexico, trained 60 American Indians annually in practical nursing skills using both classroom study and clinical experiences at the Santa Fe Indian hospital. Advanced training was available in Rapid City, South Dakota, and Shiprock, New Mexico. Graduates were virtually guaranteed employment in an Indian hospital. Training was also available at three Indian and Alaska Native schools, which trained thirty dental assistants per year, most of whom found employment in the Indian dental program. Other programs provided training for environmental health (sanitarian) aides, health record technicians, laboratory and radiologic technicians, social work associates, and food service supervisors.[25]

The use of aides increased the number of opportunities for direct American Indian and Alaska Native involvement in the delivery of health services. By 1968 the Indian Health Service trained and employed more than 1,600 American Indians and Alaska Natives. These para-professionals increased the availability of services provided by the Indian Health Service and increased the frequency of American Indian utilization of services. In fact, greater acceptance of preventive services and Indian participation reduced by two full days the average daily patient length of stay between 1960 and 1968. While inpatient care levels were plateauing, the level of outpatient care increased, reflecting greater participation and better preventive services.[26]

American Indian and Alaska Native involvement at the administrative and management level remained the most difficult of the levels of involvement. One administrator opined that "five generations of [the] Federal practice of deciding what was best for the Indians created traditional management barriers for . . . the Indian people." Nonetheless, Rabeau developed, piloted, and presented a number of health service management and supervisory leadership programs and workshops for tribal and program employees at all levels of administration. He also contracted with Arrow, Inc., an Indian training organization, to provide a series of management institutes held throughout the country to teach American Indians and Alaska Natives management principles. Tribes were assisted through the training of tribal health committee members, area advisory boards of health, and sundry supervisory and coordinating positions. Under the expanding programs of tribal involvement, and as an exercise of the rising demand for Indian self-determination, tribes developed and enforced health, sanitation, and safety codes and regulations. To carry out these programs, tribal health committees, advisory boards, and boards of health were established to represent tribal governments on health matters.[27]

Most tribal health boards exercised little or no authority and more often than not the Indian Health Service ignored their input. "Many health boards felt frustrated seeing the Indian Health Service accept or reject their input when desired." Taylor McKenzie, a Navajo physician and director of the Shiprock Service Unit, argued for Indian health boards controlling their own institutions because there were "certain decisions about medical and health services relating to and affecting Navajos that only Navajos can make." If made by outside institutions, McKenzie argued, they would "engender resentment and suspicions." By 1970, Indian tribes within the Aberdeen and Phoenix area offices had established Indian advisory boards and all service units in Oklahoma had advisory boards.[28]

## Management Information Systems

Surgeon General Leroy E. Burney emphasized the importance of medical research in the context of Indian health, viewing it "as a method of developing better techniques, of improving service, of gaining additional and medical information about the extent of health problems, and of developing yardsticks for evaluating methods of handling these problems." This was true for epidemiology, nutrition, infant care, prenatal toxemia, microbiology, sanitation, mental health, health education, and others. In short, the Indian Health Service recognized a fertile field for research in the development of preventive and rehabilitative programs.[29]

Program planning, introduced in 1964, was useful as a management tool for determining priorities and allocation of finite medical resources. Rabeau envisioned bringing tribal representatives and IHS staff together to establish operational and strategic objectives. To implement such a program required tribal health organizations that could plan, implement, and conduct preventive health programs, and systematic, scientific methodologies that could determine the extent of disease and the effectiveness of medical approaches combating those diseases.

To realize these objectives medical professionals had to conduct operational research with the intent of determining which approaches were useful and which were not. This was especially important as the demand for health services mounted and the gap between services and resources increased. By devising systematic approaches to ensure optimal use of such resources, the gap between services and finite resources could be reduced. To implement such a program required creating a research unit capable of developing programs that would improve the delivery and management of Indian healthcare. The development of a management information system would ensure that health and health-related information was readily available to community health planners and to system practitioners. To gain the involvement of tribes, the Indian Health Service needed to train tribal officials and health personnel to carry out these new functions.[30]

The Indian Health Service was unique in this endeavor in that it had the unusual opportunity of examining the complete dynamics of a comprehensive, federally-supported healthcare system. Encouraged by medical associations and public health agencies, the Indian Health Service, with Congressional recognition and approval, established the Health Program Systems Center in July of 1967.[31] With the creation of an operations research unit to develop a systems analysis module applicable to community health programs, the Indian Health Service entered a new phase in the delivery of healthcare. With the research unit housed in the former Tuberculosis Sanitarium on the San Xavier Indian Reservation south of Tucson, Arizona, the Systems Analysis Module, or Operation SAM, studied the "complete universe" of the Tohono O'odham and the delivery system serving them to produce statistically significant and accurate research. The module also provided an evaluation system that reflected the results of community health programs. The Indian Health Service strengthened its management component by providing scientific methods applicable throughout the service population, believing Operation SAM would facilitate community medicine without separating preventive, curative, and rehabilitative services.[32]

Operation SAM was politicized in the 1968 Indian healthcare appropriation hearings. Rabeau sought to assemble an interdisciplinary staff of researchers and scientists, a venture that required fiscal resources. While the complexities of administering the program were significant, scattered information was already available regarding some of the "variables involved in planning and implementing a comprehensive healthcare program." Most of this data was fragmented, Rabeau argued, "having been gained through studies conducted by and for monodiscipline groups" that were "designed to eliminate or hold constant the interaction of other professional disciplines."[33]

The interdisciplinary approach to healthcare and management research was not accidental. The idea fostered by Rabeau in establishing a research component hinged on the philosophy that no one academic discipline could contribute all potentially useful information. On the other hand, a team mind might be able to do so. By 1969, Operation SAM included a multidisciplinary team of three research specialists and physicians; two statisticians, health administrators, and information specialists; one mathematician, anthropologist, research nurse, research director, social science analyst, program analyst, management specialist, systems analyst; and sundry clerical staff. Rabeau encouraged the team to determine how much time should be spent on specific health challenges.[34] By creating a program that could "develop, test, refine and demonstrate" the most efficient way of "planning, budgeting, implementing and evaluating" health programs, Rabeau hoped to accelerate the campaign against ill-health and achieve healthcare parity with non-Indians. The Sells Service Unit west of Tucson was attached to the research component as the developmental grounds for all systems studies and to anchor the unit to reality. Among the first projects completed were health concepts and attitudes, a computerized analysis of the family planning program, a comprehensive environmental health methodology, a demographic and sociocultural characteristics study, an impact study of the Sanitation Facilities Construction Act, and an evaluation of maternal and infant healthcare. Once the procedures and methodologies were proven practical and effective within the Sells Service Unit, they were to be recommended for use throughout Indian Country. In 1969, the research unit was renamed the Office of Program Development.[35]

Committed to American Indian involvement in the planning and delivery of Indian health services, Rabeau advocated for Indian participation. But to Rabeau, the training of American Indian and Alaska Native health workers was just one avenue of preparing them to control their own health programs. At the annual appropriation hearings for fiscal year 1966, Rabeau sounded the familiar ring of tribal involvement. "Lack of knowledge and understanding of what causes disease and how disease is spread underlies the Indian health problem." Some management officials advocated building an IHS staff college, while others advanced the idea of a national training center. When Rabeau opened the Desert Willow Training Center southeast of Tucson, in July of 1968, he adopted the latter course to train "American Indians to man and manage their own health delivery systems [by aiding] in the transition of program decision making and operation from non-Indian health professionals to the Indian people." Training included clinical and hospital management, and for the first time emphasized the technical, medical, and managerial skills Indians needed to administer their own programs.[36]

Desert Willow served as the training center for all new management and operations programs developed by the Health Program Systems Center. As it developed new management concepts and methodologies, the center put them into service-wide practice. This required the center to develop training courses in management principles, problem-solving, resource allocation, and program planning. Its importance to the larger goal of training Indian leadership was significant.[37]

Rabeau had personal reasons for establishing a centralized center in Tucson. For one, Desert Willow consolidated the existing fragmented research and training resources, materials, facilities, personnel, and services. It was more efficient and effective in conducting research, conferences, workshops, and seminars than scattered facilities, and theoretically it would alleviate disparities "between the needs of the individual training programs and the services which their allotted funds . . . provide[d]." Once the program was established in Tucson, Rabeau stepped down as head of the Indian Health Service to lead it. While an important step in providing training, such a paradigm did little to make the Indian Health Service more culturally relevant to the people it served.[38]

## Establishing a Cooperative Relationship

The Indian Health Service has always been charged with a task no other single health organization in the United States has ever been given: Combining direct (curative and rehabilitative) and public (preventive and environmental) health services. Out of this combination of responsibilities grew the concept of community healthcare. In order for the Indian Health Service to achieve the goal of elevating Indian health to the "highest possible level," the Public Health Service identified several Indian health objectives, one of which was fostering and promoting full and equitable utilization of all available resources, public and private, with a focus on state and local government responsibility for American Indian and Alaska Native citizens.[39]

Although curative, preventive, and rehabilitative services were offered at most health facilities, where such services were not available or could be provided more economically at non-service facilities, or where specialized care could not be provided by the program, the Indian Health Service utilized outside facilities via contractual agreements. In 1968, for example, over 200 community, tuberculosis, and mental hospitals made beds available for American Indians and Alaska Natives under contractual agreements. In addition, 250 pharmacies, 450 physicians, 200 dentists, and over 100 other healthcare professionals were brought under contract agreements. The Indian Health Service signed twenty-six contracts with state and local health agencies. Contract medical care, consuming 19 percent of the annual Indian health appropriations, represented nearly 27 percent of all patient admissions, as seen in Table 4.3. Service units ensured the quality of care received from third party vendors met the standards of the program.[40]

Table 4.3

*Contract Medical Care: 1964-1970*

| Year | IHS Funding | CMC Funding | Percent CMC | Percent Total Admissions |
|------|-------------|-------------|-------------|--------------------------|
| 1964 | $58,960,750 | $11,029,177 | 18.7 | 26.7 |
| 1965 | $62,940,000 | $11,815,000 | 18.7 | 26.2 |
| 1966 | $66,193,000 | $12,861,000 | 19.4 | 27.0 |
| 1967 | $76,323,703 | $14,106,000 | 18.5 | 26.9 |
| 1968 | $84,327,260 | $15,537,000 | 18.4 | 26.1 |
| 1969 | $91,710,000 | $17,779,000 | 19.4 | 26.3 |
| 1970 | $101,529,000 | $20,095,000 | 19.8 | 26.8 |

(Source: *Annual Appropriation Hearings & Annual Statistical Review*, 1970)

Contract medical care did not always meet the need. The Indian Health Service allocated service units a percentage of funds to be used for contract medical care each year. These funds were appropriated on the principle of the more one spent this year, the more one would get next year. Yet, such resource allocation worked to the disadvantage of Indian beneficiaries. A patient needing specialized care, for instance, might be referred to an external care provider at one point during the year and not at another, depending on the solvency of the contract medical care fund. Another scenario might prevent a patient from receiving contract care early in the fiscal year for fear of insolvency at the close of the year. On the other hand, as the fiscal year wound down, any potential surplus might be expended on patients who were less ill than those who needed care earlier in the year. For all intents and purposes, contract healthcare was rationed.

To minimize the likelihood of having contract medical care funding reduced the following fiscal year, it was not unusual for funds to be spent when they need not have been. Former Service Unit director Robert Kane assessed the contract medical care funding formula as a "spend-when-you-can, save-when-you-have-to, and hunt-for-external-funds" game. Not surprisingly, he scoffed at how contract care funds were used to treat acute medical needs with the remainder being expended on chronic health problems such as corrective ear surgery or open-heart surgery. The result was little money remained to mitigate chronic problems that yielded well to medical treatment.[41]

To elevate health services to an acceptable level also required the cooperation of other federal agencies. While the Indian Health Service worked with a number of executive departments in discharging its responsibilities, cooperation was most intimate with the Bureau of Indian Affairs, primarily because many of the latter's functions involved health. Boarding schools, for instance, were planned and constructed with the provisioning of health services in mind. Likewise, the Indian Health Service planned the construction of health facilities in relation to the Bureau's immediate and long-range objectives regarding road construction and water and waste disposal facility sites.

As tribes became eligible for federal housing funds, under the Department of Housing and Urban Development (HUD), the Indian Health Service ensured its sanitation health objectives were not infringed upon. In 1968, for example, Rabeau went to Congress seeking supplemental appropriations to provide 3,700 new or improved individual sanitation units when Indian demand for HUD homes increased. President Johnson proposed increases for 1969 to correct the shortages but newly constructed homes sat empty due to lack of existing funds. A sympathetic Congress feared additional HUD and BIA houses would be constructed without sanitation facilities, meaning additional unoccupied new houses. At an average per unit cost of $1,900, the agency sought a $4,238,000 increase to provide the additional facilities.[42] Overall, the Indian Health Service was less than diligent in working with other federal departments to ensure that Indian communities were provided with adequate housing. While technically not an IHS responsibility, cooperation was important to public health.

## Health Services for California Indians

While the Indian Health Service fell short of providing a level of healthcare comparable with the general population, it did make important gains by 1970. The experiences of the Indian Health Service providing comprehensive health services to a rural, isolated, and culturally diverse people, and its ability to cultivate community health in Indian Country was put to international use in the 1960s when the agency provided consultative and training assistance to a number of international health organizations. Under agreements consummated between the Public Health Service and the Agency for International Development, for example, the Indian Health Service provided administrative, technical, and consultative services to the National Public Health Service of Liberia to assist the northern African nation in implementing a comprehensive health program of its own. Under additional contracts, Peace Corps volunteer community health aides were trained for assignments in Korea and Malawi at the Desert Willow Training Center.[43]

But while the expertise of the agency served foreign health agencies, there was much work to be done at home. One glaring need was in California. Prior to the transfer act, there were two federal Indian hospitals in California, where most Indian healthcare since the 1930s was provided through contracts with private and county health facilities. In the midst of the termination fervor of the 1950s, the Bureau of Indian Affairs began withdrawing services from the state in 1958. Federal facilities were closed when the State of California agreed to assume responsibility for health services. Over the next decade, no system of healthcare replaced the withdrawn federal services, despite assurances by the state, and few funds were available from local sources. The already beggared health conditions among the state's Indian population deteriorated rapidly.[44]

Health conditions of California Indians grew intolerable. Tuberculosis, cirrhosis of the liver, influenza, pneumonia, congenital malformations, and early infant diseases plagued tribal communities, especially the scattered Indians in southern California. Poor housing and sanitation facilities made matters worse, as did inadequate medical facilities near reservations, lack of transportation, and delays in receiving services from local health facilities. Life expectancy in California for American Indians was just forty-two years, versus sixty-two years for the general population.[45]

The California Bureau of Maternal and Child Health reported appalling conditions. In a survey of ten reservations, more than 70 percent of the households earned less than $3,000 annually. Mothers had inadequate prenatal care and nearly one-third had only third trimester or no prenatal care, compared with 8.5 percent of all California mothers. The probability was greater that California Indians experienced accidental death or died of cirrhosis of the liver than non-Indians.

Medical care on the Hoopa Reservation in northern California was "fragmented, episodic, and almost exclusively crisis oriented." In 1967, the State of California initiated a health project specifically for Indians within the state.[46]

At that time the California State Legislature approved of a resolution requesting the federal government reassume responsibility for the healthcare of the 150,000 California Indians, approximately 40 percent of whom were scattered over 70 small reservations, rancherias, and individual allotments. Public health nurses near the Morongo Reservation outside of Banning requested a team from the University of California, Riverside, to conduct multi-phasic screening to determine the needs of the community. The UC Riverside team examined ninety-six participants from the Morongo, Soboba, and San Manuel reservations, with diabetes, lactic dehydrogenase, parasitic infections, and bacteria prevalent. A diet "disproportionately dependent on starches and carbohydrates, and almost completely lacking in fresh fruits or vegetables" was common. When the UC Riverside team informed state and federal officials, they concurred there was a healthcare problem but each felt the other was responsible.[47]

As a result of the state legislature's resolution, the Public Health Service granted $150,000 to the state to conduct a rural Indian demonstration health project. Governor Ronald Reagan then requested the California Department of Public Health to evaluate nine rural areas and recommend four for the project. When all nine expressed interest in the project, the state requested additional money, with the Public Health Service providing $95,000 to the grant. The charge not only included an examination of healthcare but also an evaluation of "the possibility of Indian administration of their own health projects."[48]

The demonstration projects provided essential services and exhibited successful tribal control of health programs, prompting Yokut tribal leader Joe Carrillo to form the California Rural Indian Health Board in 1969, as a pan-Indian health group serving rural California Indian communities. While the project was initially funded by a grant from the Department of Health, Education and Welfare, after 1970 federal health programs were applicable to all California Indians, including those served by the California Rural Indian Health Board. Four years later, urban Indians in the San Francisco Bay area established the California Urban Indian Health Council to provide services for urban Indians. Since services for California Indians were funded through contracts with nonprofit Indian and tribal organizations, the Indian Health Service did not maintain facilities in the state, although it did provide limited sanitation and domestic water services.[49]

## A Medical Yardstick

As the 1960s grew to a close, the status of American Indian and Alaska Native health improved, although in the Southwest tribes experienced increased incidence rates of certain diseases. Diabetes, for instance, increased and was becoming associated with congenital anomalies in children. Perhaps the most dynamic example of improving health was the declining number of tuberculosis admissions, which represented 58 percent of the average daily patient census in 1955. The use of chemotherapy for ambulatory patients reduced the need for hospitalization and, by 1968, the average daily tuberculosis patient census had dropped to 9 percent. As the number of tubercular patients declined, the number of tuberculosis sanitaria and hospital wards waned. By 1969, only the Albuquerque, New Mexico, and Rapid City, South Dakota, sanitaria remained. The 400 bed Tacoma, Washington (1960), 35 bed San Xavier, Arizona (1965), and 167 bed Talihina, Oklahoma (1967), tuberculosis hospitals were closed and converted into general hospitals (Tacoma and Talihina) or a health center (San Xavier). Table 4.4 highlights the declining tuberculosis rates.[50]

Table 4.4

*Tuberculosis Death Rates for Select Years, 1955-1967*
(Per 100,000 Population)

| Year | American Indian | Alaska Native | U.S. General |
|------|-----------------|---------------|--------------|
| 1955 | 47 | 158 | 9.1 |
| 1957 | 34 | 83 | 7.8 |
| 1959 | 28 | 42 | 6.5 |
| 1961 | 25 | 35 | 5.4 |
| 1963 | 25 | 28 | 4.9 |
| 1965 | 19 | 16 | 4.1 |
| 1967 | 16 | 17 | 3.5 |

*Indian and Alaska Native rates are three year averages while the U.S. general population rate is for a single year.

(Source: *Indian Health Trends and Services*, 1969)

Successful immunization programs were instrumental in reducing preventable diseases among the 415,000 American Indians and Alaska Natives. Vaccinations, while not universally accepted, were important in fighting whooping cough, diphtheria, and measles. American Indians remained sixty-five times as likely to experience dysentery and eight times as likely to contract hepatitis. Table 4.5 shows the incidence rates for various infectious diseases.

More American Indians utilized health services in the 1960s. During fiscal year 1968, there were more than 92,000 admissions to IHS contract hospitals, a 60 percent increase over fiscal year 1956. An additional 1.6 million outpatient visits were made to clinics, health centers, and field stations. And, despite high infant mortality rates, new studies indicated that improved sanitation facilities, particularly water systems, made a positive impact on infant diarrhea.[51]

For all its progress, the Indian Health Service remained crisis-oriented. Sanitation remained a challenge in the Southwest. Among the Navajo, nine of ten families lived in crowded wood or adobe hogans, and 75 percent had inadequate or non-existent waste facilities. Eight of ten families carried their domestic water a mile or more and a random survey found barrel contamination universal. "These gross deficiencies of sanitation and housing, so essential for elemental hygiene," John Irvine, physician at the Public Health Service Indian hospital in Crown Point, New Mexico, wrote in 1970, "contribute to the high incidence of death from communicable diseases." In 1968, the Pan American Health Organization and the International Biological Program of the National Academy of Sciences sponsored a program in Washington, D.C., to research the biomedical enigma of American Indians throughout the Western Hemisphere. American Indians were afflicted with modern diseases, yet retained a "genetic heritage which permitted his survival through ages past." In other words, American Indians suffered, but survived.[52]

Table 4.5

*Incidence Rates for Select Infectious Diseases, 1952-1965*
(Per 100,000 Population)

| Disease | American Indians 1952-1954 | 1965 | Percent Change | All Races 1955 | 1965 | Percent Change |
|---|---|---|---|---|---|---|
| Tuberculosis | 643.3 | 175.9 | -72.7 | 60.1 | 25.3 | -57.9 |
| Syphilis | 385.3 | 113.4 | -70.6 | 74.9 | 58.2 | -22.3 |
| Dysentery | 857.2 | 365.9 | -57.3 | 10.5 | 5.7 | -45.7 |
| Whooping Cough | 128.2 | 17.8 | -86.1 | 38.2 | 3.5 | -90.8 |
| Measles | 842.5 | 761.3 | - 9.6 | 337.9 | 135.1 | -60.0 |
| Chicken pox | 248.7 | 553.7 | +122.6 | 198.9 | 127.6 | -35.8 |
| Mumps | 213.3 | 291.6 | + 36.7 | 159.5 | 108.7 | -31.8 |
| Hepatitis | 125.5 | 139.1 | + 10.8 | 19.5 | 17.5 | -10.3 |
| Trachoma | 279.2 | 1,478.4 | +429.5 | N/A | N/A | N/A |
| Influenza | 1,600.5 | 1,103.1 | -31.1 | N/A | N/A | N/A |
| Pneumonia | 1,306.5 | 4,023.1 | +207.9 | N/A | N/A | N/A |
| Gastroenteritis | 860.0 | 6,078.8 | +606.8 | N/A | N/A | N/A |

(Source: *American Indians and Federal Aid*, 1968)

The overall health status of American Indians and Alaska Natives remained unacceptable. In Alaska, pediatric caseloads were high, representing 40 percent of all patients seen in IHS facilities. Furthermore, 70 percent of pediatric discharges from all Indian hospitals in the United States represented children under the age of five. An inadequate number of pediatricians, insufficient sanitation facilities, malnutrition, and exposure to infections all contributed to the high recidivism rates among this age group.[53]

Among the more sensational of childhood diseases was otitis media, which struck especially hard among Alaska Native infants. The number of cases increased dramatically in 1961, with epidemiological studies identifying children under the age of two as most at risk for this inner ear disease. More than six out of ten otitis media episodes in 1967 were in children under the age of five. Some episodes resulted in permanent damage, such as "badly scarred or punctured eardrums" that required major reconstructive surgery or special facilities for treatment and hospitalization. By the time these children reached school age, their hearing was "severely damaged."[54]

Otitis media was just one of many health challenges facing Indian children. By the latter 1960s, the incidence rate for infectious or viral hepatitis nearly doubled, increasing from 139 to 264 cases per 100,000, while the comparable non-Indian rate increased only slightly, to 21 per 100,000. Among American Indians and Alaska Natives, 78 percent of all cases of hepatitis were children under the age of 14, again demonstrating the challenging health obstacles faced by American Indian children.[55]

Periodontal disease and dental caries also taxed the well-being of American Indians. Although the ratio of dentists to patients in the overall population stood at 1:1,900 in 1969, it was nearly double that for American Indians and Alaska Natives (1:3,700). A variety of factors dictated whether or not someone received treatment for dental complications, including transportation, cultural attitudes, and availability of services. Consequently, just 32 percent of American Indians and Alaska Natives received dental care in 1969, with only 62 percent of the required treatments available. The backlog of work and IHS's continuing inability to increase dental resources to keep up with growing demands magnified dental problems. While children remained the priority for services, adults received care during the summer months when schools were not in session but only if resources were available. A nationwide shortage of dentists and physicians in the 1960s had an especially acute impact in Indian Country. To combat unmet dental needs, the Indian Health Service provided topical fluoride applications and fluoridation of community water systems, but not without controversy. Since many American Indian and Alaska Native communities were without community water systems, potential benefits of such preventive services were bypassed.[56]

The leading causes of death in Indian Country changed little in the 1960s. The top five causes of mortality included accidents, heart disease, malignant neoplasms (cancer), influenza/pneumonia, and infant diseases. Table 4.6 shows the incidence rates for the leading notifiable diseases in 1968. Perhaps the most startling changes were the increasing rates of alcoholism, suicide, dysfunctional families, child neglect, and mental illness. The suspected causal factors included poverty, cultural clashes, unemployment, geographic isolation, and lack of education, all of which combined to create an atmosphere of frustration, dependency, and hopelessness. Cultural stress brought on by industrialization and changing cultural roles contributed to the burgeoning mental health problems, including child neglect and abuse.[57]

The mental health needs of American Indians and Alaska Natives were inadequately met and then only through state mental health programs. In 1965, the Indian Health Service initiated its first mental health project on the Pine Ridge Oglala Sioux Reservation. Additional programs were started in Alaska (1966), Albuquerque and Window Rock (1968), and Phoenix, Portland, and Billings (1969). The number of funded positions, however, never equaled demand or need. By the end of the decade one could argue that the greatest need of the Indian Health Service was a mental health program that reflected tribal values. The suicide rate of American Indians and Alaska Natives increased in the 1960s, rising from 11.7 to 13.6 per 100,000, while the comparable non-Indian rate increased from 10.6 to 10.9.[58]

Table 4.6

*Incidence Rates of Leading Notifiable Diseases in 1968*
(Per 100,000 Population)

| Disease | American Indian and Alaska Natives | General U.S. |
|---|---|---|
| Otitis media | 9,115.2 | * |
| Gastroenteritis | 6,031.2 | * |
| Streptococcus infection | 3,742.8 | 217.6 |
| Pneumonia (except newborn) | 3,665.8 | * |
| Influenza | 3,318.7 | * |
| Gonorrhea | 912.5 | 232.4 |
| Trachoma | 871.0 | * |
| Chicken Pox | 413.1 | 80.0** |
| Mumps | 376.2 | 76.1 |
| Dysentery (amoebic & bacillary) | 217.7 | 7.5 |
| Hepatitis | 174.0 | 25.3 |
| Syphilis | 158.0 | 48.1 |
| Tuberculosis | 145.0 | 21.3 |
| Rubeola | 79.0 | 11.1 |

*not reported
**43 states reporting

(Source: *Indian Health Trends and Services*, 1969)

As the Indian Health Service prepared to move into the 1970s, it elevated the health status of American Indians and Alaska Natives. But while health status improved, it remained below that of the rest of America. The life expectancy of American Indians remained far below the general population (see Table 4.7). At birth an American Indian could expect to live 45.7 years in 1967 (but 53 years if the child lived past the first year). A white American could expect to live 66.3 years (or 68.7 years if the child lived past the first year). Despite increasing utilization of hospital services (Indian hospitals experienced a greater percentage of hospital occupancy than non-Indian community hospitals), diseases and health challenges controlled or no longer a challenge in the rest of the nation remained all too common and frequent among American Indians and Alaska Natives. Further improvements depended as much on tribal involvement in determining the scope and manner of the health program as the services provided. American Indian voices across the country were growing louder: they desired improved health but wished to control their own programs in order to mold them to fit the needs of their community. [59]

Table 4.7

*Longevity of American Indians at Birth and One Year, 1955-1967*

| | *Average age of death* | | | *Average age of death after 1 year* | | |
|---|---|---|---|---|---|---|
| *Year* | *Indian* | *White* | *All* | *Indian* | *White* | *All* |
| 1955 | 37.7 | 63.0 | 61.4 | 50.2 | 67.1 | 66.0 |
| 1960 | 40.3 | 64.3 | 62.6 | 57.6 | 68.0 | 66.9 |
| 1961 | 41.3 | 64.5 | 62.9 | 52.6 | 68.2 | 67.2 |
| 1962 | 42.1 | 64.9 | 63.3 | 53.1 | 68.4 | 67.4 |
| 1963 | 42.7 | 65.2 | 63.6 | 53.3 | 68.5 | 67.5 |
| 1964 | 42.9 | 65.2 | 63.6 | 57.5 | 68.4 | 67.3 |
| 1965 | 43.4 | 65.7 | 64.1 | 53.2 | 68.5 | 67.5 |
| 1966 | 44.0 | 66.0 | 64.5 | 52.8 | 68.6 | 67.6 |
| 1967 | 45.7 | 66.3 | 64.7 | 53.0 | 68.7 | 67.6 |

(Source: *Measure of Longevity of American Indians*, 1970)

# Notes

1. Rabeau served in Nome, Barrow, Tanana, and Kotzebue before becoming Deputy Area Director of the Alaska Native Health Service. Copy of Resolution Passed by the Inter-Tribal Council of the Five Civilized Tribes adopted October 11, 1968, in *To the First Americans: Third Annual Report of the Indian Health Program of the U.S. Public Health Service* (Washington, D.C.: Government Printing Office, 1969), 15. Todd, "Interview with Dr. Erwin S. Rabeau."

2. *Annual Report of the United States Department of Health, Education and Welfare,*

1966, x-xi. Congress legislatively established four new assistant secretary positions and a special post for the Assistant Secretary for Civil Rights. Rabeau told the House that he expected little impact from the Medicare program on the Indian Health Service because there were so few elderly affected. "Department of the Interior and Related Agencies Appropriations for 1967," *Hearings before a Subcommittee of the Committee on Appropriations House of Representatives* 89th Congress, 2d session, part 3, March 2, 1966, 554. *Annual Report of the Department of Health, Education and Welfare*, 1968, xii-xiii.

3. Robert and Rosalie Kane, *Federal Healthcare (With Reservations!)* (New York: Springer Publishing Company, 1972), chapter VII "A Service Unit in Search of a Program." Kane provides a case study from his personal experience as director of the Shiprock Service Unit, illustrating how too much centralized control inhibited the work at the operational level. Robert L. Kane, "Community Medicine on the Navajo Reservation," *Health Services and Mental Health Administration Health Reports* (86:8) August 1971, 733-740. Irving Schlafman, "Health Systems Research to Deliver Comprehensive Services to Indians," *Public Health Reports* (84:8) August 1969, 698.

4. Kane, *Federal Healthcare*, 122. Chapter X ("M.D. or Not M.D." 121-129) of Kane's essay provides an overview of the question of who should administer the Indian Health Service and how physicians responded to non-physician administrators. "Department of the Interior and Related Agencies Appropriations for 1970," *Hearings before a Subcommittee of the Committee on Appropriations House of Representatives* 91st Congress, 1st session, part 3, March 24, 1969, 396.

5. Cahn, *Our Brother's Keeper*, 56, argued, "the fundamental health indices among the Indians do not depend solely on more doctors, more treatments, more pills and serums." If the Indian Health Service continued to preoccupy itself with this type of approach, its goal of elevating Indian health standards to that of the general population would fail. Kane, *Federal Healthcare*, 19.

6. Cahn, *Our Brother's Keeper*, 18.

7. Training was provided in internal medicine, pediatrics, obstetrics, preventive medicine, surgery, gynecology, general medical management, and health administration. *General Practice Residency Program* (Department of Health, Education and Welfare, Public Health Service, 1966).

8. "Department of the Interior and Related Agencies Appropriations for 1968," *Hearings before a Subcommittee of the Committee on Appropriations House of Representatives* 90th Congress, 1st session, part 2, March 8, 1967, 555. Sorkin *American Indians and Federal Aid*, 57. Arthur Owens, "The New Surge in Physicians' Earnings and Expenses," *Medical Economics* (46:12) December 1969, 85. "Department of the Interior and Related Agencies Appropriations for 1970," 409. Rabeau urged Congress to increase contract care funding because contract physicians, having once provided the agency with lower rates, now were charging "usual and customary" fees.

9. Kane, *Federal Healthcare*, 21-33.

10. Sorkin, *American Indians and Federal Aid*, 58, noted that at the Pine Ridge hospital the nursing shortage necessitated the closing of the surgery unit. The Indian hospitals on the Tohono O'odham (vacant head nurse position), Zuni (five vacancies), Blackfeet (three of ten positions vacant) and Pine Ridge (twelve of twenty-five positions vacant) reservations all had difficulty in securing and retaining nurses.

11. Kane, "Community Medicine on the Navajo Reservation," 735-736. Sorkin,

*American Indians and Federal Aid*, 60. Some physicians argued for an increase in the number of examining rooms, which would allow them to see more patients per hour without rushing patients out of the hospital. Interestingly, many Navajo resisted pharmacists dispensing drugs, preferring to wait for a physician to examine them for minor illnesses, such as colds. Kane, "Community Medicine on the Navajo Reservation," 737.

12. At the Navajo Shiprock Service Unit in 1969, for example, just 4 of 18 registered nurses were Navajo and there were no Navajo sanitarians, pharmacists, or dentists. Yet, all the LPN nursing aides and custodians were Navajo.

13. To the First Americans: First Annual Report on the Indian Health Program of the U.S. Public Health Service, 1966 (Washington, D.C.: Department of Health, Education and Welfare, Public Health Service), 1. Kane, *Federal Healthcare*, 34, argued that the oft-stated goal of Indian participation to the "fullest possible extent" was too often defined by employees at the local level "aided and abetted by local tribal politicians" who did not want to lose their connections to Washington politicians who handed out money and power.

14. Irving Schlafman, "Indian Management of Indian Health Programs," Presented at the Fifth Joint CS-COA Meeting, Washington, D.C., April 2, 1970, 2.

15. Personal Interview conducted by the author with Dr. Stanley Stitt, Tucson, Arizona, February 14, 1990. Schlafman, "Indian Management of Indian Health Program," 1.

16. Henry J. Keneally, "The Philosophy of Good Tribal Relations," *Journal of American Indian Education* (1:3), May 1962, 1.

17. Charles S. McCammon, "The Terms of Partnership: IHS and the Indian People," Presented at the 13th Annual Tribal Leaders Health Conference, April 24, 1970, Tucson, Arizona. Kane, *Federal Healthcare*, 33. Kane was amazed at "how many different kinds of aides" could be created for Indians. "No matter how worthwhile the goals of the Washington office, a work force like this (careerist) will have difficulty uniting to put them into effect."

18. Erwin S. Rabeau, "The Division of Indian Health: Current and Future Program," Seminar on Indian Health, Tucson, Arizona, November 9-11, 1967, 17.

19. Richard B. Uhrich, "Tribal Community Health Representatives of the Indian Health Service," *Public Health Reports* (84:11) November 1969, 968-969. Uhrich describes how well baby visits, chest, influenza, diabetes, and other screening clinics were considerably more successful once the CHR began working. More than 85 percent of one northwestern reservation community turned out for immunizations and examinations and 350 Southwestern Indians attended an alcoholism conference largely because of the work of the CHRs. As importantly, the CHRs stimulated "health agencies to take greater interest in Indian citizens of the communities for which they have responsibility."

20. Uhrich, "Tribal Community Health Representatives," 965-967. CHRs were trained in socio-cultural affairs (to see both the Indian and non-Indian value system and how it impacted healthcare); communication; concepts of disease and health (and how cultural background influenced a people's attitude toward health and disease); and basic technical skills (taking temperatures, blood pressure, pulse, etc.).

21. Kane, *Federal Healthcare*, 39.

22. Most of the CHR programs were stimulated and funded by the Office of Economic Opportunity. *To the First Americans: The Third Annual Report of the Indian Health Program of the US Public Health Service*, 1968. Nadine Rund, *Community Health Representative: A Changing Philosophy of Indian Involvement* (Washington, D.C.: Office

of Program Development, Indian Health Service, 1970), 4. Kane, *Federal Healthcare*, 39.

23. Rund, *Community Health Representative: A Changing Philosophy of Indian Involvement*, 1.

24. Uhrich, "Tribal Community Health Representatives," 966. Contracts were negotiated with thirty-seven Indian contractors representing Indian communities in fourteen states, exclusive of Alaska.

25. Sanitation training was provided at Sandia Pueblo, New Mexico, and health record technicians were trained at a number of community colleges in Arizona, including Phoenix College and Central Arizona College. Dental training courses were offered at Brigham City, Utah; Lawrence, Kansas; and Mt. Edgecumbe, Alaska. *To the First Americans: Third Annual Report of the Indian Health Program of the U.S. Public Health Service*, 1969, 6-7. In 1968, the Indian Health Service sponsored training for one Indian physician and two registered nurses and provided an internship for an Indian pharmacy assistant each summer while he earned his degree.

26. "Department of the Interior and Related Agencies Appropriations for 1970," 393.

27. Schlafman, "Indian Management of Indian Health Programs," 4.

28. *Task Force Six: Report on Indian Health*, American Indian Policy Review Commission (Washington, D.C.: Government Printing Office, 1976), 132. Quoted in Kane, *Federal Healthcare*, 41. *To the First Americans: The Third Annual Report of the Indian Health Program of the US Public Health Service*, 1969, 8. Kane, "Community Medicine on the Navajo Reservation," 739, raised an interesting question related to health boards in general: "The question of health boards raises issues not unique to the Navajo but which may have implications for all federally financed medical care. The appropriate role of consumer representatives in healthcare planning is the subject of a long debate. In the context of a system which is dependent on Federal lump-sum financing, the need for a consumer advocate becomes dual. He must not only represent the consumer to the providers of care, but he must also be prepared to justify the providers' needs for funds. This aspect has particular relevance to the Navajo and must influence the feelings of both providers and consumers toward the need for a health board."

29. *Health Services for American Indians*, 139.

30. In December 1968 and, again, in March 1969 the Office of Program Planning and Evaluation initiated a series of workshops for field workers and American Indians in planning service unit health programs. The training was held at the Desert Willow Training Center in Tucson and enabled participants to "develop guidelines for planning day-by-day activities at community levels."

31. The Indian Health Service established two objectives with the creation of the program: The training of staff in using "epidemiology as a scientific tool in decision-making in program management" and the development of a health records system. "Department of the Interior and Related Appropriations for 1968," 617.

32. "Interior Department and Related Agencies Appropriations Bill, 1967," *Senate Report 233* 90th Congress, 1st session, May 15, 1967, 2004. Rabeau argued before the Senate that Tucson was chosen because it provided a typical service unit, was close to the University of Arizona allowing easy access to consultants, and the Bureau of Ethnic Research at the University of Arizona had complete demographic information on all Papago, allowing the agency to conduct research with "considerable ease." Schlafman, "Health Systems Research to Deliver Comprehensive Services to Indians," 697. Schlafman argued

that as the demand for services increased and the gap between services and available resources widened, "systematic management, training, and research are mandatory to assure the wise use of such resources." Kane, "Community Medicine on the Navajo Reservation," 740, argued that for community medicine to work the IHS had to treat all aspects of the problems at once: patient care, teaching, research, and the local dynamics of the individual communities.

33. *Justifications of Appropriation Estimates for Committee on Appropriations*, fiscal year 1968, IHA-21.

34. *Justifications of Appropriation Estimates for Committee on Appropriations*, fiscal year 1968, IHA-23. "Interior Department and Related Agencies Appropriations Bill, 1968," 2002.

35. Nadine Rund, "Application of the Social Compass to the Study of Health," (Health Program Systems Center, Indian Health Service, September 1968), iii. The Sells, Arizona, Service Unit was the home of some 8,000 Tohono O'odham living on a 2.8 million acre reservation west of Tucson. Schlafman, "Health Systems Research to Deliver Comprehensive Services to Indians," 698.

36. Schlafman, "Health Systems Research to Deliver Comprehensive Services to Indians," 698, opined that such a staff college would "undoubtedly strengthen the quality and continuity of Indian Health Service services and personnel and facilitate the training of Indian leaders in the ultimate management and direction of their own health programs." *Task Force Six: Report on Indian Health*, 114. One of the unique aspects of the Desert Willow Training center was that when it opened it was funded by the Indian Health Service for the benefit of American Indians and Alaska Natives before Congress mandated such assistance in the Indian Self-determination Act and Indian Healthcare Improvement Act. "Interior Department and Related Agencies Appropriations Bill, 1968," 2007.

37. For an overview of the programs and training offered by Desert Willow see *Indian Health Service Office of Research and Development* (U.S. Department of Health, Education and Welfare, Health Services and Mental Health Administration, Public Health Service, Indian Health Service, 1973), 14-18.

38. The Desert Willow Training Center was not the first training facility in the Indian Health Service. Over the course of years there had been numerous training facilities in or near Indian Country. There had been a training center located in Phoenix, Arizona, for example, which briefly provided training in epidemiology, environmental health, and health records management. The Phoenix training center, however, was chronically understaffed, underfunded and lacked the necessary physical resources. With the establishment of the Health Program Systems Center in Tucson, where operational research was at hand, Rabeau moved the Phoenix facility south, where training and research analysis could complement each other. In 1968 the facility was expanded into a nucleus of twelve professionally trained personnel. In addition to the twelve trained personnel, professional staff from the San Xavier Health Center provided training or training materials needed to meet existing and future needs within the Indian Health Service. *Justifications of Appropriation Estimates for Committee on Appropriations*, fiscal year 1968, IHA-55-56. The Office of Program Development combined the Desert Willow Training Center, Sells Service Unit, and the Health Program Systems Center. OPD became a significant research branch of the Indian Health Service.

39. G. P. Carlyle Thompson, "Coordination of Health Programs for American Indians and Alaska Natives," Presented at the Seminar on Indian Health, November 9-11, 1967, Tucson, Arizona, 23.

40. This was largely done on a case-by-case study rather than through any collaborative auditing system. Kane, "Community Medicine on the Navajo Reservation," 738.

41. Kane, *Federal Healthcare*, 96, 99.

42. "Supplemental Appropriations Bill, 1969," *Senate Report 1667* 90th Congress, 2d session, October 6, 1968, 421. "Second Supplemental Appropriation Bill, 1968," *Senate Report 1269* 90th Congress, 2d session, June 19, 1968, 42.

43. *The Indian Health Program of the United States Public Health Service* (Department of Health, Education and Welfare, Public Health Service, 1969), 15. "Department of the Interior and Related Agencies Appropriations for Fiscal Year 1969," *Hearings before a Subcommittee of the Committee on Appropriations United States Senate* 90th Congress, 2d session, part 2, March 6, 1968, 1688.

44. L. J. Bean and Corrine Wood, "The Crisis in Indian Health: A California Example," *The Indian Historian* (2:3), Fall 1969, 29-32, 36.

45. David D. Castillo, "The Impact of Euro-American Exploration and Settlement," in *Handbook of North American Indians: California* (Washington, D.C.: Smithsonian Institution, 1978), 124.

46. *Task Force Six: Report on Indian Health*, 163-164. "American Academy of Pediatrics Committee of Indian Health Report," 1974, in *Task Force Six: Report on Indian Health*, 161.

47. Bean and Wood, 31, pointed out that one state official responded: "We already know there is a problem; don't tell us about it. There is nothing we can do and if you tell people they are sick and you don't have the facilities for caring for them, what service have you done? You make them worse."

48. "American Academy of Pediatrics Committee of Indian Health Report," 161.

49. Volunteer physicians and dentists staffed the California Rural Indian Health Board facilities but eventually most of the facilities found funds to allow payment for services rendered. Each facility was governed by a local all-Indian board and was nearly autonomous. The California Rural Indian Health Board, which today is made up of project representatives, provided statewide support. Most of the rural facilities provided transportation to medical and other health facilities, with most providing limited healthcare services. Castillo, "The Impact of Euro-American Exploration," 124.

50. L. J. Comess, P. H. Bennett, M. B. Man, T. A. Burch and Max Miller, "Congenital Anomalies and Diabetes in the Pima Indians of Arizona," *Diabetes* (18:7), July 1969, 471-477.

51. "Effects of Improved Sanitary Facilities on Infant Diarrhea in a Hopi Village," 1093-1097.

52. Kane, *Federal Healthcare*, 79, argued that the shortage of personnel played a role in this continuing crisis. "While the United States per capita health expenditure is reported in excess of $300, Shiprock spends only $65 per capita. In Shiprock, there are 92 professional nurses per 100,000 people as compared to 331 per 100,000 for the nation. Similarly, the Shiprock ratio of physicians is 48 per 100,000 compared to 125 nationally. Not surprisingly, those laboring under such scarcities feel, like the Red Queen, that all their energies are required just to remain in the same place." John Irvine, "The Navajo," *Journal*

*of the American Medical Association* (213:1) July 6, 1970, 17. The infant death rate was three to seven times the national rate (depending on the location of the 16,000,000 acre reservation one was on), the tuberculosis incidence rate was 7 times greater and the rates for trachoma, syphilis, septic sore throat, gonorrhea, dysentery, measles, and chicken pox were all 3 to 10 times the national average. "Genetic Lag Plagues Indian Survival," *Journal of the American Medical Association* (205:3) July 15, 1968, 26-27. Gall bladder disease struck the Pima especially hard, with 37.5 percent of adult men and 67.6 percent of adult women afflicted with the disease. Thomas Burch of the Clinical Field Studies Unit of the National Institute of Arthritis and Metabolic Diseases, in Phoenix, Arizona, argued the high rate among the Pima was possibly due to their low levels of serum cholesterol. It was possible, Burch noted, that the Pima's "unusually efficient mechanism for clearing serum cholesterol" could be medicated through "exaggerated biliary excretion of cholesterol" and therefore reduce the likelihood of gall bladder disease. The Pimas' high rate of diabetes and obesity likely resulted from the fact that their "insulin-production system" had not yet "adjusted to a steady and plentiful diet."

53. *Justification of Appropriation Estimates for Committee on Appropriations*, fiscal year 1967, IHA-24. *Annual Report of the Department of Health, Education and Welfare*, 1966, 87. In 1965 the Indian Health Service initiated a family planning program as a means of improving the health of mothers and children. The objectives of the program were sometimes controversial, especially as the program matured in the 1970s. For an overview of the family planning program see Erwin S. Rabeau and Angel Reund, "Evaluation of PHS Program Providing Family Planning Services for American Indians," *American Journal of Public Health* (59:8) August 1969, 1331-1338.

54. *Annual Statistical Review*, 1969, 35. R. D. Zonis, "Chronic Otitis Media in the Arizona Indian," *Arizona Medicine* (27:6) June 1970, 1-6.

55. *Annual Statistical Review*, 43. Helen M. Wallace, "The Health of American Indian Children," *Health Services Reports* (87:9) November 1972, 867-876. Wallace, "The Health of American Indian Children," *American Journal of Disabled Children* (125:3) March 1973, 449-454. Wallace, "The Health of American Indian Children: A Survey of Current Problems and Needs," *Clinical Pediatrics* (12:2) February 1973, 83-87. Wallace, "Childhood Tuberculosis with Reference to the American Indian," *Public Health Reports*, 30-34. G. L. Portney and S. B. Portney, "Epidemiology of Trachoma in the San Xavier Papago Indians," *Archives of Ophthalmology* (86:9) September 1971, 260-262.

56. *Dental Services for American Indians and Alaska Natives* (Department of Health, Education and Welfare, Public Health Service, Indian Health Service, 1974), 12. In 1969, there were ninety-six permanent dental facilities within the Indian Health Service: seventeen in the Aberdeen Area; seven in Albuquerque; ten in Alaska; nine in Billings; seventeen in Navajo; thirteen in Oklahoma City; thirteen in Phoenix; and ten in Portland. *The Dentist in Indian Health* (Department of Health, Education and Welfare, Public Health Service, Indian Health Service, 1969). *Justification of Appropriation Estimates for Committee on Appropriations*, fiscal year 1970, IHS-29. Felix Bronner "Fluoridation—Issue or Obsession?" *The American Journal of Clinical Nutrition* (22:10) October 1969, 1346-1348. The prevalence of oral clefts in American Indians was actually declining, approximating the rate among the white population. Jerry D. Niswander and Morton S. Adams, "Orals Clefts in the American Indian," *Public Health Reports* (82:9), September 1967, 807-812. J.

Abramowitz, "A Children's Dental Program for American Indians," *Journal of the American Dental Association* (81:8) August 1970, 395-405.

57. L. Oakland and R. L. Kane, "The Working Mother and Child Neglect on the Navajo Reservation," *Pediatrics* (51:5) May 1973, 849-853. Kane, "Community Medicine on the Navajo Reservation," 739.

58. Sorkin, *American Indians and Federal Aid*, 64. Larry Dizmang, "Suicide among the Cheyenne Indians," (2177-2181); Sol Goldstein and Philip R. Trautmann, "Report on the Quinault Indian Consultation," (2343-2350); and Robert L. Leon, "Mental Health Considerations in the Indian Boarding School Program," (2203-2208) all in "Indian Education" *Hearings before the Special Subcommittee on Indian Education of the Senate Committee on Labor and Public Welfare United States Senate* 90th Congress, 1st and 2nd session, 1969, part 5. Michael Ogden, Mozart I. Spector and Charles A. Hill, "Suicide and Homicide among Indians," *Public Health Reports* (85:1) January 1970, 75-80. "Department of the Interior and Related Agencies Appropriations for Fiscal Year 1970," 1459. Maurice L. Sievers, "Cigarette and Alcohol Usage by Southwestern American Indians," *American Journal of Public Health and the Nation's Health* (58:1) January 1968, 71-81.

59. Charles A. Hill, "Measure of Longevity of American Indians," *Public Health Reports* (85:3) March 1970, 233-239. After the age of 5, an Indian child could expect to live 55.6 years while an Anglo child could expect to live 69.1 years.

# CHAPTER FIVE

## The Era of Self-Determination

In March of 1968, President Lyndon B. Johnson issued a call for Indian self-determination. "Our goal must be a policy of maximum choice for the American Indians," the president declared, "a policy expressed in programs of self-help, self-development and self-determination." Tribal participation was to be part of all federal programs for Indians. The goal, Johnson informed Congress, was to "narrow, then to close" the gulf between the health of American Indians and other Americans.[1] Two years later, President Richard M. Nixon pledged his support for Indian self-determination. "There is no reason why Indian communities should be deprived of the privilege of self-determination," Nixon asserted, "merely because they receive monetary support from the federal government." To this end, the president encouraged Congress to enact legislation authorizing tribes and tribal communities to assume control over all federally supported and administered programs within the departments of Interior and Health, Education and Welfare.[2]

Notwithstanding improvements in the fifteen years since the Indian Health Transfer Act, the health of American Indians remained twenty-five years behind that of the general population. Infectious diseases that disappeared among mainstream Americans continued to haunt American Indians. Mitigating the effects of alcoholism, promoting mental health, and controlling otitis media remained challenges in Indian Country. Reduction of these and other diseases could be realized only if American Indians administered and took responsibility for their own health.

## Decentralizing the Indian Health Service

The task of implementing the policy of Indian self-determination in the Indian Health Service fell upon a forty-year-old Sioux Falls, South Dakota, native and University of Minnesota–educated family practice physician named Emery Johnson. A former deputy director under Rabeau, Johnson entered the Public Health Service in 1955 with the intention of fulfilling his two-year obligation under the doctor-dentist draft law. He not only stayed with the Public Health Service for thirty years but he also remained as director of the Indian Health Service longer (1969-1981) than any other director.[3]

Guided by the principles of President Nixon's address to Congress, Johnson decentralized the Indian Health Service operations by delegating authority to area offices and, increasingly, to the service units, where tribal input was most meaningful. The Indian Health Service reorganized itself, establishing three offices (Tribal Affairs, Research and Development, and Program Support) four divisions (Program Formulation, Program Operation, Resource Coordination, and Indian Community Development). Johnson also modified the area office structure, adding three program areas to the eight area offices. In 1975, he created the Bemidji Program Area, originally part of the Aberdeen Area Office, to serve American Indians in Minnesota, Michigan, and Wisconsin. That same year he established the Nashville, or United South and Eastern Tribes (USET), Program Area. Originally a small field office in Sarasota, Florida (in the Oklahoma City Area Office), the Nashville Program Area served twenty-one tribes in the eastern United States. In 1977, Johnson separated the California Program Area from the Phoenix Area Office.

The program and area offices differed only in administrative structure. Area offices provided financial management, program planning and evaluation, tribal affairs/community development, environmental health, and medical, nursing, mental health, pharmacy, and other services. The California Program Area differed from all others in that there was no IHS facilities, with all healthcare provided through contracts. The Tucson Program Area, established in 1969 as the home of the Office of Research and Development, was unique in that, while providing services to the Tohono O'odham Nation, it combined research and development with program training for all area and program offices and the headquarters office in Rockville, Maryland.

Johnson believed that medical challenges and health needs differed among tribes and that no single policy or structural model could meet the unique situations in the field. By vesting authority in the service units, he believed meaningful tribal control would be more practical.[4] For the time, this level of authority was a revolutionary concept.

The Indian Health Service turned over much of the non-policy decision-making authority to the area offices, especially in terms of management, planning and budgeting, administration of the contract health program, and identifying services to be delivered. Alaska Native village corporations established under the 1971 Alaska Native Claims Settlement Act assumed responsibility over their own health programs in collaboration with the Alaska Area Native Service and the State of Alaska. IHS headquarters retained its liaison authority with Congress and the Department of Health, Education and Welfare, and established long-range planning, budget preparation and data, and information collection. Changes in fiscal management gave service units limited discretion in allocating funds at the local level and authority to implement health programs necessary to meet the needs of individual tribes.[5]

Increasingly, the Indian Health Service advocated for federal, state, and local health services for American Indians and Alaska Natives. For nearly a century, first under the Bureau of Indian Affairs and then as part of the Public Health Service, the Indian Health Service viewed itself as the sole source of medical services for American Indians and Alaska Natives. As state and federal agencies established new health or health-related programs, government officials believed American Indians and Alaska Natives were excluded from such services since they received medical care through the Indian Health Service. Medicare and Medicaid, for instance, had little impact on Indian Country since most American Indians and Alaska Natives lived far from available services. For reservation-based Indians the only available services were in IHS facilities, but they were prohibited from seeking Medicare and Medicaid reimbursements. Because American Indians and Alaska Natives lived within the confines of a unique legal and historical relationship with the United States Government based on treaties, court decisions, and federal statutes, they received federal health services. By virtue of their American citizenship, American Indians and Alaska Natives were entitled under the 14th Amendment of the Constitution and Title VI of the 1964 Civil Rights Act to all state, local, and federal health programs if otherwise eligible.[6]

The Indian Health Service rarely adhered to the concept of dual entitlement. Such entitlement frequently resulted in denial of services rather than ensuring access to such services. State and local agencies viewed the Indian Health Service as having primary responsibility for Indian healthcare and, therefore, referred American Indians to that agency. The Indian Health Service with its finite resources was unable to provide all needed services, with the patient ultimately caught between the two systems and frequently receiving no care at all.[7]

When the Department of Health, Education and Welfare abolished its Office of Indian Affairs, the Indian Health Service assumed the role of tribal advocate and became actively involved in the political process of impacting legislation to protect Indian rights. After 1970, it became the leading agency for "identifying, selecting and coordinating efforts to benefit American Indians and Alaska Natives in the area of health services [and locating] all potential resources which might be focused on increasing health services." In 1974, the Indian Health Service signed a tri-agency memorandum of agreement with the Office for Civil Rights and Social Rehabilitation Services, requiring state and local agencies to publicize the availability of services to and for American Indians. The Social Rehabilitation Services agreed to inform state agencies that no health service or program permitted denial of services to American Indians simply because of the existence of the Indian Health Service.[8]

## The Indian Self-Determination Act

To increase tribal involvement in the healthcare process and foster Indian control over health programs, the Indian Health Service contracted with tribes for health services. While contracting did not equate into self-determination, it was one aspect of the self-determination process. Tribes employed Community Health Representatives after contracting with the Indian Health Service for services. Under the prevailing contracting mechanism, the Buy Indian Act, tribes assumed all the responsibilities and liabilities of the Indian Health Service in administering the program, much like any federal contractor did. However, since Community Health Representatives were contractually responsible to service unit directors, the letting of the contract did not advance the idea of self-determination as tribes viewed it. This was largely because a majority of contracts described the scope of work to be furnished by the contracting tribe.[9]

The Buy Indian Act was the only means available prior to 1975 for tribes to assume control over federal programs. The law originated with the 1908 Indian Appropriation Act, which provided that whenever possible Indian labor was to be employed and "purchase in the open market made from Indians, under the direction of the Secretary of the Interior." The Indian Appropriation Act of 1910 modified the act by repealing the language "under the direction of" and amending it to "in the discretion of" the secretary. The amendment made it lawful for the federal government to make noncompetitive awards to Indian tribes or organizations to provide American Indians with opportunities to benefit from "appropriation based procurements to the extent that their labor could be employed in the products or services purchased."[10]

Buy Indian contracts for Indian labor and services were essentially the same as any other federal contracting mechanism except that they did not require formal advertising. The act, however, did not provide any method for tribes to assume control of programs, since federal agencies were prohibited from contracting away any of their legislatively delegated authority without statutory authorization. Without authority to control such programs, Buy Indian contracts were simply methods of employing Indians and an alternate way of providing services that would otherwise be provided through the Indian Health Service. Lucy Covington, Vice-President of the Northwest Affiliated Tribes, told Congress in 1973 that without a contracting mechanism authorizing tribal control of programs "tribes might well find themselves merely contracting the frustration of Public Health Service administrators."[11]

President Nixon encouraged Congress to enact legislation that would allow tribes, at their own request, to assume control over all federal programs for their benefit. Under-Secretary for Health, Education and Welfare Frank Carlucci expressed the sentiments of the department when he urged the Senate to support such legislation and remain "sensitive to the need for maintaining Federal support and concern for Indian people." Self-determination needed to reinforce, rather than undermine, the federal-Indian relationship.[12]

While Congress limited the scope of contracting the President advocated, it did enact legislation similar to what Nixon proposed. On January 4, 1975, in large measure due to American Indian demands for self-determination, President Gerald Ford signed into law the Indian Self-Determination and Educational Assistance Act (Public Law 93-638). Under the act, the secretary of Health, Education and Welfare (subsequently the secretary of Health and Human Services) was authorized "upon the request of any Indian tribe, to enter into a contract or contracts with any tribal organization or any such Indian tribe to carry out any or all of his functions, authorities, and responsibilities" under the Indian Health Transfer Act, as amended. The secretary was also authorized to make grants to any tribe or tribal organization for the development, construction, operation, provision, and maintenance of health facilities and services, including the training of personnel for such work.[13]

Congress asserted a new policy direction in the preamble of the act. Federal agencies were "to respond to the strong expressions of the Indian people for self-determination by assuring maximum Indian participation in the direction of . . . Federal services to Indian communities so as to render such services more responsive to the needs and desires of those communities." Congress reaffirmed its commitment to maintaining the federal-Indian relationship by permitting the "orderly transition from Federal domination of programs for and services to Indians to effective and meaningful participation by the Indian people in the planning, conduct, and administration of those programs and services."

Table 5.1

*Contracts and Grants under Public Law 93-638: Fiscal Year 1977*

|                     | Contracts | | Grants | |
| *Area/Program Office* | *Number* | *Funding* | *Number* | *Funding* |
| Aberdeen | 3 | $683,482 | 15 | $1,046,530 |
| Alaska |  | n/a | 1 | $48,448 |
| Bemidji | 2 | $700,000 | n/a | |
| Billings |  | n/a | 6 | $603,052 |
| Oklahoma City | 2 | $450,000 | n/a | |
| Phoenix |  | n/a | 9 | $785,210 |
| Navajo | 5 | $2,334,299 | n/a | |
| Portland | 29 | $2,024,896 | 1 | $30,000 |
| Total | 41 | $6,192,677 | 32 | $2,513,240 |

(Source: 1977 *Indian Self-Determination Oversight Hearings*)

With the passage of the Indian Self-Determination Act, Congress created a mechanism for tribal assumption of health programs. Unlike the Buy Indian Act, the Indian Self-Determination Act allowed the secretary to contract away his legislatively delegated authority. However, partially because of the federal fiduciary responsibility, the secretary of Health, Education and Welfare was empowered to approve or reject tribal contracts. Consequently, the secretary retained authority over funding and planning, as well as "the right to decide to his satisfaction, and without consultation . . . the dimensions and characteristics of a fundable program." Any contract awarded to a tribe or tribal organization could be retroceded by the tribes to the Indian Health Service.[14]

Following passage of the law, the Indian Health Service promulgated rules and regulations governing the self-determination process, taking steps to develop the infrastructure to carry out the law. Johnson told Congress in 1977 oversight hearings "that, like other IHS program activities, [this infrastructure] would be highly decentralized. In this way responsibilities and commensurate authorities . . . are placed in the IHS area [offices] . . . as close to the tribes as possible." Under adopted rules and regulations, contracts exceeding $100,000 required the approval of headquarters; otherwise contracting authority was exercised by the area and program offices. Table 5.1 shows self-determination contracts and grants issued for fiscal year 1977.[15]

In the years following passage of the law, contracts far exceeded the use of grants since most tribes were more familiar with the contracting system, having already used Buy Indian contracts. Perhaps more importantly, tribes perceived grants as reflecting a subordinate relationship with the federal government, while contracting fostered equality among parties. But while contracting became the predominate method of transferring IHS functions to tribes and tribal organizations, many tribes were reluctant to initiate contracts, fearing the law to be "termination by contract." Navajo Nation president Peter MacDonald, an early outspoken critic of the contracting process, described the law as "a bad joke." He argued that it "gave to the same bureaucrats whose conspicuous failures had led to the act, the responsibility for determining how Tribes might try to accomplish what these same officials had already failed at. . . . We don't need the Indian Health Service to be tolerant about our running programs that they have administered for years," MacDonald concluded. "That's not self-determination."[16]

MacDonald was not alone in his concerns. In 1978, the General Accounting Office (GAO) concluded that the agency "met the intent of PL 93-638 in a weak manner." One of the challenges with implementing self-determination contracts was that the Indian Health Service developed policies that required its personnel to respond to tribal contract initiatives but not to encourage or facilitate such actions. On the other hand, the GAO opined that for the Indian Health Service to encourage contracting would be "contrary to the concept of self-determination" since Indian tribes also had the right to not enter into contracts.[17]

Because the self-determination act required the Indian Health Service to promulgate rules and regulations for implementing the law, the Congressional intent of the law was skirted by administrative policies. In 1986, a second GAO study concluded that tribes and the Indian Health Service differed in their view of what self-determination meant. Tribal contractors perceived the law "as giving them the opportunity to determine for themselves the manner in which healthcare services should be delivered." Tribes viewed the Indian Health Service restricting this freedom via contracting regulations. The Indian Health Service, on the other hand, viewed self-determination as tribes "being able to operate IHS activities through contracts as stated in the law."[18]

The law established high expectations, but as carried out it did not foster self-determination. Questions such as the extent to which tribes could modify programs to fit their unique needs were unanswered. The limitation placed on tribes to perform contracted services as the Indian Health Service would was also a concern. "In theory and in legislative history, the Indian tribes are correct in their view that Congress intended to permit redesign and local control of Federal functions, programs, and services," one policy official concluded. In terms of administrative law, the Indian Health Service was correct that the regulations governing the law were lawful. While both views were correct, there was "a certain irony to the fact that Indian tribes correctly interpret[ed] the law, and the Indian Health Service correctly interpret[ed] the regulations."[19]

While nearly 90 percent of eligible Indian tribes operated some portion of the health program by 1980, few tribes assumed control of them. Several, including the Seneca Nation of New York, the Menominee tribe of Wisconsin, and two Alaska Native corporations (Bristol Bay and Norton Sound) assumed fully functioning health programs. The Creek Nation, the Navajo Nation, Bristol Bay, and Norton Sound also ran their own hospitals. All together Indian tribes ran 252 health clinics and stations, while the Indian Health Service operated 202.[20]

## The Indian Healthcare Improvement Act

To implement a successful policy of Indian self-determination required an American Indian and Alaska Native population that was healthy and trained in the healthcare professions. Despite incremental improvement, much work remained to bring Indian health to a parity level with the nation at-large. Forty percent of the IHS hospitals in 1978 failed to meet standards of accreditation (see Table 5.2) due to insufficient staffing and poor physical plants, and nearly half were obsolete, with sixteen requiring replacement. Incidence rates for tuberculosis, malnutrition, diarrhea, otitis media, and pneumonia all remained greater among American Indians and Alaska Natives than among other Americans, with infant mortality rates 50 percent higher.[21]

Such discrepancies did not escape attention. A majority of American Indians lived in environments characterized by inadequate and understaffed health facilities, improper or nonexistent waste disposal and water supply systems, and the dangers of deadly or disabling diseases. As a result, American Indians and Alaska Natives experienced "a health status below that of the general population," and dealt with "health concerns other American communities have forgotten as long as 25 years ago."[22]

Table 5.2

*Accredited and Non-Accredited IHS Hospitals, 1979*

| *Two Year Accreditation* | *One Year Accreditation* | *Non-Accreditation* |
|---|---|---|
| Cass Lake | Belcourt | St. George |
| Rapid City | Pine Ridge | St. Paul |
| Red Lake | Alaska Native M.C. | Eagle Butte |
| Albuquerque | Phoenix | Ft. Yates |
| Zuni | Sacaton | Rosebud |
| Barrow | Harlem | Sisseton |
| Bethel | | Wagner |
| Kanakanak | | Winnebago |
| Kotzebue | | Mescalero |
| Mt. Edgecumbe | | Santa Fe* |
| Tanana | | Crownpoint |
| Browning | | Claremore* |
| Crow | | Clinton |
| Ft. Defiance | | Pawnee |
| Gallup | | Ft. Yuma |
| Shiprock | | Owyhee* |
| Tuba City | | Parker |
| Lawton | | Schurz |
| Tahlequah | | Cherokee |
| Talihina | | Acomita# |
| Keams Canyon | | |
| San Carlos | | |
| Whiteriver | | |
| Sells | | |
| Philadelphia | | |

*Newly replaced and not yet surveyed for accreditation
# New facility not yet surveyed for accreditation

(Source: *Department of the Interior Appropriations*, 1979)

With the Indian Self-Determination Act already law, Congress proposed to enact additional legislation to facilitate self-determination. Senator Henry Jackson (D-WA) argued that American Indians and Alaska Natives were the most "depressed group of citizens in our Nation. . . . Nowhere is the discrepancy between Indians and other citizens as glaring as in the field of health." While Congress recognized that medical inadequacies and poor facilities were short-comings in themselves, it also believed inadequate health resources were a constraint on self-determination. Successful self-determination over the delivery of health services was problematic without adequate resources and properly trained health professionals.[23]

Congress responded to these unmet health conditions by enacting into law the Indian Healthcare Improvement Act (Public Law 94-437), in 1976. While proclaiming a national goal of ensuring "the health status of the Indians is raised to the highest possible level," Congress encouraged "maximum participation of Indians in the planning and management of these services." To bring Indian health conditions to the highest possible level, Congress committed the United States to a policy of providing "existing Indian health services with all resources necessary to effect that policy."[24]

The Indian Healthcare Improvement Act established an ambitious national goal of "rais[ing] the status of healthcare for American Indians and Alaska Natives, over a 7-year period, to a level equal to that enjoyed by other citizens." Congress authorized funds to recruit American Indians for healthcare professions, train Indian healthcare professionals, update services provided by the Indian Health Service, construct healthcare facilities, assist urban Indians, and improve sanitation. While the original bill called for $1.6 billion in appropriations over a seven-year period, the approved version of the bill pledged $475 million for a three-year period beginning in fiscal year 1978 and called for reauthorizing legislation for the final four years (1981-1984). The act contained seven titles with provisions to increase the number of Indian health professionals (Title I); eliminate unmet Indian health needs by authorizing funds for specific purposes (Title II); construct and renovate hospitals, health facilities, and sanitation facilities (Title III); amend the Social Security Act to remove prohibitions against the Indian Health Service receiving Medicare and Medicaid reimbursements for services provided to eligible members (Title IV); provide health services for urban Indians (Title V); conduct a feasibility study to determine the need for an American Indian School of Medicine (Title VI); and allocate funds for miscellaneous reports and regulations (Title VII).[25]

In 1980, Congress enacted Public Law 96-537 to amend and reauthorize the Indian Healthcare Improvement Act. In the amended act, Congress reaffirmed its commitment to elevate the health status of the American Indians and Alaska Natives to a level equal that of the general population. In addition to increasing appropriations for the programs spelled out in the original act, the amendment provided additional resources to implement a child sexual abuse program on the Hopi and Fort Peck reservations.[26]

The Indian Healthcare Improvement Act did not usher in a new era in healthcare overnight. Indeed, the law was intended to improve health conditions over a span of seven years. Nonetheless, Kiowa physician Everett Rhoades argued the law was important because the Indian Health Service had been unable to develop "a coherent program" due to funding constraints and division of uncoordinated Indian programs throughout the federal government. Rhoades argued the Department of Health, Education and Welfare acted in an antagonistic manner toward the Indian Health Service by ordering the agency to not request additional funds for hospitals between 1969 and 1975. The result was just one hospital was constructed, the Claremore Indian hospital in Oklahoma, and that in 1975. With the passage of the act, Rhoades believed a well-defined legislative policy of providing American Indians and Alaska Natives with the highest possible health status and supporting "existing Indian health services with all resources necessary to effect that policy" would enable the Indian Health Service to accomplish its mission of health parity.[27]

## Indian Preference

To implement self-determination also required tribal programs administered by and staffed with Native Americans. The policy of granting American Indians employment preference in the Indian Service (BIA and IHS) stemmed from the 1834 trade and intercourse act. A century later, Congress reaffirmed its commitment to Indian preference in the 1934 Indian Reorganization Act by directing the secretary of the interior to "establish standards of health, age, character, experience, knowledge, and ability for Indians who may be appointed, without regard to civil service laws, to the various positions maintained now or hereafter, by the Indian Office, in the administration of functions or services affecting any Indian tribe." Qualified Indians were to have preference for any vacancies within the Bureau of Indian Affairs. When the Branch of Indian Health was transferred to the Public Health Service, the Indian Health Service retained this policy.[28]

In the 1970s, Indian preference laws became a contentious issue. In 1972, Enola Freeman brought a class action suit against Secretary of the Interior Rogers C. B. Morton, alleging that the Indian Reorganization Act gave her preference over non-Indians in all initial hirings, promotions, transfers, reassignments, and any other personnel movements, including training programs. In 1974, the U.S. Court of Appeals affirmed a lower court ruling that American Indians indeed had preference because the Indian Reorganization Act stated qualified American Indians "*shall* hereafter have" preference not "*may* have preference." Had Congress intended to give discretionary authority to federal agencies, the court opined, it would have done so.[29]

That same year, the United States Supreme Court affirmed Indian preference in *Morton v. Mancari*, a case involving non-Indian employees of the Bureau of Indian Affairs who initiated a class action suit against secretary Morton alleging that Indian preference laws were contrary to the 1972 Equal Employment Opportunity Act, which prohibited racial discrimination in federal employment. The District Court of New Mexico concurred with the plaintiffs, opining that such preference laws were "implicitly repealed" by section 11 of the 1972 law. In the summer of 1974, the Supreme Court reversed the District Court, holding Indian preference laws were not racially motivated but were intended "to further the cause of Indian self-determination and make the (Indian Service) more responsive to the needs of its constituent groups." The Court opined that despite the transfer of the

Indian Health Service to the Department of Health, Education and Welfare, Indian preference had "continuing application."[30]

Although the *Mancari* decision clarified and confirmed the federal government's policy of Indian preference as a method of enhancing self-determination, federal agencies frequently neglected the implementation of this policy. Rhoades argued there was a need to define "precise regulations" for both the Bureau of Indian Affairs and the Indian Health Service and a need for special personnel to monitor and enforce implementation of Indian preference. Less than a year later, the District Court for the District of Columbia found the Indian Health Service "in derogation of the Indian preference laws." In *Tyndall v. United States* the Court ordered the Indian Health Service to implement "absolute preference for qualified Indian applicants in the filling of all present and future vacancies" no matter how they were created. The court directed the Indian Health Service to adopt the same Indian preference policies of the Bureau of Indian Affairs and publish them in the *Federal Register*. In May 1977, Emery Johnson issued Circular 77-2, which provided "absolute preference, without exception," to all qualified American Indian and Alaska Native applicants who were members of a federally recognized tribe.[31]

## A New Approach to Mitigating Professional Staff Shortages

The chronic shortages of medical professionals hampered the Indian Health Service and threatened to undermine self-determination. Johnson blamed the shortage of physicians for the higher rates of emergency and urgent needs patients admitted for care. Due to staffing shortages, Johnson closed 262 beds in twelve Indian hospitals in 1977 (see Table 5.3). More of a concern, Johnson feared the increased challenges tribes would face in assuming control over Indian Health Service facilities. Foremost among his concerns was that tribes would be unable to operate facilities that were already inadequately funded. Even if they could operate such facilities, there were too few American Indians in the health professions. Johnson was keenly aware that the Indian Health Service did not have the technical staff to train tribes that wanted full authority over their own programs.[32]

In light of the Congressional mandate of self-determination, the shortages of physicians, especially American Indian and Alaska Native physicians, was alarming. While the sophistication of American Indians was rising, the number of health professionals remained low, prompting Congress to provide educational funding for prospective American Indian health professionals in the Indian Healthcare Improvement Act.[33] Because of the chronic shortages, the Public Health Service continued detailing Commissioned Corps officers to the Indian Health Service. Under the doctor-dentist draft law, thousands of physicians and dentists entered the Commissioned Corps, with many eventually serving time in the Indian Health Service. By 1971, nearly 70 percent of the physicians and dentists in the Indian Health Service served in lieu of military service. The flip side of this influx was that most Commissioned Corps officers fulfilled their required tenure then left the program to enter private or clinical practice. A good many physicians left the Indian Health Service because of the great challenges that overwhelmed them or due to the frustration of making so little headway in decreasing crisis care.[34]

Table 5.3

*Indian Hospital Beds Closed for Lack of Staff, 1977*

| Hospital | Reduced Beds | Staff Needed to Reopen |
|---|---|---|
| Alaska Native Medical Center | 93 | 249 |
| Crownpoint, NM | 10 | 27 |
| Ft. Defiance, AZ | 24 | 64 |
| Gallup Medical Center, NM | 26 | 71 |
| Winslow, AZ | 20 | 54 |
| Talihina, OK | 14 | 37 |
| Tahlequah, OK | 9 | 24 |
| Pawnee, OK | 18 | 47 |
| Lawton, OK | 8 | 20 |
| Clinton, OK | 12 | 34 |
| Sells, AZ | 10 | 27 |
| Phoenix Indian Medical Center | 18 | 47 |
| Totals | 262 | 701 |

(Source: *Department of the Interior Appropriation Hearings*, 1978)

The 1970s differed little from preceding decades in that the Indian Health Service faced chronic shortages of physicians, nurses, and other professional staff. When Congress ended the military draft on June 30, 1973, these shortages became more acute as the primary vehicle through which most physicians entered the Indian Health Service ended. With the draft, the Indian Health Service enjoyed an application rate of about three physicians per vacancy; when the draft ended the agency experienced an immediate shortage of 200 physicians. In 1972, for example, the Indian Health Service received one hundred applications for twenty-two vacancies. In 1969, it received over 700 applications. Added to the challenge of ending the draft was a lack of financial security, professional growth, and cultural amenities that made "Indian communities less than competitive" for attracting new doctors. In an effort to alleviate the shortage, Congress established the National Health Service Corps to provide medical professionals for rural and underserved areas, including Indian reservations.[35]

Table 5.4

*Services Provided by the Indian Health Service for Select Years, 1955-1974*

| Type | 1955 | 1970 | 1974 |
|------|------|------|------|
| Inpatient | 50,143 | 92,710 | 103,853 |
| Outpatient* | 455,000 | 1,786,920 | 2,361,654 |
| Dental | 180,000 | 646,580 | 927,701 |
| *Hospital and Clinic | | | |

(Source: *Trends in Indian Health*, 1989)

With an increasing number of hospital admissions, outpatient treatments, and dental services, IHS medical staff labored under great demands. As Table 5.4 shows, patient utilization rates suggested an increased number of medical personnel at a time when such staff was difficult to attract due to the cessation of the doctor-dentist draft law.

While the Indian Health Service was handicapped by inadequate funding, it mitigated such shortages. One vehicle by which it did this was emphasizing a team approach to health services. This team approach extended the capacity of team members "to provide high quality services." For example, community health medics were an important component of the healthcare delivery team, relieving physicians of tasks that were accomplished equally as well by someone with less training. This was also true of the community health representatives and village aides.[36]

An equally challenging issue was that medical professionals working with American Indians and Alaska Natives were trained to practice medicine in urban settings, which differed from rural and reservation settings. Moreover, the Indian Health Service attracted a large number of Commissioned Corps officers resulting in high turnover rates at the operational level. This made it difficult to establish and maintain program continuity. Furthermore, there were cultural and linguistic gaps between the consumers of health services and the providers.[37]

One solution to this challenge was the introduction of the community health medic program. The brainchild of Dr. James Justice, who was stationed in Alaska, the community medic was premised on the idea that it was better to have someone "with practical experience" who was willing to live and work in a rural setting than someone who was better trained but unwilling to do so.[38] In collaboration with the University of Arizona School of Medicine, the Indian Health Service implemented a community health medic program at the Phoenix Indian Medical Center in March of 1971, after a two-week introductory course at the Desert Willow Training Center in Tucson. Ten candidates from a field of nearly 200 applicants participated in the two-year program. While the first year was spent in didactic training and in field training experiences, the second year included an internship that focused on clinical skills. A month after initiating the course, the Indian Health Service began a second

class at the Ft. Wingate and Gallup (New Mexico) Indian hospitals. By the summer
of 1971, thirty American Indians were enrolled in the programs.[39]

One of the most unique features of community medics was that they were
American Indians and Alaska Natives who lived in and intended to serve their
community. This was important as tribal members working in their tribal
community had a better "understanding of the needs, the expectations, and the
attitudes" of the tribe and they spoke the language of the people they served.[40]

Community health medics, like community health representatives, played an
important role in bridging the gap between tribal communities and the Indian
Health Service. Nonetheless, this did not put American Indians and Alaska Natives
in levels of authority, as most community health medics worked under the
supervision of physicians. Because of inferior educational opportunities, cultural
and linguistic barriers, apathy, and/or discrimination, there were just thirty-nine
American Indian and Alaska Native physicians (a ratio of 1:20,513) in the United
States, while there were 340,000 non-Indian physicians (a ratio of 1:618). Out of
14,000 doctors of osteopathy, none was Indian; of 120,000 dentists one was Indian;
of 25,000 doctors of veterinary medicine, only two were Indian; of 18,000
optometrists, just one was Indian; and out of 120,000 pharmacists, just six were
Indian. Of the nearly 2 million nurses, aides, and orderlies in the United States,
fewer than 500 were American Indian or Alaska Native.[41]

Not surprisingly, many American Indians and Alaska Natives agreed with
community health medic Larry Thomas, who described the need of Indian America
for "[role] model[s] for the youth, so they won't think that all Indians who work in
healthcare are clerks or janitors." Arlie Beeson, a Hopi, affirmed Thomas' remarks
by adding, "Indian children must be taught early in life about the possibilities of
such a [medical] career." As George Blue Spruce, the first American Indian dentist
in the United States, argued, most Indian children never saw an Indian physician,
dentist, nurse supervisor, health administrator, or pharmacist. "Consequently, in
their minds, [Indian] health professionals do not exist."[42]

In response to this concern, Everett Rhoades helped form the Association of
American Indian Physicians (AAIP) in May of 1971. The mission of AAIP was to
bring American Indians into the field of medicine. Rhoades, who was then director
of infectious and communicable diseases at the Veterans Administration Hospital
in Oklahoma City, was selected as the first president. The foremost objective of the
AAIP was to identify American Indians in medical (or premed) school and pair
them in a "buddy system" with an Indian physician. This would encourage
American Indian medical students as well as provide such students with someone
with whom to identify. The AAIP also consulted with state and federal agencies
that dealt with Indian health, particularly the Indian Health Service.[43]

With the number of applicants for physicians decreasing, the Indian Health
Service searched for new methods of attracting physicians. Programs such as the
Commissioned Officer Student Training and Extern Program (COSTEP) and the
Commissioned Officer Residency Deferment Program (CORD) were established in

the 1960s as recruitment mechanisms. By subsidizing students during their medical programs, the Indian Health Service required a payback of two years for both programs. But these programs and others like them did not cure the shortage of physicians. Consequently, in the fall of 1972 the Indian Health Service initiated a national recruitment effort using mass media and other means of communication to sell medical students and physicians on "the health needs, adventure, challenge, and personal fulfillment the Indian Health Service offered."[44]

Although the media blitz secured sixty-nine new physicians in 1974, few Indians were among the recruits. In an era of rising Indian fervor for self-determination, Johnson encouraged and emphasized professional training for American Indians and Alaska Natives. "Indian participation and involvement," Johnson opined, "is clearly necessary to properly identify problem areas." Professional training for American Indians in all areas of healthcare, including administration, public health nursing, sanitary science, education, nursing, and medicine was the backbone of self-determination.[45]

American Indian and Alaska Native physicians were needed not only as role models but also as caregivers who understood the unique needs of Indian communities. While there were few American Indians trained as physicians, change was coming, as colleges, including prestigious eastern colleges, recruited American Indians and Alaska Natives. In the fall of 1971, Dartmouth College, in what was billed as "a literal and symbolic reversal" of western removal, opened its doors to American Indian medical students. Funded by the Indian Health Service and private contributions (up to $5,000 per student per year), three American Indians were selected to attend the medical school, which envisioned itself as the preeminent training center for American Indian physicians east of the Rocky Mountains. The three medical students at Dartmouth represented 14 percent of all American Indian medical students in the United States. Thirteen other medical schools enrolled Indian students, with the University of Minnesota having the largest Indian population with four. By 1974, there were ninety-seven American Indians and Alaska Natives in medical school, representing 0.2 percent of the total medical school enrollment.[46]

To encourage American Indians and Alaska Natives to enter the medical profession (and provide them with support once they were in training), the Indian Health Service in 1973 established INMED (Indians into Medicine) to replace the community medic program. While INMED was funded by the Health Manpower Opportunity program of the National Institutes of Health, the Office of Economic Opportunity stepped in and provided INMED students with scholarships and other assistance since the National Institutes of Health covered only administrative costs, leaving Indian students with limited financial support. In 1979, INMED began receiving funding from Title I of the Indian Healthcare Improvement Act. While a regional program serving the five state northern Plains area and based in North Dakota, INMED provided professional training for American Indians across the United States. By training physicians to respect and work with, not against, cultural attitudes, values, and beliefs, INMED increased the number of practicing American

Indian physicians, turning out twenty-eight physicians and one dentist by June 1980. In 1976 the INMED program was moved into the Indian Health Service, which provided two years of support and a fixed monthly stipend ($453) for students.[47]

## An American Indian Medical School?

The need for American Indian physicians was so great that healthcare professionals argued for an American Indian School of Medicine to train American Indians and Alaska Natives in a culturally meaningful way and in a manner that incorporated Indian values into the practice. Largely a result of the Navajo Nation and the progressive Navajo Health Authority led by executive director Taylor McKenzie, the proposed $38 million facility would train American Indian physicians to work in Indian Country. Many tribes and tribal health authorities supported the medical school believing that such an institution dedicated to the unique health challenges and circumstances facing American Indians was fundamental to self-determination. Furthermore, because of the shortage of medical schools (demand exceeded the supply), many American Indians failed to gain entry into medical programs.[48]

In 1976, Title VI of House Bill 2525 (forerunner to the Indian Healthcare Improvement Act) proposed to construct an American Indian School of Medicine, with $16 million to be appropriated over a seven year period. Although Congress scaled down the provision in the final bill to provide for a feasibility study, the Department of Health, Education and Welfare concluded that an American Indian medical school was feasible. Selling Congress on the idea and the costs associated with constructing and maintaining the school were difficult. Ultimately, Congress rejected the school on the grounds that it would not open in time to impact Indian healthcare within the seven year period identified in the Indian Healthcare Improvement Act and there was no guarantee Indian students would prefer to attend such a school over other medical schools.[49]

But while an American Indian medical school did not open, the National Institute of Mental Health provided a grant to the Rough Rock (Navajo) Demonstration School to establish a medical school for traditional healing practices and ceremonies. Because of the years associated with learning the ceremonies and songs, few Navajo youth could afford to become "singers." Opening in the fall of 1969, six Navajo healers were each assigned two apprentices to learn "the letter perfect performance of 50-100 hours of ritual" associated with sand paintings, recitation of ceremonial myths, and management techniques. The opening of a school for traditional healers was important to the Navajo Nation, as the Navajo believed Western medicine treated the symptoms of disease but did not always deal with its root cause, something they believe only a traditional healer could discover and cure.[50]

The need for American Indian and Alaska Native administrative and management leaders was as acute as the need for physicians. While Erwin Rabeau encouraged American Indians to seek advanced degrees, it was not until 1971 that the University of Oklahoma created a graduate program in public health. Housed in the Health Sciences Center and initiated by the university's Department of Health Administration, with funds from the Office of Economic Opportunity, the graduate program provided American Indians with the planning, administrative, and personnel skills necessary to operate Indian health programs. By 1984, fifty American Indians received Masters of Public Health degrees and two earned doctorate degrees. Despite such changes, Indian graduates rarely were given responsibility over budgetary approval.[51]

To encourage American Indians and Alaska Natives to enter the field of medicine, Title I of the Indian Healthcare Improvement Act provided for recruitment programs specifically targeting American Indians and worked to remove entrance barriers to the health professions in the Indian Health Service and private practice. Grants, scholarships, and loans were available for American Indians and Alaska Natives to enroll in schools of medicine, osteopathy, pharmacy, public health, nursing, and other allied health professions. The Indian Health Service also established extern programs to provide summer employment for students. By 1980, the Indian Health Service shifted attention to training and educating American Indians and Alaska Natives for the medical professions.

## Urban Indians

In the 1970s the Indian Health Service also expanded its services to include urban Indians. The Bureau of Indian Affairs, and the Indian Health Service after 1955, operated on the belief that once an Indian left his reservation he forfeited rights to any services unless he returned to the reservation. By the nation's bicentennial, nearly half of all American Indians and Alaska Natives lived in urban areas, with many arriving via the 1950s relocation program, which encouraged and assisted American Indians to seek employment and educational opportunities in America's urban areas and which was an integral part of Congress's termination policies of midcentury. As the number of urban Indians increased, and their low economic status, limited work experiences, unfamiliarity with urban health services, and cultural differences became apparent, urban health challenges became acute. Inadequate academic or vocational training, as well as the difficult adjustment from kin-based reservation systems to highly de-personalized urban settings exacerbated health issues.[52]

As American Indians left reservation communities for urban life, many state and local medical and social workers assumed the Bureau of Indian Affairs or Indian Health Service provided the needed health and social services. The reality was that many urban Indians lacked basic health services. Urban Indian health conditions in Minneapolis, Minnesota, for instance, were worse than reservation conditions. The infant mortality rate among urban Indians (35 and 32 deaths per 100,000 in Hennepin and Ramsey counties, respectively) was higher than that of the white community (23 per 100,000) and two reservation counties (24 and 13 per

100,000 in Beltrami and Cass counties, respectively). In Oklahoma City, urban Indians faced difficulty accessing basic health services. With state and local officials mistakenly believing the Bureau of Indian Affairs took care of American Indians, the gap between services urban Indians needed and those they actually received widened.[53]

Many indigent urban Indians did not utilize Medicaid because they were either unaware of it or they found it difficult to prove eligibility because of the myth of Indian Health Service services. Some urban Indians feared the "white man's institutions" or allowed pride to interfere with choices. Cultural barriers impeded access to healthcare, as urban medical professionals typically were unknowledgeable about tribal culture, community resources, and unique Indian needs. Consequently, many Indians found the services unacceptable. Medical practices in private offices and clinics were too impersonal, with long waits for service and little explanation of medical matters. For a people accustomed to interpersonal relations, such treatment was culture shock.[54]

With urban Indians receiving little or no care, American Indians formed organizations in cities across the nation to provide an array of services. Initially, small volunteer clinics opened on an ad hoc basis. As the number of Indian patients increased and the extent of the need became known, urban Indian health organizations became more sophisticated, until eventually they were able to search out and secure federal grants or funding from state and philanthropic sources to operate their clinics. Not until 1967 did Congress appropriate funds ($321,000) for an urban Indian health clinic (in Rapid City, South Dakota). Two years later, the Kinatechitapi Indian Council was formed in Seattle, Washington, and in 1971, it received grants and donated clinic space from the Seattle Public Health Service Hospital to establish the first urban Indian health clinic in the city.[55]

Despite the absence of federal legislation prohibiting urban Indians from receiving federal health services, Congress only slowly recognized its responsibility to these Indians. Authority under the 1921 Snyder Act (the main statutory authority for the Indian Health Service) made no distinction between urban and reservation Indian entitlement. When urban Indians demanded resources, Congress in 1972 appropriated $150,000 for the Indian Health Service to evaluate urban Indian health issues in Minneapolis. From this appropriation (and using the authority of the Snyder Act) the Indian Health Service established an outreach program to assist American Indians living in Minneapolis in gaining access to public or private health services. Within a year, and only after Congress appropriated funds for urban Indians, the Indian Health Service established three additional urban Indian organizations, with one in Oklahoma City, Seattle, and San Francisco (with nine urban projects forming the California Urban Indian Health Council).[56]

The funding of urban Indian health centers did not alleviate unmet health needs. With large American Indian populations in most American cities, expanded urban health programs were essential lest urban Indians "fall through the cracks." As a matter of budgetary policy, the Indian Health Service did not provide services to urban Indians unless they were eligible and returned to the reservation, which many did in order to secure basic health services.[57]

When Congress approved the Indian Healthcare Improvement Act in 1976, it established a goal of providing urban Indians with healthcare. "The American Indian has demonstrated all too clearly," the Senate subcommittee on Indian Affairs explained, "despite his recent move to urban centers, that he is not content to be absorbed in the mainstream of society." Having exhibited strong cultural and social ties, American Indians aspired to the same goal of other citizens, namely to live a healthy life and remain self-sufficient. To ensure this goal was achieved, Congress authorized the Indian Health Service to enter into contracts with urban Indian organizations. Contracts with urban programs emphasized increasing access to existing services funded by other public or private sources rather than providing or paying for services directly. As a result, most urban Indian funding was for community assistance and various non-medical programs, rather than for urban Indian medical needs. Since urban Indian health programs received funding from Medicare, Medicaid, Maternal and Child Health, Women, Infants and Children, as well as state, local, and private sources, urban health centers by law opened their doors to non-Indians.[58]

## The Housing Crisis

While urban Indians experienced unique health needs, many reservation-based Indians faced health complications exacerbated by inadequate housing. In 1969, the Indian Health Service attempted to improve reservation conditions by initiating a series of memorandum of understanding with the Bureau of Indian Affairs (Department of the Interior) and the Housing Assistance Administration (Department of Housing and Urban Development). The memorandum defined the objectives of the Indian housing program and the responsibilities of each agency, which agreed to an ambitious goal of eliminating substandard Indian housing by 1980. The Department of Housing and Urban Development (HUD) agreed to construct 30,000 Indian homes between 1970 and 1974, while the Bureau of Indian Affairs and tribal housing authorities committed to building an additional 1,000 homes each. The task was formidable: 60 percent of existing Indian houses were substandard and two-thirds of the housing backlog required new construction. At the existing rate of improvement, it would take fifty years to complete the job.[59]

Two years later there was no progress in eliminating substandard housing. The General Accounting Office informed Congress that the lack of progress meant American Indians remained in an environment that was "seriously detrimental to their health and well-being." The main difficulty in providing adequate housing was the lack of interagency enforcement and accountability. While HUD was responsible for planning, funding, and developing Indian housing, the Bureau of Indian Affairs provided access roads to housing projects and approved site leases. The Indian Health Service was responsible for providing water and sanitation facilities. Before any housing start could begin, HUD required flood plain clearances from the Army Corps of Engineers. The Bureau of Indian Affairs, in collaboration with the National Park Service, required new projects to follow the antiquities act of 1906 to ensure that they were not constructed on archaeological sites or sites eligible for the National Historic Register. Added to this was the Department of Transportation, which approved the construction of all access roads and financed improved road programs provided to the Bureau of Indian Affairs. The bureaucracy and red tape virtually ensured a lack of accomplishment.[60]

There were an estimated 63,000 American Indian families living in substandard homes in 1970. Despite the tri-agency cooperation, there were 86,500 Indian families living in substandard houses six years later. While there were 17,161 new housing starts and 13,542 homes completed of the 30,000 homes promised to be constructed by 1974, the pace failed to keep up with population demands. If Indian health conditions were to be brought up to the highest possible level, American Indian living standards had to be improved.[61]

In an effort to improve departmental responsibilities and communication, a new tri-agency agreement was consummated in 1976 between the secretaries of Interior, Housing and Urban Development, and Health, Education and Welfare. Following two years of negotiations, the new memorandum of understanding defined more clearly the functions of each participating agency. Under the new agreement the agencies established guidelines requiring preliminary interagency meetings to review housing plans and schedules. Delays in any agreed upon schedule was to be justified in writing. No one agency, however, had authority to remedy delays, with the result that the new agreement maintained its old weaknesses.

In practice, the new agreement retained their old weaknesses. No one agency was accountable for coordinating housing projects through to completion. Budgeting caused additional challenges, especially since the Indian Health Service budgeted in three-year cycles. The Bureau of Indian Affairs and HUD, on the other hand, budgeted annually. The Indian Health Service was disadvantaged in that it was often unsure where HUD or the Bureau of Indian Affairs would construct houses. Such disjointed activities and responsibilities all but ensured that the goal of eliminating substandard Indian housing during the 1970s would not be accomplished.[62]

## Hospital Construction

Indian hospitals also were in need of repair or replacement. In 1955, more than one-quarter of IHS hospitals had been built before 1925 and just one was less than ten years old. Most were fire hazards and lacked modern amenities. By 1969, 40 percent of all Indian hospitals were accredited and twelve new hospitals had been built, with seven of the oldest demolished. But the need for additional hospitals remained. Rabeau argued that modern, up-to-date facilities were a prerequisite for efficient and effective medical care. "Despite continuous improvement in this direction, many of the present Indian health facilities . . . are inadequate, are not functionally arranged nor properly equipped, involve hazardous conditions, or require comprehensive repair and thereby represent a major deterrent to efficient use of personnel and the practice of modern medicine."[63]

By the 1970s, a growing number of IHS hospitals were outdated and inadequate to meet the needs of a growing American Indian and Alaska Native population. Just twelve hospitals met fire and safety regulations and even these would have been forced to close if under state fire codes. Despite fire hazards, the needs in Indian Country were so great that the Indian Health Service could not close any facilities despite of the lack of safety. Of fifty hospitals, three were more than thirty-five years old. While nearly two dozen were built or modernized by 1975, just twenty-five were accredited. Thirty-three needed complete replacement or major modernization, and new facilities were needed in locations where hospitals had never been constructed.[64]

In September 1978, in response to yet another General Accounting Office report, Congress placed a moratorium on the construction of IHS hospitals until the agency reevaluated its inpatient bed needs for all hospitals planned and for which construction funds were available. That same year, a House appropriations committee prohibited construction of new hospitals until the size and bed assessments for proposed hospitals were resolved. Funding levels for hospital construction and planning plummeted from $41 million in 1978 to just $8 million in 1980.[65]

Table 5.5

*Public Law 94-437 Hospitals and Health Centers Constructed, 1978-1989*

| *Hospitals* | *Health Centers* |
|---|---|
| Acomita, New Mexico | Lummi, Washington |
| Santa Fe, New Mexico | Poplar, Montana |
| Whiteriver, Arizona | Lawrence, Kansas |
| Bethel, Alaska | Chemawa, Oregon |
| Ada, Oklahoma | Cibecue, Arizona |
| Cherokee, North Carolina | Lodge Grass, Montana |
| Red Lake, Minnesota | Inscription House, Arizona |
| Chinle, Arizona | Ft. Duchesne, Utah |
| Tahlequah, Oklahoma | Tsaile, Arizona |
| Browning, Montana | Huerfano, New Mexico |
| Kanakanak, Alaska | Ft. Thompson, South Dakota |
| Crownpoint, New Mexico | Kyle, South Dakota |
| Sacaton, Arizona | |
| Rosebud, South Dakota | |

(Source: *Office of Environmental Health and Engineering*, 1990)

To comply with the General Accounting Office report and to encourage Congress to lift the moratorium, the Indian Health Service proposed a methodology for determining future acute care hospital bed needs. This methodology projected utilization rates eight years into the future using average daily patient loads with sundry adjustments. These projections were then compared with several health barometers to determine a reasonably efficient facility. The General Accounting Office, however, recommended that Congress continue the moratorium because the revised methodology used assumptions that increased the agency's bed totals. The GAO believed bed needs at the Chinle, Arizona (Navajo Nation) hospital could be reduced if the Indian Health Service increased its use of unused beds at referral hospitals, improved transportation, and emphasized the construction of outpatient health facilities. When the Indian Health Service satisfied Congress in 1981, funding for new construction projects commenced, with Indian hospital construction and renovation increasing to nearly $650 million.[66] Using the authority of the Indian Healthcare Improvement Act, the Indian Health Service constructed fourteen hospitals and twelve health centers by 1989, as shown in Table 5.5.

## Healthcare Progress?

In March of 1981, Emery Johnson went before Congress and argued that investments made in Indian healthcare were showing "sound dividends." Part of the credit could be attributed to the Indian Healthcare Improvement Act, which gave the Indian Health Service its first quantifiable goal of "rais[ing] the status of healthcare for American Indians and Alaska Natives . . . to a level equal to that enjoyed by other American citizens." To ensure the success of this goal, the Indian Health Service provided a comprehensive healthcare delivery system and sought to deliver the highest qualitative health services with the finite resources appropriated by Congress. These services included hospital and ambulatory care, preventive and rehabilitative services, and community environmental health programs. In keeping with its commitment to seek alternative resources, the Indian Health Service in 1979 assisted the Pasqua Yaqui Tribe of Arizona in becoming the first tribe to enter into a tri-party Health Maintenance Organization agreement, the first time the Indian Health Service provided service via an HMO.[67]

Despite inadequate housing, deficient sanitation facilities, and antiquated hospitals, the Indian Health Service eliminated some of the backlog of disease by 1980. But as with the nation at-large, the American Indian and Alaska Native patterns of disease were changing and there was a growing distinction between health challenges and medical challenges. Health challenges were predicated on "socio-cultural and physical-environmental" factors that negatively impacted the physical and emotional well-being of people. This included poor housing and nutrition, lack of job and educational opportunities, and insufficient recreational activities. Medical challenges included diseases and levels of ill-health that required clinical solutions. These issues were increasingly symptomatic of health challenges, and as health challenges changed so too did the medical. The major medical challenges are illustrated in Table 5.6, which provides the age-adjusted mortality rates for select causes of death among American Indians and Alaska Natives in 1975.[68]

Table 5.6

*Age-Adjusted Mortality Rates: 1975*

| Cause of Death | American Indian/Alaska Native | | United States | Ratio |
| | Number | Per/100,000 | Per/100,000 | Indian: U.S. |
|---|---|---|---|---|
| All Causes | 5,774 | 824.8 | 638.3 | 1.3 |
| Accidents | 1,256 | 170.5 | 44.8 | 3.8 |
| Heart Disease | 965 | 147.4 | 220.5 | 0.7 |
| Malignant Neoplasm | 508 | 79.8 | 130.9 | 0.6 |
| Cirrhosis of Liver | 355 | 61.4 | 13.8 | 4.4 |
| Cerebrovascular | 291 | 43.5 | 54.5 | 0.8 |
| Influenza/Pneumonia | 281 | 36.1 | 16.6 | 2.2 |
| Homicide | 185 | 26.5 | 10.5 | 2.5 |
| Suicide | 180 | 26.0 | 12.6 | 2.1 |
| Diabetes | 145 | 23.8 | 11.6 | 2.1 |
| Tuberculosis | 64 | 9.9 | 1.2 | 8.3 |

(Source: *Illness Among Indians and Alaska Natives*, 1979)

Technology was also aiding the Indian Health Service in overcoming distance barriers. In 1972, the Indian Health Service developed the Applications Technology Satellite-6 (or ATS-6) in Alaska to connect rural Alaska villages in Galena and Fort Yukon (principally Athapaskans) with physicians in Tanana and Anchorage. Due to the harsh Alaska environment, radio transmissions between rural villages and medical centers functioned only 30 percent of the time. Using ATS-6 technology allowed community health workers to send video transmissions to physicians and receive audio instructions. While initially limited to three hours of satellite time per week, the ATS-6 showed promise in improving Alaska Native healthcare by allowing treatment to be administered in a timely manner.

Two years later, the Office of Research and Development worked with NASA to create STARPAHC (Space Technology Applied to Rural Papago Advanced Healthcare). Using a mobile van clinic, computer center, and television-voice data transmission equipment, the Indian Health Service linked the 2.8 million acre Tohono O'odham Nation to medical facilities in Sells, Santa Rosa, and Phoenix. The Office of Research and Development also teamed up with Bell-Aerospace Company to develop a controversial prototype health information system (or HIS) for the Tohono O'odham Nation. Using a computerized central data base, with remote terminals for information retrieval, medical workers gained instant access to complete and up-to-date patient, family, and community health information. The computerized system allowed the Indian Health Service to maintain comprehensive medical records that prior to HIS were fragmented, with information available to schools, clinics, hospitals, and other health offices. Medical, environmental, and socio-economic information on every tribal member was stored in a central data bank in Tucson and up-dated with each health team contact. HIS, however, was controversial as the Tohono O'odham feared their lives would be "put on public display."[69]

While the Indian Health Service managed to attack the backlog of health challenges, agency protocol was the same as it was in 1955: "Crisis intervention care must come first." With the utilization of new and modernized hospitals and clinics, as well as additional community hospitals, of which there were twenty by 1981, and the construction of additional sanitation facilities (more than 50,000 American Indian and Alaska Native homes still lacked or had inadequate water and waste disposal facilities) the morbidity and mortality rates for disease decreased. But diseases that had all but disappeared in the general population, only slowly declined in Indian Country. And as life expectancy increased, new diseases surfaced, as shown in Table 5.7.[70]

Table 5.7

*Notifiable Diseases among American Indians, 1970-1978*
(New Cases per 100,000)

| Disease | 1978 | 1970 | Percent Change |
|---|---|---|---|
| Otitis Media | 11,099 | 9,745 | +13.9 |
| Strep Throat | 6,200 | 4,699 | +31.9 |
| Gastroenteritis | 6,039 | 5,060 | +19.4 |
| Impetigo | 3,942 | 3,445 | +14.4 |
| Pneumonia | 3,197 | 3,059 | +4.5 |
| Influenza | 2,134 | 2,569 | -17.0 |
| Dysentery | 442 | 256 | +72.9 |
| Trachoma | 119 | 617 | -80.6 |
| Syphilis | 89 | 172 | -48.3 |
| Tuberculosis | 66 | 154 | -57.2 |
| Measles | 41 | 263 | -84.5 |
| Scarlet Fever | 17 | 13 | -35.9 |

(Source: *Illness Among Indians and Alaska Natives*, 1979)

In the 1960s one of the more severe diseases among American Indian and Alaska Native children was otitis media, an inner ear disease. It was especially prevalent in Alaska, Oregon, and parts of the Southwest, but could be found throughout Indian Country. Because of the severity of the disease (and possible genetic predisposition of Native Americans), Congress appropriated funds in 1971 to establish the first otitis media program. Combined with additional funds made available as a result of President Nixon's address to Congress, the Indian Health Service instituted yet another program to control the disease.[71] The Indian Health Service emphasized the treatment of acute cases of otitis media as the primary means of containing the spread of the disease and preventing it from reaching the more advanced and chronic stages. Among the Navajo upwards of 50 percent of the children in certain parts of the reservation suffered from chronically perforated eardrums. The Indian Health Service provided preferential treatment to children under the age of two since they were the age group most likely to contract the disease.[72]

Mental health issues and the relationship of mental wellness and good health also were better understood in the 1970s. Of the top ten causes of death in 1971, four—accidents, cirrhosis of the liver, homicide, and suicide—were either directly or indirectly related to mental health issues. In 1973, an Indian Health Service task force opined that good mental health resulted from proper sanitation, adequate housing, nutritional food, and available healthcare, all of which remained inadequate for many American Indians. Three years later, another study found a nexus between health and mental well-being. American Indians lost much of their land and economic base, and their culture was undermined. Many believed they were "inferior and that their most precious values were false." Decades of epidemics and social upheavals disrupted their family and community institutions. On top of this, "two centuries of autocratic, uncoordinated federal control, substandard living conditions, insufficient diets, poor physical health, meager employment opportunities and inappropriate education" compounded these cultural clashes.[73]

The loss of self-esteem had a devastating effect. Confronted with a struggle for identity and control of personal destiny from an early age, many Indian youth struggled with self-worth, which had a direct and adverse impact on their mental well-being. Between 1976 and 1980, 75 percent of suicides among Alaska Natives resulted from self-inflicted gunshot wounds, with alcohol a contributing factor in most cases. In 1979, 70 percent of all services provided by the Indian Health Service through its hospitals and clinics, or purchased from contract providers, were for alcohol-related conditions. This extraordinary phenomenon manifested itself in an age-adjusted American Indian suicide rate 1.2 times higher than that of the general population and a homicide rate 1.7 times greater.[74]

The federal government devoted limited funds to Indian alcohol and substance abuse programs prior to 1970, with tribes having few resources of their own to devote to such programs. After 1970, several federal departments and agencies allocated $10,000,000 to support Indian health initiatives. Of these funds, $1.2 million came from the Office of Economic Opportunity, while the National Institute of Mental Health provided an additional $750,000. While none of the programs was under the control of the Indian Health Service, interagency cooperation led to the creation of thirty-nine Indian alcoholism programs. When Congress enacted the Comprehensive Alcohol Abuse and Alcoholism Prevention, Treatment, and Rehabilitative Act, it established the National Institute on Alcohol Abuse and Alcoholism. Within two years, all federally supported alcohol programs, including fifty Indian programs funded by the Office of Economic Opportunity and one Indian counselor training program were transferred to the new Institute, which created an Indian desk for additional support. Having assumed control of all federally funded Indian alcohol programs, the Institute was the sole mechanism for funding Indian alcohol treatment and prevention programs.[75]

The National Institute on Alcohol Abuse and Alcoholism had authority and responsibility for administering federally supported alcohol programs. The Indian Health Service, although charged with carrying out the responsibilities for Indian healthcare, lacked authority to establish alcohol treatment or prevention programs. The Indian Healthcare Improvement Act changed this. Title V of the act funded the establishment and support of programs for urban Indians. Consequently, with alcohol abuse identified as a health challenge under the jurisdiction of the Indian Health Service, Congress in 1978 directed all Indian alcohol programs be transferred to the agency. Congress did so because the National Institute on Alcohol Abuse and Alcoholism had authority to fund demonstration projects, not long term projects. Over the next six years, 158 federally supported programs were transferred to the Indian Health Service.[76]

The real test of the effectiveness of the Indian Health Service was whether there was progress in elevating the Indian health status. While the major diseases of the nineteenth and early twentieth centuries were less threatening to American Indians and Alaska Natives, they had not disappeared by the latter twentieth century. Over 50 percent of the thirty-seven reported cases of plague in 1983 were among American Indians (and all in the Southwest). While the old nemeses declined, new diseases took their place. Diabetes mellitus was one such disease, rivaling in some aspects the twin scourges of tuberculosis and trachoma. Diabetes rapidly increased among American Indians and, by the 1960s, grew to epidemic proportions in some tribal communities. It became a leading cause of morbidity and mortality for most tribes, with the exception of some Athabaskans and the Inuits in Alaska. Among the Pima of Arizona nearly 50 percent of all adults over the age of 35 were diabetic, nearly fifteen times the national average. By 1981, diabetes was the second leading cause of adult outpatient visits to Indian health facilities and was frequently responsible for limb amputations. It was a significant factor in fetal and neonatal congenital malformations.[77] Table 5.8 shows the rates of diabetes by Indian Health Service area office.

Nutritional deficiencies, such as kwashiorkor, affected many American Indians and Alaska Natives, contributing to or complicating a variety of health challenges. American Indians and Alaska Natives still lacked nutritious and sufficient food and, because of poverty, many lacked the economic resources to mitigate improper nutrition. Particularly at risk were infants and children, women of childbearing age, elderly, and the chronically ill. Malnutrition resulted in anemia, increased the chances of acquiring an infectious or communicable disease, affected maternal and infant morbidity, and affected mortality and underweight or obesity.[78]

Table 5.8

*Age-Adjusted Mortality Rates for Diabetes by IHS Area: 1980-1982*

| Area | per 100,000 | Area | per 100,000 |
|------|-------------|------|-------------|
| U.S. All Races | 10.4 | Nashville | 22.5 |
| IHS (excluding CA) | 21.4 | Portland | 17.2 |
| Aberdeen | 42.2 | Albuquerque | 15.4 |
| Billings | 36.4 | Navajo | 15.0 |
| Phoenix | 35.5 | Oklahoma City | 12.5 |
| Alaska | 25.5 | Bemidji | 11.9 |
| Tucson | 23.8 | | |

(Source: *Office of Technology Assessment*, 1986)

The U.S. Department of Agriculture provided American Indians and Alaska Natives with surplus commodities, many of which were low in protein, vitamins, and minerals. These commodity foods tended to exacerbate malnutrition and its related challenges. Due to the poor nutritional values in commodity foods and the physiological differences in American Indians, most commodities complicated health matters. Commodity milk, for example, created problems for the lactose intolerant. Processed rice, beans, potatoes, and corn meal were high in carbohydrates and fat content and were poor replacements for traditional diets.[79]

Infant health and dental care were two additional challenges complicated by poor nutrition. Improved pre- and postnatal care decreased infant morbidity and mortality rates so that by 1982, the Indian infant mortality rate was lower than the national average (10.6 vs. 11.5 deaths per 1,000 live births). Nonetheless, post-neonatal deaths occurred more frequently among American Indians than non-Indians, due in part to inadequate sanitation facilities, inadequate housing, and poor maternal diets. Sudden infant death syndrome (SIDS) was another cause of infant mortality, with congenital anomalies also increasing.

Despite the introduction of fluoridation, periodontal disease was common and dental care failed to meet needs. In 1977, just 35 percent of American Indians and Alaska Natives received the recommended dental care for proper hygiene. As late as 1984, 81 percent of Indian youth had known dental caries, compared to 63 percent of non-Indian youth. Despite shortcomings, dental services escalated, climbing from 703,000 services in 1969 to over 1.8 million in 1981.[80]

## Critics Remain

While the Indian Health Service made progress in the fight against disease and ill-health, it did not escape public criticism. The activities of former director and then head of the Office of Research and Development (ORD) Erwin Rabeau were at the center of the criticisms. Rabeau established ORD in Tucson in 1969 as a premier IHS research facility. By 1976, ORD was accused of being a "small club of commissioned public health officers" researching programs that were "worth far less than they cost." While none of the charges was ever substantiated, a number of senior officials argued that the Congressional mandate of yielding control of the Indian Health Service to the tribes was flouted by the same commissioned corps officers that established the agency. Rabeau was personally charged with attempting to build an empire seeking to control the Indian Health Service.[81]

The Office of Research and Development was particularly condemned for creating programs that, some IHS officials—including Sacramento Area Office director Robert McSwain—believed were technically sound but not in tune with the needs of Indian Country. Not everyone agreed. Montana Area director Jimmy Smith and Phoenix program officer Gordon Aird both considered ORD's programs to be excellent. While the Tohono O'odham benefited from STARPAHC and HIS, the cost of expanding these services out of the Tucson area was not always cost-efficient.[82]

An especially sensitive criticism was the allegation that the Indian Health Service involuntarily sterilized Indian women. Choctaw physician Connie Uri, working at the Claremore, Oklahoma, Indian hospital, initiated a General Accounting Office investigation of the Indian Health Service after discovering large numbers of sterilization surgeries in the hospital records. When the GAO completed its investigation of four area offices, including Aberdeen, Albuquerque, Oklahoma City, and Phoenix, it uncovered more than 3,000 sterilizations. In most cases, the Indian Health Service failed to comply with government regulations requiring informed consent. One-third of the procedures took place in contract facilities that were not technically subject to federal guidelines. When the GAO notified Johnson of the report in August of 1976, he disputed neither the observations nor the recommendations of the report.[83]

While the GAO estimated 3,400 Indian women had been sterilized, Uri placed the number at more akin to a quarter of all Indian women, a number never substantiated. Physicians allegedly told Indian women it was time they "quit having babies" and if they did not submit to sterilization they would lose federal aid. The GAO recommended the Indian Health Service clarify its consent forms and stress to patients that at no time could benefits be withdrawn or withheld for refusing sterilization. When the report was submitted to Senator James Abourezk (D-SD) in November, the U.S. Information Agency issued a report and denied the allegations. The National Council of Churches condemned the policy of sterilization and asked the Department of Health, Education and Welfare to further investigate the extent to which the Indian Health Service may have incorporated the practice into their policy. Studies among a number of Indian tribes substantiated the rising number of sterilizations, but concluded they were due more to Indian women's "involvement in the wage economy" than to coerced sterilization.[84]

The GAO report also raised the question of inappropriate use of American Indians in medical research. Between 1967 and 1973, during a time when trachoma flared in the Southwest, the University of California's Proctor Foundation for Research in Ophthalmology (San Francisco) conducted trachoma research at three Indian boarding schools comparing the effects of oral triple sulfa, tetracycline, and placebos. Proctor did not utilize consent forms until its fifth year, when, for political reasons, the Indian Health Service requested they be obtained. Proctor acted on the premise that consent was not needed since the Indian Health Service was the legal guardian of the children while they attended boarding schools. While technically not medically harmful, the delay in services (four to five months for those on the placebo) and the lack of consent placed Proctor in an awkward light. In July of 1975, Proctor abandoned the research due to fears that a case could be made they were using "defenseless minority children to study an immunological problem."[85]

As the new decade dawned in 1980, the Indian Health Service reflected on important steps made in improving Indian healthcare. The Indian Self-Determination Act enabled tribes to assume control over their health programs and the Indian Healthcare Improvement Act established a goal and the means for elevating Indian health to a level equal with the overall U.S. population. After 25 years of IHS responsibility for healthcare, diseases and causes of death differed significantly from those of 1955. Injuries, violence, diabetes, and mental health were now prominent challenges among American Indians and Alaska Natives. But as the Indian Health Service matured into a full-fledged bureaucracy, it continued to face scrutiny. Mounting criticisms increased as the voices of American Indians and Alaska Natives seeking to control their own destinies grew louder. When Kiowa physician Everett Rhoades succeeded Emery Johnson as director in 1981, the Indian Health Service entered a new phase. For the first time it had an American Indian heading the agency.

# Notes

1. Special Congressional Message on "The Forgotten Americans," Delivered by President Lyndon Baines Johnson, March 6, 1968, *Public Papers of the Presidents of the United States: Lyndon Baines Johnson, Containing the Messages, Speeches and Statements of the President 1968-1969*, Vol. 1 (Washington, D.C.: Government Printing Office, 1970), 336 and 340.

2. Special Message to the Congress on Indian Affairs, Delivered by President Richard M. Nixon, July 8, 1970, *Public Papers of the Presidents of the United States: Richard M. Nixon, Containing the Messages, Speeches and Statements of the President 1970*, Vol. 1

(Washington, D.C.: Government Printing Office, 1971), 572.

3. Johnson was born April 16, 1929, and graduated from Hamline University in St. Paul, Minnesota, with a Bachelor of Science degree in 1951; his doctor of medicine degree was from the University of Minnesota Medical School in 1954. He earned a Master of Public Health degree from the University of California, Berkeley, in 1964. Todd, *Interview with Dr. Emery Johnson*.

4. *A Study of the Indian Health Service and Tribal Involvement in Health*, Prepared by Urban Associates, Inc., (Washington, D.C.: Government Printing Office, 1974), 101.

5. Within Alaska there were seven service units. The Indian Health Service operated the Alaska Area Native Service. *Alaska Area Native Health Services: A Description of the Program* (Department of Health, Education and Welfare, Public Health Service, Indian Health Service, Alaska Area Native Health Service, 1978). *A Study of the Indian Health Service and Tribal Involvement in Health*, 102.

6. "Indian Healthcare Improvement Act," *Hearings before the Subcommittee on Indian Affairs of the Committee on Interior and Insular Affairs House of Representatives on H.R. 2525 and related bill* 94th Congress, 1st session, May 23-24, 1975, August 5, 1975, and September 25-26, 1975, 69. Public Law 88-352, 78 Stat. 241.

7. Everett R. Rhoades, "Barriers to Healthcare: The Unique Problems Facing American Indians," *Civil Rights Digest* (10:1) fall 1977, 29-30. Rhoades argued that the Indian Health Service met the needs of roughly 50-75 percent of the people they served. When funds ran out services were "abruptly discontinued."

8. The agency helped create local Indian health boards to set policy and evaluate the program, trained personnel, and used community health representatives as grassroots organizers for seeking out county, state, or local health, hospital, and social services. "Department of the Interior and Related Agencies Appropriations for 1974," *Hearings before a Subcommittee of the Committee on Appropriations House of Representatives* 93d Congress, 1st session, part 4, April 11, 1973, 7. "Message to Congress by President Richard M. Nixon," 572. Rhoades, "Barriers to Healthcare," 30.

9. Although tribes might specify the service(s) to be provided they were always in accordance with the directives of the Indian Health Service. Consequently, the ultimate decision-making body remained the Indian Health Service. From the Indian Health Service's viewpoint, the government was obligated to maintain a high level fiduciary responsibility on behalf of Indian communities and therefore justified in making the ultimate decisions.

10. 35 stat. 71. 36 stat. 861. *Indian Healthcare*, Prepared by the Office of Technology Assessment (Washington, D.C.: Government Printing Office, 1986), 43.

11. Johnson argued before a Senate subcommittee on Indian Affairs that the Buy Indian Act was inadequate for contracting because of its prohibitive procurement regulations and requirement for advanced payments. The Indian Health Service needed greater flexibility in contracting to fulfill tribal desires for self-determination. "Indian Self-Determination and Education Program," *Hearings before the Subcommittee on Indian Affairs of the Committee on Interior and Insular Affairs United States Senate on S.R. 1017* 93rd Congress, 1st session, June 1 and 4, 1973, 75 and 201.

12. *Hearings before the Subcommittee on Indian Affairs of the Committee on Interior and Insular Affairs United States Senate on S.R. 1017*, 162-163.

13. 88 stat 2203, (Section 103 (a) and 104 (b)). "Indian Self-Determination and

Education Assistance Act," *Hearings before the Subcommittee on Indian Affairs of the Committee on Interior and Insular Affairs House of Representatives on S.B. 1017,* (93rd Congress, 2d session, May 20-21, 1974).

14. Guy Senese, "Self-Determination and American Indian Education: An Illusion of Control," *Educational Theory* (36:2) spring 1986, 157.

15. "Indian Self-Determination and Education Assistance Act Implementation," *Hearings before the Select Committee on Indian Affairs United States Senate* 94th Congress, 1st session, (Washington, D.C.: Government Printing Office, 1977), 207, 219. *The Federal Register* (40:221) published its Department of Health, Education and Welfare Indian Self-Determination Act regulations (Title 42) on Friday, November 14, 1975.

16. "Indian Self-Determination and Education Assistance Act Implementation," 234, 329.

17. *Many Obstacles Remain to be Overcome in Implementing the Indian Self-Determination Act,* Report to the Congress by the Comptroller General of the United States, January 1978. National Indian Health Board and American Indian Technical Services, *Evaluation Report: The Indian Health Service's Implementation of the Self-Determination Process* (Department of Health and Human Services, 1984), 12. The response of the IHS is in "Department of the Interior and Related Agencies Appropriations for 1979," *Hearings before a Subcommittee of the Committee on Appropriations United States Senate* 95th Congress, 1st session, part 2, March 23, 1978, 142-148.

18. *Indian Health Service: Contracting for Health Services under the Indian Self-Determination Act,* (Washington, D.C.: Government Printing Office, 1986), 3.

19. *Technical Comparative Analysis of Statutory, Regulatory, Jurisdictional Policy and Health Industry Entry Requirements Limiting Tribal Participation in Alternative Healthcare Delivery Systems,* Systems Resource Management, Inc., (Bethesda, Maryland, 1988), 20.

20. "Department of Interior and Related Agencies Appropriations for 1982," *Hearings before a Subcommittee of the Committee on Appropriations House of Representatives,* part 9, 97th Congress, 1st session (Washington, D.C.: Government Printing Office, 1981), 2.

21. "Department of the Interior and Related Agencies Appropriations for Fiscal Year 1979," *Hearings before the Subcommittee of the Committee on Appropriations United States Senate,* part 4, 95th Congress, 2nd session, (Washington, D.C.: Government Printing Office 1978), 336. Additional reasons for non-accreditation included inadequate separation of patients with infectious diseases, lack of utilization review program and medical audits, safety hazards, deficiencies in radiology services, anesthesia services, medical record-keeping, and poor emergency care rendered.

22. "Indian Healthcare Improvement Act," *Hearings before the Subcommittee on Health and the Environment of the Committee on Interstate and Foreign Commerce House of Representatives on H.R. 2525,* 94th Congress, 2d session, April 27-28, 1976.

23. "Indian Healthcare Improvement Act," *Hearings before the Subcommittee on Indian Affairs of the Committee on Interior and Insular Affairs United States Senate* 93rd Congress, 2d session, 1974, 1-2. By 1974, there were 150 American Indians and Alaska Natives in professional and administrative positions within the Indian Health Service. There were also 484 Indian nurses, 35 pharmacists and 108 pre-med students supported by the Indian Health Service or the Bureau of Indian Affairs. There were a total of 1,085 American Indians and Alaska Natives in health-related training in 1974. "Department of the Interior

and Related Agencies Appropriations for 1974," 18.

24. "Indian Healthcare Improvement Act," *Hearings before the Subcommittee of the Committee on Interior and Insular Affairs House of Representatives on H.R. 2525 and related bills* 94th Congress, 1st session, May 23 and 24, 1975, August 5, 1975, and September 25-26, 1975. Five separate bills were introduced, with H.R. 2525 the preferred bill. 90 stat. 1400.

25. "House Report 94-1026," *United States Code and Administrative News*, vol. 3 (Washington, D.C.: Government Printing Office, 1976), 2652. *House Report 94-1026*, "Indian Healthcare Improvement Act," 94th Congress, 2d session, and "Senate Report 94-133," 94th Congress, 1st session. *Congressional Record*, November 25, 1974, 37100. Prucha, in *The Great Father, The United States Government and the American Indians* vol. 2, 1152, argued the original amount was reduced because the Ford administration was worried about inflation, thus the initial three-year authorization and the subsequent four-year reauthorization. The House minority report outlines additional reasons for the reduction: Namely the IHS being unable to "comprehend a variety of unforeseen developments" that would "by-pass Congressional oversight." "Indian Healthcare Improvement Act," *House Report 94-1026*, part 3, 94th Congress, 2d session, May 12, 1976, 29. The original bill authorized $123,880,000 for fiscal year 1977 but was reduced to $67,180,000 for fear of a presidential veto. The House Committee on Ways and Means opposed the Medicare and Medicaid provision, arguing it would shift the "financial burden from general revenue financing through the appropriation process to a narrower social security based tax paid by individuals who already bear an inordinately large payroll tax burden."

26. 94 stat. 3173.

27. *Hearings before the Subcommittee on Health and the Environment of the Committee on Interstate and Foreign Commerce House of Representatives on H.R. 2525*, 67. Rhoades, "Barriers to Healthcare," 31.

28. 4 stat. 729. 48 stat. 984.

29. *Freeman v. Morton*, 499 F2d 497 (1974). Indian preference in training programs was denied, however, as the federal court held that although Congress intended for Indian employees to be trained when it enacted the Indian Reorganization Act, such training was to be governed by the legislation creating the program rather than through Indian preference laws.

30. *Morton v. Mancari*, 359 F. Supp. 585. *Morton v. Mancari*, 417 US 535 (1974). Justice Harry Blackmun, writing the opinion of the court argued: "As long as the special treatment can be tied rationally to the fulfillment of Congress' unique obligation toward the Indians, such legislative judgments will not be disturbed."

31. *Task Force Six: Indian Health*, 130. *Tyndall v. United States*, Civil Action no. 77-0004 (1977). *Indian Health Service Circular No. 77-2*, issued May 22, 1977.

32. "Department of the Interior and Related Agencies Appropriations for Fiscal Year 1978," *Hearings before the Subcommittee of the Committee on Appropriations United States Senate*, part 3, 95th Congress, 1st session, 528, 572-573.

33. Rhoades, "Barriers to Healthcare," 31. The American Indian Nurses Association and the organization of urban Indians attested to the rising sophistication of Indians in the 1970s. George Blue Spruce, "Needed: Indian Health Professionals," *Health Services Reports* (88:8) October 1973, 692-695, argued the IHS too often trained Indians in health

occupations or allied health professions but not in the health professions. This was largely due to the lack of support American Indians received while in primary, secondary, and post-secondary schools. Congress would have to overhaul the Indian educational system so that Indian children could be tapped, motivated and directed into the health professions.

34. "House Report 94-1026," 2666. See "Life on an isolated Indian reservation not Perfect, but . . . ," *Journal of the American Medical Association* (230:6) November 11, 1974, 805. Physician John Lewin argued that two or three physicians serving the Kayenta Service Unit (the size of Connecticut) meant long days and night duty every other day. In three years at Kayenta, Lewis worked with fifteen different physicians who were "here and gone." Many left because they thought nurses should do much of the prep work and cleanup, something Lewin argued was not feasible when nurses already had their own long days.

35. "Legislative History of the Indian Healthcare Improvement Act," *United States Code and Administrative News*, vol. 3 (Washington, D.C.: Government Printing Office, 1976), 2671. "Indian Health Recruitment Problems," *Hearings before the Subcommittee on Indian Affairs of the Committee on Interior and Insular Affairs, United States Senate*, November 19-20, 1972, 93rd Congress, 1st session, 1-2. Rhoades testified on behalf of the Association of American Indian Physicians, arguing that the problem with attracting physicians to some remote reservation hospitals was based on physicians' need for financial security, cultural amenities, professional growth and a respectable standard of housing, all of which the IHS could not offer. "Emergency Health Personnel Act Amendment," *Senate Report 92-1062* 92d Congress, 2d session, August 16, 1972.

36. "Legislative History of the Indian Healthcare Improvement Act," 2673.

37. Kane, "Community Medicine on the Navajo Reservation," 738, provides a description of some of the difficulties, including physicians trying to make medical decisions on the basis of interpreted data.

38. "Indian Aide Helps Reservation Physician," *Journal of the American Medical Association* (224:8) May 21, 1973, 1084. "Substitute Doctors Are on the Way to Aid the Indian Health Service," *Journal of the American Medical Association* (218:5) November 1, 1971, 671-672.

39. Medics were rotated through five major health areas: maternal health, child health, mental health, infectious and communicable diseases, and accidents. Training in pharmacology, anatomy, laboratory and X-ray procedures, program planning, management, and epidemiology was provided. The second community health medic program also used the campus of Navajo Community College and was the result of the Navajo Nation's desire to be self-sustaining and determine its own future. When the Navajo Nation founded the Navajo Health Authority, it established goals for the creation of a health manpower training program and assessment of the feasibility of an American Indian medical school, both of which would be sensitive to the needs of the Indian people it would serve. "American Indians Trained as Physician Assistants," *Health Services and Mental Health Administration Health Reports* (86:7) July 1971, 596.

40. Jerry Bathke, "The Community Health Medic in Indian America," *World Health Association Public Health Paper No. 60* (Geneva, Switzerland, 1974), 73.

41. Blue Spruce, "Needed: Indian Health Professionals," 693-694. Bathke, "The Community Health Medic," 70.

42. "Indian Aide Helps Reservation Physician," 1086. "Medicine's Door Opens Wider

to Indians," *Journal of the American Medical Association* (218:5), November 1, 1971, 674. Blue Spruce, "Needed: Indian Health Professionals," 695.

43. Interestingly, Rhoades, as an American Indian, never joined the physician corps of the Indian Health Service prior to becoming its director in 1981. When asked about his decision to not join the health program, Rhoades replied he didn't join because his interest was in clinical research, which required a university setting. If he had joined the Indian Health Service, Rhoades noted, he would be unable to speak out against government policies on behalf of the Indian community. "Indian Health Recruitment Problems," 10. "Medicine's Door Opens Wider to Indians," 674.

44. C. L. Hostetter and J. D. Felsen, "Multiple Variable Motivators Involved in the Recruitment of Physicians for the Indian Health Service," *Rural Health* (90:4) July-August 1975, 319.

45. Statement by Emery Johnson on "Indian Health Services and Indian Health Facilities," to the Health Services and Mental Health Administration, March 1972 (Indian Health Service mimeograph), 6.

46. "Medicine's Door Opens Wider to Indians," 673. "Nearly 100 Indians in Medical School," *Journal of the American Medical Association* (230:6), November 11, 1974, 806. The Office of Health Resources Opportunity made grants to a number of organizations to support native medical students. These included the Alaska Federation of Natives, American Indians into Medicine, Hopi Indian Agency, Seattle Indian Center, Eastern Oklahoma Indian Healthcareers Project Cherokee Nation, United Tribes of Kansas and Southeast Nebraska, and the University of Nevada, Reno. Contracts for career motivation were concluded with the Association of American Indian Physicians, Association of Native American Health Professionals, United South and Eastern Tribes, Oklahoma City Area Indian Health Service Advisory Board, California Rural Indian Health Board, and the North Central Intertribal Health Council.

47. Lois Steele, director of the INMED program argued that the two year stipend was insufficient as, on the average, Indian students needed 5.1 years to graduate. "Reauthorization of the Indian Healthcare Improvement Act," *Hearings before the Select Committee of Indian Affairs United States Senate* 96th Congress, 2d session, April 21-22, 1980, 135. Steele's testimony is on 131-132.

48. "Navajo Health Authority Is Planning Pan-Indian Medical School," *Health Services Reports* (89:5) September-October 1974, 488-489. "House Report No. 94-1026," 119. "Undergraduate Medical Education," *Journal of the American Medical Association* (234:13) December 29, 1975, 1333-1351.

49. "Indian Healthcare Improvement Act," *House Report no. 94-1026* part III, 94th Congress, 2d session, May 12, 1976, 22. The American Medical Association opposed the construction of such a facility arguing there was already a surplus of doctors in the United States. Personal interview with Jennie Joe, Native American Research and Training Center, Tucson, Arizona, April 5, 1990. Congress was apprehensive about such a facility, believing the per student cost (estimated at $200,000) too costly. "Department of the Interior and Related Agencies Appropriations for Fiscal Year 1979," *Hearings before a Subcommittee of the Committee on Appropriations*, House of Representatives, Part 4, 95th Congress, 2nd session, March 2/3, 1978, 372.

50. "Indian Healing Ceremonies Get New Lease on Life," *Journal of the American*

*Medical Association* (221:9) August 28, 1972, 962. "Indian Health Service Modernizes Medical Care on Reservations," *Journal of the American Medical Association* (218:4) October 25, 1971, 512. In Navajo culture, religion and medicine are interrelated and traditional healers believe any illness, physical, emotional, or mental, is caused by a transgression by the ill or someone in his family, resulting in disharmony between the individual and the supernatural. For an overview of some aspects of Indian healing in the Northwest see Morgan Martin, "Native American Medicine: Thoughts for Post traditional Healers," *Journal of the American Medical Association* (245:2) January 9, 1981, 141-143, and Sisvan W. A. Gunn, "Totemic Medicine and Shamanism Among the Northwest American Indians," *Journal of the American Medical Association* (196:8) May 23, 1966, 700-706.

51. Mitchell V. Owens, "Graduate Education Program in Public Health for American Indians," *Public Health Reports* (94:3) May-June 1979, 287. Mitchell V. Owens, Charles M. Cameron, Jr., and Patti Hickman, "Job Achievements of Indian and Non-Indian Graduates in Public Health: How Do They Compare?" *Public Health Reports* (102:4) July-August 1987, 372-376.

52. In California, over 80 percent of American Indians lived in urban areas, most of who arrived as a result of termination. Testimony of Leonard Smith, California Urban Indian Health Council, Inc., "Department of the Interior and Related Agencies Appropriations for Fiscal Year 1978," part 9, 69.

53. C. McCreary, C. Deegan, and D. Thompson, "Indian Health in Minnesota," *Minnesota Medicine* (2:56), October 1973, 87-90. Willy De Geyndt, "Health Behaviors and Health Needs of Urban Indians in Minneapolis," *Public Health Reports* (88:4) April 1973, 360-366. Rhoades, "Barriers to Healthcare," 27-28. Rhoades argued urban Indians in Oklahoma would be "willingly treated if they can get to an IHS facility" but the Indian Health Service limited contract care funds and did not provide any urban Indian facilities. Tony Castro, "Crisis of the Urban Indian," *Human Needs* (1:2) August 1972, 29.

54. *Health of the American Indian: Report of a Regional Task Force* (Department of Health, Education and Welfare, Public Health Service, Indian Health Service, April 1973), 19.

55. *Task Force Six: Indian Health*, 143.

56. Funding authorization often denied services to urban Indians. The Indian Health Service believed this justified the denial of services to urban Indians since they were not on or near reservations. The Indian Health Service argued funding urban Indian programs shifted the government-to-government relationship (under which services were part of the fiduciary responsibility) to a racial one (since urban Indians mythically lost their political connection to their tribe once they left the reservation, a view the BIA used in the 1950s with relocation). 42 Stat 208 (1921). "House Report 94-1026," 2753.

57. "Indian Healthcare Improvement Act," *Hearings before the Subcommittee on Indian Affairs of the Committee on Interior and Insular Affairs United States Senate*, 279.

58. "House Report 94-1026," 2754. *Indian Healthcare*, 194. *Urban Indian Health Programs Evaluative Report Fiscal Year 1983: A Report to the Director, Indian Health Service* (Indian Health Service, Office of Research and Development, Division of Health Systems Development, February 1984), 10. As a result over 40 percent of the fiscal year 1984 users were non-Indians. Urban Indian health centers offer a variety of services, many of which are not directly medical in nature but contributed to mental and physical well

being. The programs provided through urban health centers included health education (i.e., well baby, diabetes and prenatal clinics), job assistance and training, nutrition, outreach (i.e., referrals, transportation, liaison with governmental agencies) and various social services (alcohol and drug abuse recovery, counseling and family support). By 1980, there were forty-one urban Indian health centers funded in twenty states and according to the 1980 census over 50 percent of American Indians and Alaska Natives were living in urban areas.

59. *Indian Housing in the United States*, A Staff Report on the Indian Housing Effort in the United States (Washington, D.C.: Government Printing Office, 1975), 153. George W. Rucker, "Indian Housing: A Background Paper," Presented to the 8th Annual Meeting of the Rural Housing Alliance (Rapid City, South Dakota, October 1973), 1.

60. *Slow Progress on Eliminating Substandard Indian Housing: Report to Congress by the Comptroller General of the United States* (Washington, D.C.: Government Printing Office, 1971), 16. "Towards an Indian Housing Delivery System," Prepared by the Housing Assistance Council, Inc., November 1974, in *Indian Housing in the United States*, 171-172.

61. "Report on Indian Housing," *Hearings before the Select Committee on Indian Affairs United States Senate*, 1.

62. "Department of the Interior and Related Agencies Appropriations for 1979," *Hearings before a Subcommittee of the Committee on Appropriations House of Representatives* part 4, 396. "Report on Indian Housing," 136.

63. In February of 1978 the Indian Health Service drew up and presented to Congress a wish-list for 18 replacement and 2 new hospitals and a list of 14 hospitals needing major modernizations, totaling over $451,000,000. "Department of the Interior and Related Agencies Appropriations for 1979," part 4, 320. Sorkin, *American Indians and Federal Aid*, 61-62. *Justification of Appropriation Estimates for Committee on Appropriations*, fiscal year 1970, 51.

64. "Department of the Interior and Related Agencies Appropriations for 1974," part 4, 115-116. "House Report no. 94-1026," 2728. Appropriations never matched the authorizations set forth in the Indian Healthcare Improvement Act. For example, in 1978 the Indian Health Service was authorized to spend $178,000,000 on hospital and health facilities construction, yet appropriations were less than one-quarter that amount, or $43,760,000. "Department of the Interior and Related Agencies Appropriations for Fiscal Year 1978," part 4, 141, and part 4, fiscal year 1979, 320.

65. The Indian Health Service sought to construct a new hospital in Chinle, Arizona (Navajo Area), but the General Accounting Office believed the agency's methodology for determining bed needs was too high and consequently recommended Congress not fund the hospital. Since the agency used the same methodology for all its hospitals, the GAO suspected similar problems existed throughout the agency. The GAO reported to Congress in May of 1977 and Congress soon after approved a moratorium on construction. Johnson disagreed, informing Congress that the agency had a need for a greater volume of beds than the GAO acknowledged because the Indian Health Service provided a "comprehensive and integrated healthcare system." Three criteria were used to justify bed needs: the Indian population and its demography; disease characteristics; and the statistical process of needs (IHS bed needs were calculated to be lower than the general community and statistically there was a fixed amount beyond which care and planning needs could not exceed). "Department of the Interior and Related Agencies Appropriations for 1979," part 4, 246-252.

66. *Congressional Monitoring of Planning for Indian Healthcare Facilities Is Still Needed*, Report to the Congress by the Comptroller General of the United States, April 16, 1980, 10.

67. "Department of the Interior and Related Agencies Appropriations for 1982," *Hearings before a Subcommittee of the Committee on Appropriations House of Representatives*, part 9, 97th Congress, 1st session, March 2-3, 1981, 1. "House Report No. 94-1026," 2652. *The Indian Health Program* (Department of Health, Education and Welfare, Public Health Service, Indian Health Service, 1978), 2. Such authorization for the Indian Health Service to contract with an HMO was provided via the Indian Health Maintenance Act, Title VIII, Section 6, 87 stat. 935 (1973).

68. Patricia D. Mail, "Hippocrates Was a Medicine Man: The Healthcare of Native Americans in the Twentieth Century," *The Annals of the American Academy* (436:3) March 1978, 43.

69. "Satellite Helps to Bring Healthcare to the Indians," *Journal of the American Medical Association* (230:6) November 11, 1974, 807. Testimony of Helen Christy Cannon, Medical Officer of the Alaska Native Health Service, in "1976 NASA Authorizations" *Hearings before the Committee on Science and Technology, United States House of Representatives on H.R. 2931*, February 4, 1975, 94th Congress, 1st session, 18-28. "A Truly Remote Place," *Journal of the American Medical Association* (230:6) November 11, 1974, p, 808. Brint Dillingham, "Indian Health Service and the Health Information System," *American Indian Journal* (3:4) fall 1977, 16-18. Dillingham expressed apprehension over the Health Information System, believing it could be used to generate lists for unscrupulous uses since it included emotional, social, environmental, and educational data. Virginia B. Brown, William B. Mason and Michael Kaczmarski, "A Computerized Health Information Service," *Nursing Outlook* (19:3), March 1971, 158-160. For an overview of HIS see the *Indian Health Service Office of Research and Development* and *A Summary of the Initial System Designs* (Health Program Systems Center, Indian Health Service, 1969).

70. "Medical News: Progress Report: Some Gains, but a Lot Remains to be Done," *Journal of the American Medical Association* (218:4) October 25, 1971, 518. McCammon argued that until there were gains in community health programs, the sick would have to be treated and clinicians would be unable to "guide efforts to improve the conditions that created the medical problems in the first place."

71. *Programs and Problems in Providing Health Services to Indians*, Report to Congress by the Comptroller General of the United States (Washington, D.C.: Government Printing Office, 1973), 24-31. Maurice L. Sievers and Jeffrey R. Fisher, "Diseases of North American Indians," in Henry Rothschild, ed., *Biocultural Aspects of Disease* (New York: Academic Press, 1981), 238.

72. E. A. Mortimer, "Indian Health: An Unmet Problem," *Pediatrics* (51:6), June 1973, 1065.

73. *Alcoholism a high priority health problem: A Report of the Indian Health Service Task Force on Alcoholism* (Department of Health, Education and Welfare, Health Services and Mental Health Administration, Indian Health Service, 1972). *Health of the American Indian: A Report of a Regional Task Force*, 2. *Task Force Six: Indian Health*, 68.

74. Sievers and Fisher, "Diseases of North American Indians," 222. Brian L. Kost-Grant, "Self-Inflicted Gunshot Wounds Among Alaska Natives," *Public Health Reports*

(98:1) January-February 1983, 72-78. Of thirty-four suicides between 1976 and 1980, twenty-eight were male with twenty using alcohol at the time of death. Kost-Grant concluded that most suicides were impulsive rather than premeditated. James M. Andre, *The Epidemiology of Alcoholism among American Indians and Alaska Natives* (Albuquerque: Indian Health Service, Office of Alcohol Programs, 1979), 5-6.

75. 84 Stat. 1848. American Indians were not specifically named as a targeted group until the 1976 reauthorization of Public Law 94-371. Prior to this time there was no statutory authority for allocating funds for American Indians as members of tribal entities, although funds were available through the American Indians' and Alaska Natives' status as American citizens. The reauthorization act specifically called for "treatment and preventive services with special emphasis on currently underserved populations, such as ... Native Americans." 90 stat 1035.

76. *Indian Health Service Alcoholism/Substance Abuse Prevention Initiative* (Department of Health and Human Services, Public Health Service, Health Resources and Services Administration, 1989), 23.

77. Bruce Chelikowsky, "Half of the 1983 Plague Cases Reported in the United States Occurred in Indians," *Public Health Reports* (99:1) January-February 1984, 104. Of the 19 Indian cases, 15 were from the Navajo Nation. The 37 cases of plague were the most reported in the United States since 1924. Sievers and Fisher, 198-199, 204. Diabetes among other Southwestern tribes was also high, with 24.5 percent of the Cocopah over age fifteen suffering from diabetes. R. E. Henry, Thomas A. Burch, Peter H. Bennett and Max Miller, "Diabetes in the Cocopah Indians," *Diabetes* (18:7) July 1969, 33-37. Studies among the Paiute and Washoe showed both tribes with very high hyperglycemia rates. Gregory W. Bartha, Thomas A. Burch and Peter H. Bennett, "Hyperglycemia in Washoe and Northern Paiute Indians," *Diabetes* (22:1) January 1973, 58-62. Studies among the Pima show that traditional starchy foods (mesquite pods, acorns, white and yellow tepary beans and a strain a corn long cultivated by the Pima) slowed the digestion of carbohydrates and lowered the production of insulin and blood-sugar levels. Ron Cowen, "Seeds of Protection: Ancestral menus may hold a message for diabetes-prone descendants," *Science News* (137) June 2, 1990, 350-351.

78. B. Y. Iba, J. D. Niswander and L. Woodville, "Relation of Prenatal Care to Birth Weight, Major Malformations, and Newborn Deaths of American Indians," *Health Services Reports* (88:8) October 1973, 697-701. Gary Ruggera, "Diet Counseling to Improve Hematocrit Values of Children on the Blackfeet Reservation," *Health Services Reports* (88:8) October 1973, 722-725. Ashley Foster, Alice M. Haggerty and Edwin O. Goodman, "Use of Health Services in Relation to the Physical Environment of an Indian Population," *Health Services Reports* (88:8) October 1973, 715-721.

79. *Task Force Six: Indian Health*, 64.

80. *Indian Healthcare*, 106. The Indian age classification was five to nineteen while the non-Indian age group was five to seventeen. *Justification of Appropriation Estimates for Committee on Appropriations*, fiscal year 1976, IHS-6.

81. "Cronyism Within IHS Alleged," *The Arizona Daily Star* (135:292), Tucson, Arizona, October 18, 1976, A-1. "Empire Building Charged in Moving ORD Here," *The Arizona Daily Star* (135:291), Tucson, Arizona, October 17, 1976, A-4. It was alleged that Rabeau's original plan in stepping down as director of the Indian Health Service and

heading up ORD was to move key program evaluation sections to Tucson. That would have left Johnson a figurehead director in Washington. Rabeau countered the claims by arguing he left because he was "sick of Washington." Apparently, when Rabeau left for Tucson, many ranking officials had already moved or were in the process of moving to Tucson when Forrest Gerard, head of the Office of Indian Affairs in the Department of Health, Education and Welfare, heard the complaints and notified higher-ranking officials who stopped the move. Rabeau was further alleged to have provided lucrative teaching contracts at Desert Willow or ORD consultant contracts for retired Indian Health Service commissioned corps officers.

82. "Critics Assail Indian Health Research Efforts," *The Arizona Daily Star* (135:291), Tucson, Arizona, October 17, 1976, A-1. The Tohono O'odham benefited because ORD implemented all new technology on the San Xavier and Tohono O'odham reservations, both of which were attached to the research unit. STARPAHC was criticized because the cost of providing mobile health set-ups and microwave communications nationwide would be astronomical. As for HIS, although everyone agreed it was the most advanced health data system in the world, the concern was where the area offices would get the funding to plug into it.

83. There were 3,406 total sterilizations of which 3,001 were among women of child-bearing age (15-44). There were also 142 male sterilizations reported. "Medical Research Using American Indians as Subjects," Report of the Comptroller General of the United States to Senator James Abourezk, November 4, 1976, enclosure I, 18 and 23. Comptroller General Lewis B. Staats informed Abourezk that three different consent forms were used. The most widely used form did not indicate that consent had been presented orally to the patient, contain written summaries of the oral presentations and did not contain a statement notifying the patients of their right to withdraw consent from the services. Brint Dillingham, "Indian Women and IHS Sterilization Practices," *American Indian Journal* (3:1) January 1977.

84. Brint Dillingham, "Sterilization of Native Americans," *American Indian Journal* (3:7), July 1977, 16. In August of 1977 a coalition of Democrats and Republicans asked the GAO to conduct a nationwide investigation to determine the extent of sterilization. Dillingham, "Sterilization Update," *American Indian Journal* (3:9) September 1977, 25. Janet Karsten Larson, "And Then There Were None: Is federal Policy Endangering the American Indian 'Species?'" *Christian Century* (94) January 26, 1977, 61. Larson describes how many Indian women were fearful of filing a lawsuit due to the high costs and more importantly "the risk of losing one's place in the Indian community, where sterilization has particular religious resonance." Some Indians accused the Indian Health Service of making genocide a part of its policy, a claim the agency called unwarranted, pointing out that consent documents were on file. "Oversight Hearings on Indian Health," *Hearings before the Select Committee on Indian Affairs, United States Senate* 96th Congress, 2d session, August 2, 1979, 59-63. Helena Temkin-Greener, Stephen J. Kunitz, David Broudy and Marlene Haffner, "Surgical Fertility Regulation among Women on the Navajo Indian Reservation, 1972-1978," *American Journal of Public Health* (71:4) April 1981, 403-407. Margot Liberty, David V. Hughney and Richard Scaglion, "Rural and Urban Omaha Indian Fertility," *Human Biology* (48:1) February 1976, 59-71. Stephen J. Kunitz and John C. Slocumb, "The Use of Surgery to Avoid Childbearing among Navajo and Hopi Indians," *Human Biology* (48:1) February 1976, 9021.

85. "Medical Research Using American Indians as Subjects," Enclosure I, 1, 12, 14 and 18. Students involved in the project were from Stewart (Carson City, Nevada), Intermountain (Brigham City, Utah), and Tuba City (Navajo) boarding schools. Proctor issued the statement after a meeting with the Children's Defense Fund and abandoned the project in September 1974. The research projects investigated included an evaluation of prediabetics among the Pima; low density lipoprotein metabolism among Southwestern Indians; the use of Phoenix Indian Medical Center pharmacists as providers of primary medical care; pediatric pulmonary disease among White Mountain Apaches; and a vaccine trial of pneumococcal pneumonia among Navajos. The Indian Health Service subsequently adopted these and other recommendations.

# CHAPTER SIX

## An Agency of the Public Health Service

In 1982, President Ronald Reagan named a strong advocate for Indian healthcare as director of the Indian Health Service. Everett R. Rhoades was a fifty-year-old Kiowa physician appointed to replace the retiring Emery Johnson. Born in an IHS hospital in Lawton, Oklahoma, on October 24, 1931, Rhoades was the first American Indian to lead the agency. While new to the Indian Health Service, Rhoades was no stranger to Indian healthcare, having served as professor of medicine at the University of Oklahoma's School of Medicine and as chief of infectious diseases at the Oklahoma City Veteran's Hospital. An outspoken critic of the Indian Health Service and supporter of Indian health issues, Rhoades supported the agency's health promotion and disease prevention program, having served on the Kiowa Health Board and the Oklahoma Area Advisory Board.[1]

The 1980s were a time of transition for the Indian Health Service, as more tribes assumed control over the health programs serving them. At the same time, the Indian Health Service reoriented its management and health programs to meet the changing needs and desires of American Indians and Alaska Natives, but did so with great difficulty. As tribes were federally recognized (or re-recognized after having been politically terminated in the 1950s), and as the American Indian and Alaska Native population increased, the Indian Health Service evaluated and modified its eligibility requirements. It also devised new means of allocating scarce resources. Although its budget nominally increased during the 1980s, it remained static when considering population and service growth (see Table 6.1).[2]

The 1980s also reflected a continuance of the government-to-government relationship between the United States and tribal nations, with one-third of the IHS budget under tribal auspices by 1989. By 1994, tribes operated 8 of 49 hospitals, 114 of 184 health centers, 233 of 277 health stations and clinics, and 70 service units. All tribally controlled hospitals were accredited by the Joint Commission on Accreditation of Health Care Organizations, with all but one of the 41 IHS facilities accredited. In addition, tribal organizations operated 34 urban

Indian programs. By 1989, there were 350 self-determination contracts totaling over $350 million.[3]

Table 6.1

*IHS Service Population and Appropriations, 1980-1989*

| Year | Population | Appropriations | 1982 dollars | Per capita |
|------|-----------|----------------|--------------|------------|
| 1981 | 849,315 | $677,172,000 | $704,653,485 | $797.32 |
| 1982 | 871,167 | $657,997,000 | $657,997,000 | $755.31 |
| 1983 | 902,701 | $719,283,000 | $707,955,708 | $796.81 |
| 1984 | 936,942 | $824,003,000 | $794,602,700 | $879.46 |
| 1985 | 961,881 | $855,362,000 | $816,916,660 | $889.26 |
| 1986 | 986,551 | $864,859,000 | $838,041,666 | $876.65 |
| 1987 | 1,011,837 | $907,364,000 | $860,876,660 | $896.75 |
| 1988 | 1,038,121 | $1,005,808,000 | $931,303,703 | $968.87 |
| 1989 | 1,073,886 | $1,081,774,000 | $953,104,845 | $1,007.35 |

(Source: *Trends in Indian Health*, 1990, 1991, 1992, and 1990 *Justification for Appropriations*)

## Becoming an Agency of the Public Health Service

As tribes assumed greater control over their own health programs and sought health parity with other Americans for their people, President Reagan elevated the Indian Health Service to the agency level with direct access to the secretary. Since 1968, the Indian Health Service had been a bureau within the Health Services and Mental Health Administration. In 1982, it was transferred to the newly formed Health Resources and Services Administration and the following year President Reagan called for the elevation of Indian healthcare to a priority level, indicating that tribal involvement in healthcare required the Indian Health Service to be at a higher organizational level within the federal bureaucracy.

Tribes concurred with the president, noting that the Indian Health Service was too buried within the Department of Health and Human Services and, therefore, faced policy-decision delays and obscured budget and resource assistance. The Health Resources and Services Administration, however, advocated retention of the existing level of organization. Robert Graham, director of the Health Resources and Services Administration, opined that elevating the Indian Health Service to a level equal with the Social Security Administration and Health Care Financing Administration would politicize the agency, and therefore sever program management continuity and lead to a loss of visibility.[4]

Table 6.2

*American Indian and Alaska Native Household Characteristics: U.S. General and IHS Service Areas: 1980*

| Area | Median Income | Percent below Poverty Line | Percent Lacking Plumbing | Percent Employed |
|---|---|---|---|---|
| United States | $16,841 | 12.4 | 2.7 | 93.0 |
| All IHS areas | $11,471 | 31.1 | 15.6 | 53.3 |
| Aberdeen | $9,625 | 42.7 | 12.5 | 49.8 |
| Alaska | $15,750 | 25.1 | 40.3 | 44.9 |
| Albuquerque | $12,226 | 30.2 | 14.2 | 57.3 |
| Bemidji | $10,464 | 26.9 | 7.3 | 50.5 |
| Billings | $10,967 | 34.0 | 7.6 | 51.0 |
| California | $13,235 | 20.4 | 3.2 | 55.2 |
| Nashville | $11,471 | 27.4 | 6.8 | 59.1 |
| Navajo | $8,412 | 43.7 | 49.1 | 47.2 |
| Oklahoma | $11,579 | 23.1 | 3.5 | 61.4 |
| Phoenix | $12,295 | 31.6 | 11.1 | 56.0 |
| Portland | $13,563 | 24.8 | 2.4 | 55.1 |
| Tucson | $9,432 | 38.7 | 27.3 | 52.4 |

(Source: *Organization of Health Services for Indian People*, 1987)

While Congress considered elevating the Indian Health Service, it believed that the Health Resources and Services Administration should retain authority over the program since it was responsible for health services in areas not adequately served by the private sector. In the summer of 1987, Secretary of Health and Human Services Otis R. Bowen requested a departmental paper outlining options regarding the elevation. The department concluded that it was "essential that any proposal [for elevation] provide for maximum tribal involvement." If changes were made they were to be done "with minimal disruption of existing IHS programs and staff." Wherever the agency was located within the federal bureaucracy it was to be at an "organizational location appropriate for [its] size, scope and mission." On November 4, 1987, Bowen approved of a reorganization plan. The 100th Congress concurred, stating that IHS responsibilities were commensurate with an organizational status equivalent to the Health Resources and Services Administration. On January 4, 1988, the Indian Health Service became the seventh agency within the Public Health Service.[5]

Table 6.3

*IHS Allocation to Reservation States, 1984*

| State | Population | 1984 Allocation | Per capita |
|-------|-----------|-----------------|-----------|
| Nebraska | 4,276 | $7,249,000 | $1,695 |
| Alaska | 70,772 | $119,326,000 | $1,686 |
| Louisiana | 642 | $973,000 | $1,516 |
| Wyoming | 5,421 | $7,640,000 | $1,409 |
| Mississippi | 4,597 | $6,351,000 | $1,382 |
| Maine | 2,982 | $4,105,000 | $1,377 |
| North Carolina | 6,042 | $8,126,000 | $1,345 |
| Montana | 34,533 | $45,006,000 | $1,303 |
| Minnesota | 18,978 | $22,343,000 | $1,177 |
| South Dakota | 45,721 | $50,434,000 | $1,103 |
| Oregon | 14,298 | $14,935,000 | $1,045 |
| North Dakota | 18,382 | $18,122,000 | $986 |
| Idaho | 7,589 | $7,215,000 | $951 |
| Arizona | 169,000 | $152,980,000 | $905 |
| New Mexico | 113,007 | $98,493,000 | $872 |
| Florida | 3,966 | $3,062,000 | $772 |
| Colorado | 2,945 | $2,265,000 | $769 |
| Kansas | 3,274 | $2,404,000 | $734 |
| Michigan | 8,873 | $5,788,000 | $652 |
| Wisconsin | 18,941 | $12,138,000 | $641 |
| New York | 10,259 | $5,398,000 | $526 |
| Oklahoma | 184,325 | $94,476,000 | $513 |
| Nevada | 14,414 | $6,905,000 | $479 |
| California | 72,385 | $33,656,000 | $465 |
| Washington | 61,283 | $28,063,000 | $458 |
| Utah | 10,268 | $3,384,000 | $330 |
| Iowa | 2,070 | $655,000 | $316 |
| Total | 909,243 | $761,492,000 | $837* |

*average

(Source: *House Report 98-763*, 1984)

Despite the elevation, the hallmark of the 1980s was "ambiguity, uncertainty, and rapidity of change." American Indians and Alaska Natives "never had greater access to health care than [in the 1980s]." Static budgets and an expanding service population meant that, although American Indians and Alaska Natives had greater access to services, they were also "denied more services than ever before." American Indians remained trapped in poverty and need, as seen in Table 6.2.[6]

To alleviate this disparity, the Indian Health Service modified its resource management in an effort to ensure adequate distribution of funds to eligible American Indians and Alaska Natives. While the agency had considered modifying its antiquated allocation criteria for years, during the 1980s a federal court ordered the Indian Health Service to refine the system. The Indian Health Service historically allocated its resources to area offices based on its continuity budget approach. In 1972, the agency assembled a Resource Allocation Criteria (RAC) working group to rationalize its then-current allocation methodology. By 1975, IHS determined the annual level of available and required service minutes, both by type of service and provider, and then programmed the necessary staffing levels to provide such services under "ideal conditions." This resource allocation system, however, resulted in gaps between services required and resources available.[7]

An example from the Wind River Arapaho and Fort Peck Assiniboine reservations illustrates this disparity. While equal in population, the cost of hospital care, $325 per day at Wind River compared to $229 per day at Fort Peck (40 percent less than Wind River), was not equal. In addition, nearly 30 percent of Fort Peck patients were eligible for Medicare and Medicaid while only 3 percent of the patients from Wind River were. Despite these disparities, the RAC allocated Wind River ($2,110,000) only 25 percent more funding than Fort Peck ($1,675,000). Consequently, Arapaho Chairman Joseph Oldman argued that the Indian Health Service had "to take these factors into account, so that the present inequitable distribution of funds can be remedied." Table 6.3 shows the per capita allocation of Indian Health Service resources by state.[8]

Because the IHS historically provided services for American Indians on or near reservations, the largest share of the health budget was for clinical services provided in hospitals, clinics, and health centers. In effect, the Indian Health Service allocated resources for healthcare facilities and the staff necessary to operate them. However, as the user population increased in the 1980s, facilities and services were not comparable to existing resources. Newly recognized tribes received less-than-equitable resources than other long-standing federally recognized tribes. Because the Snyder Act of 1921 did not establish provisions regarding allocation criteria or eligibility, the Indian Health Service allocated funds according to a self-imposed priority system that included program continuity, mandatory costs, Congressional mandates, and program expansion. Program continuity represented 85 percent of the health services budget between 1970 and 1978, and was the first priority under the funding methodology. Consequently, the Indian Health Service allocated funds on the basis of what a service unit received the preceding year. Mandatory costs, which averaged 8 percent of the budget, represented expenses necessary for civil service and inflationary pay increases. Congressional mandates, representing just 2 percent of the budget, but 25 percent of the facilities budget, were funds specifically earmarked for particular facilities or programs. Program expansion, representing 5 percent of the service and 75 percent of the facilities monies, included funds that remained after all other priorities were funded.[9]

In 1974, the Rincon Band of Mission Indians in Southern California filed a class action lawsuit against the Indian Health Service alleging that the agency wrongfully denied them services because of a discriminatory system of allocating federal funds for Indian health services. While approximately 10 percent of the American Indian service population lived in California, less than 2 percent of the IHS budget went to California Indians. To show the disproportionate pattern of funding in California, just 45 of the 8,100 IHS personnel were assigned to California, with 1 of the 51 Indian hospitals and 2 of the 99 health centers in the state. Less than .4 percent of the total Indian health facilities appropriation was allocated to California tribes.[10]

In the *Rincon Band of Mission Indians vs. Califano* decision, the federal District Court of Southern California opined that the RAC was "a bureaucratic charade with respects to all IHS funds in general, and California Indians in particular." The Court ordered the Indian Health Service to adopt a program for Indians in California that was comparable to that offered eligible Indians elsewhere in the United States. In 1980, the U.S. Court of Appeals affirmed the District Court's ruling, adding that "a system that allocates funds to programs merely because the program received funds the previous year, regardless of whether the programs are ineffective, unnecessary or obsolete is not rationally aimed at an equitable division of funds."[11]

The distribution of finite resources became a political hot potato in Indian Country. The Indian Health Service for years distributed funds based on program continuity simply because it was expedient. This uneven distribution of healthcare facilities and manpower led to inequitable access to services. While the appellant court held the health allocation criteria inequitable, it did not specify how the agency should implement a new resource allocation plan. Consequently, the Indian Health Service established an equity fund centered on a needs-based formula as a method of securing an equitable allocation of funds. Fifty percent of the formula was based on demand for services, 30 percent on health status, 10 percent on unserved populations, and 10 percent on productivity. Between 1981 and 1984 Congress earmarked $32,000,000 in equity funds; once they were allocated they became recurring base funds. In 1985, the Indian Health Service set aside $5,000,000 for equity distribution and awarded these funds to tribes, through the service units or area offices, with the greatest level of deficiency. In February of 1980 there were 144 tribes 61 to 100 percent deficient in funding; by March of 1985 the number dropped to 20 percent.[12]

The agency continued to look for ways to improve resource allocation, and in 1982 convened an interagency task force to analyze issues affecting operations. The task force recommended improvements in resource allocation methods by adopting a more rational and equitable method of distribution. The following year, a second task force evaluated the Resource Allocation Methodology (RAM) and agreed to adopt changes recommended by the interagency task force. To clarify allocation, the task force defined equity as "relatively equal access of the service population to equivalent health care services." Under RAM, resources to maintain existing services continued to be allocated for the most part on an historical basis but were adjusted to "standardized manpower and other support costs." A portion of these resources were then distributed to underserved areas to compensate for their lack of access. In 1985, the Operations Analysis Project further refined RAM to allocate resources to both area offices and service units. In keeping with decentralization of management, the Indian Health Service made allocation of funds in 2 steps. The first step was from headquarters to the area offices and the second from area offices to service units and tribal contractors. Step 1, implemented in 1986, was designated the Area Resource Allocation Methodology (ARAM), while step 2, implemented a year later, was the Service Unit Resource Allocation Methodology (SURAM).[13]

The health base funding was not redistributed, as the agency feared the potential of disrupting existing services. The costs of providing comparable services still varied from service unit to service unit, as the Wind River and Fort Peck example demonstrated. Furthermore, a service unit's physical environment, the dispersed population centers, and insufficient funding all limited patient access to services. Comparisons of the per capita funding among service areas remained inequitable. Table 6.4 shows the cumulative equity allocations between 1981 and 1987.[14]

Table 6.4

*Cumulative Equity Allocations: 1981-1987*

| Area | Allocation | Percent Increase for Hospital/Clinic/Contract Services |
|------|------------|--------------------------------------------------------|
| Tucson | $2,361,000 | 16.2 |
| Albuquerque | $3,943,000 | 10.0 |
| Billings | $4,844,000 | 12.6 |
| Nashville | $5,645,000 | 30.2 |
| Bemidji | $7,152,000 | 29.6 |
| Portland | $9,468,000 | 28.9 |
| Alaska | $10,420,000 | 11.9 |
| Navajo | $10,457,000 | 14.5 |
| Phoenix | $10,557,000 | 16.5 |
| Aberdeen | $12,893,000 | 24.5 |
| Oklahoma | $13,191,000 | 22.0 |
| California | $15,917,000 | 126.3 |

(Source: *Allocation of Resources,* 1988)

With funding for healthcare and services static in the 1980s, and with the number of services required by American Indians and Alaska Natives increasing, the Indian Health Service also revisited the issue of eligibility for services. In 1989, the agency provided services to approximately 1.1 million eligible American Indians and Alaska Natives who lived on or near reservations, rancherias, and other trust holdings, or who were members of regional corporations established under the 1971 Alaska Native Claims Settlement Act. While American Indians and Alaska Natives received preventive and other health-related services through the Indian Health Service, they did not typically have access to the more technologically advanced medical care that was generally available in urban areas. Although the agency provided comprehensive services at no user cost, many services were limited by "budget constraints and by the uneven distribution of services among IHS areas." And health facilities were not "equally available and accessible to eligible populations in all parts of the country," with many of the smaller facilities providing less specialized services than those that might be found in the typical small rural community hospitals.[15]

When specialized services were not accessible, the Indian Health Service referred patients to private providers retained under the contract health service program. With limited budgets, such referrals were frequently denied. While American Indians and Alaska Natives were not directly affected by ability to pay, they faced obstacles in obtaining contract care services since funding for such services usually ran out before medical needs were met.[16]

The Indian Health Service provided services to eligible American Indians and Alaska Natives through both direct and contract care services, with the former provided by the agency or tribally operated facilities. Prior to 1990 these services were available to "persons of Indian descent belonging to an Indian community served by the local facilities and program." Individuals were eligible for services if they were regarded as Indian by the community in which they lived, as evidenced by factors such as "tribal membership, enrollment, residence on tax-exempt land, ownership of restricted property, active participation in tribal affairs, or other relevant factors in keeping with general BIA practices." Non-Indian women pregnant with an eligible Indian's child also qualified for health services through postpartum.[17]

Contract care services were more restrictive, with American Indians and Alaska Natives required to meet additional criteria. These included residency on a reservation within a contract health service delivery area or residency within a contract health service delivery area and membership in the tribe served (or maintenance of close economic and social ties with such tribe), or being an eligible student, transient, or Indian foster child. Contract health service delivery areas included counties that encompassed all or part of an Indian reservation and any county that bordered a reservation. The states of Alaska, Nevada, and Oklahoma constituted contract health service delivery areas.[18]

As the issue of eligibility came under political pressure, the Indian Health Service searched for ways to make the best use of limited resources. The agency narrowly interpreted the Snyder Act, which authorized federal agencies to spend such funds as Congress from time to time appropriated for the "conservation of [Indian] health." Even though directed by Congress to provide services to American Indians and Alaska Natives, the Indian Health Service acted as a residual health service resource rather than a primary care provider. That is, it acted as a discretionary program to deal with gaps that existed in "the availability and accessibility of health service systems serving the Indian communities." Consequently, the Indian Health Service assumed residual responsibility for contract medical care and services.[19]

This did not relieve the several states of their obligation to make services available to American Indians based on the equal protection clauses of the Constitution (5th and 14th Amendments) and Title VI of the 1964 Civil Rights Act. In fact, the federal judiciary interpreted the constitution and civil rights legislation as indicating Congress did not intend for the federal government to be expressly responsible for Indian healthcare. The 1987 *McNabb v. Bowen* decision, for instance, held that Congress "contemplated that the IHS would aid Indians in taking advantage of state and local programs, with the federal government meeting health needs not met under these programs."[20]

A year earlier, the federal District Court for Montana held that the Indian Health Service, based on the Snyder Act, the Indian Health Care Improvement Act, and the federal government's trust responsibility to tribal nations, had "the ultimate responsibility" for healthcare when two healthcare providers (IHS and state or other) both claimed residual responsibility. The District Court opined that the agency had to "assure reasonable health care for eligible members."[21]

Although the Indian Health Service was obligated to provide health services to all eligible patients, it provided such care only after all other revenue sources were exhausted. While the agency had the "ultimate responsibility" to provide American Indians and Alaska Natives with healthcare, non-IHS resources were used first, whether such services were provided in IHS or tribally operated facilities. Where possible, such services were billed to the appropriate external source (primarily Medicare and Medicaid).[22]

The Indian Health Service also created eligibility standards to restrict contract healthcare access following the provisions of the Administrative Procedures Act, which requires proposed administrative changes be published in the *Federal Register*. In 1974, the U.S. Supreme Court opined "the power of an administrative agency to administer a congressionally created and funded program necessarily requires the formulation of policy and the making of rules to fill any gaps left, implicitly or explicitly, by Congress." Consequently, the Secretary of Health and Human Services can "create reasonable classifications and eligibility requirements in order to allocate" the limited resources available. Eligibility criteria were to optimally distribute limited funds among eligible benefactors, and had to be rationally aimed at an equitable distribution of available funds. Before any patient benefits could be denied, the Indian Health Service had to publish its criteria in the *Federal Register* and solicit public input. In the months after the *Morton v. Ruiz* ruling, the Indian Health Service established and published separate eligibility criteria for contract health services.[23]

The Indian Health Service considered further eligibility changes in 1982 when Congress directed it to address the "issue of an expanding service population in terms of defining who is or should be eligible for IHS services." A year later, the Grace Commission recommended the agency limit its services to those of one-quarter or more Indian blood and who were members of federally recognized tribes. Rhoades immediately assembled a task force to evaluate the criteria, with the task force modifying the recommendation and suggesting the agency limit its services to members of federally recognized tribes and to those who met the reservation residency requirement. On June 6, 1983, the Indian Health Service proposed to revise its eligibility criteria for direct care for the first time since 1956. The 1983 general notice for eligibility criteria proposed to "strengthen the management and allocation of IHS resources to most effectively serve program beneficiaries." In 1986 a Notice of Proposed Rule Making was published in the *Federal Register*.[24]

The notice of proposed rule was a signal that the Indian Health Service intended to implement new eligibility criteria aimed at defining the service population so as to enable the agency to better allocate resources. The agency proposed providing direct care services to all persons of Indian descent who were members of, or eligible for membership in, a federally recognized tribe, one-quarter Indian or Alaska Native blood, and residents of a health service delivery area. Persons who were not members of a federally recognized tribe, but who were one-half or more Indian blood and resided in a health service delivery area, would also be eligible. Although there were no additional eligibility requirements for contract medical care, the Indian Health Service intended to establish a priority list on the basis of medical need. Such services would not be available if the patient had "alternate resources for payment" or would have such resources if applied for. In September of 1987, the Indian Health Service finalized its proposed eligibility changes in the *Federal Register*.[25]

Tribes across the country responded with an uproar to the agency's efforts to force them to create enrollment criteria based on blood quantum (tribes argued tribal membership should suffice). As a result of this political backlash—more than 16,000 individuals and tribal organizations expressed an opinion—the final proposal deleted the one-quarter American Indian or Alaska Native blood quantum for eligibility. Tribes feared the blood requirement would transform their political relationship with the federal government into a relationship defined by racial, rather than political, status. Many tribal and Congressional leaders expressed a concern that "inclusion of a specific blood quantum requirement would interfere with a tribe's sovereignty by eliminating some tribal members from eligibility based upon racial identity rather than on the political relationship that exists between tribes and the Federal Government." The provision that intended to make non-tribal Indians of one-half or more Indian blood eligible for services was also deleted due to tribal objections.[26]

The new eligibility standards were scheduled to take effect in March 1988. However, with the passage of the fiscal year 1988 Indian appropriation act, Congress delayed implementation until September 16, 1988, so as to allow Congress time to consider the impact of the proposed changes. Rhoades acknowledged that it was critical to "come to grips with who is being served" since the agency was "denying more services to the Indian people than ever before." Once the Indian Health Service completed an impact study in consultation with tribes, the new regulations were published in the *Federal Register* and called for a single set of criteria for both direct and contract care.[27]

## Indian Health Service Management Concerns

While the Indian Health Service came to grips with eligibility, its management culture was a cause for concern. Within a year of assuming the directorship, Rhoades admitted it was critical that the agency improve its fiscal management in order to meet the changing needs of Indian Country. Management deficiencies were not a new revelation, as the Institute for Government Research declared in 1928 that "practically every activity undertaken by the national government for the promotion of the health of the Indians is below a reasonable standard of efficiency." Although management improved with the Indian Transfer Act, management issues continued to hinder the program. Rhoades declared in 1989 that "the Indian Health Service serve[d] too great a mission to have it sidetracked by problems in our management of administrative functions."[28]

In March of 1990, Rhoades feared the Indian Health Service was in "serious danger of collapse." He quantified his assertion by noting that in the previous fifteen years, the agency had added fewer than three dozen full-time-equivalent employees to its administrative staff, while at the same time it had added over $200,000,000 worth of programs. Former director Emery Johnson argued that because IHS authorities were scattered throughout the Department of Health and Human Services (with the only accountability in the Office of the Secretary), it was difficult for the agency to make decisions. Just once in Johnson's eighteen years of testifying before Congress was an accountable official within the department present at a meeting on behalf of the agency. In Johnson's view, the agency was like a "mom and pop grocery store," keeping cuff accounts and using manual accounting techniques because decisions higher up in the department prohibited or delayed management improvements. The remedy according to Johnson was to create an Assistant Secretary for Indian Health.[29]

The management concerns of the Indian Health Service were underscored by the agency's elevation within the Public Health Service, which resulted in greater accountability and responsibility. With constraints on the Indian health budget,

Congress called to task the fiscal accountability and management of the Indian Health Service. Resource allocation and eligibility remained in the forefront of Indian health politics, but there were concerns with record and data management as well. None of the agency's data systems provided consistent or reliable information for national program management and reporting requirements.[30]

A larger political concern was the allegation of mismanagement regarding accountability and utilization of healthcare funding. While there was no evidence to support the assertion that mismanagement was "pervasive," there were instances of mismanagement. At the Albuquerque Area Office, administrators used memoranda of agreements contrary to federal procurement law to purchase $250,000 worth of goods and services "with little or no regards to the price or propriety of the expenditures." Administrators employed lax procurement practices to hold a conference at a resort near Santa Fe using funds appropriated for an Indian Juvenile Alcohol and Drug Abuse Prevention Program.[31]

Similar irregularities surfaced at the Bemidji Area Office, where senior administrators approved their own travel vouchers. Area director Alan J. Allery was indicted on three felony counts of filing false claims against the federal government and subsequently resigned. Funds were also illegally diverted through "improper contracts" to sponsor conferences and meetings. Among the most egregious episodes of mismanagement was when the Bemidji office hosted the quarterly Council of Assistant and Area Directors meeting at the Mission Point Resort on Mackinac Island, Michigan. Allery diverted funds for the conference from the office's Hospitals and Clinics budget and funneled them through a contract with a local Indian tribe, which then paid all conference/resort costs and retained a percentage for its administrative expenses.[32]

The Office of the Inspector General (Department of Health and Human Services) conducted seventy-five investigations of the Indian Health Service between 1984 and 1989, exposing additional management problems. When the Indian Health Service became an agency, the Department of Health and Human Services issued regulations requiring the agency to establish an Office of Program Integrity and Ethics. This office was to "investigate and resolve . . . allegations of impropriety, mismanagement of resources, abuse of authority, (and) violations of Standards of Conduct." When Robert Stakes, director of the new office, uncovered evidence of fraud and illegal contracting at the Bemidji and Albuquerque area offices, both of which raised the possibility of a criminal investigation involving top administrators, agency officials prevented him from completing the investigations. When additional allegations were raised, Stakes was prohibited from investigating them.[33]

With allegations of mismanagement, Rhoades proclaimed his top priority was to "strengthen management and overall accountability." Forthwith, he created a Quality Management Initiative and hired two independent management consulting firms to advise the agency. In September of 1989, the Quality Management Initiative team acknowledged that the Indian Health Service had serious management problems.

> It suffers from real operational deficiencies—such as the lack of criti-
> cal management information and effective direction. It also suffers
> from an almost universal perception that it is managerially inept, that
> it believes it need not follow the rules, and that it denies it has serious
> management problems. The management weaknesses that have
> caused the agency's problems must be corrected.[34]

Despite management setbacks, the Indian Health Service attained an increasingly professional culture in its healthcare delivery. While the agency devoted
energy and resources toward "conserving the health of the Indians," it
overlooked its administrative management. Consequently, while service
deliveries secured a greater degree of professionalism through accreditation,
service standards, certification, quality services, peer review, and continuing
education, administration of the agency suffered.[35]

Throughout the 1970s, the Indian Health Service experienced annual budget
and user growth, as well as a greater degree of decentralization. When budgets
leveled off in the 1980s as the user population increased, the years of benign
management neglect overwhelmed the agency. In time, an inefficient
administrative infrastructure caught up with the agency as it concentrated too
much of its effort on "identifying, promulgating and securing public support for
medical and health promotion/disease prevention services." As Rhoades
painfully discovered, the Indian Health Service could never attain its health goals
without strengthening agency management.[36]

The Quality Management Initiative team examined both internal and external agency functions. The purpose was strategic: draft a plan to create a new
management culture in the Indian Health Service. The goal was to knit together
management talent, organizational systems, and the commitment to carry out
agency responsibilities into the 1990s and beyond.[37]

It was essential that the Indian Health Service develop a strong, responsive,
and accountable management infrastructure. By assessing strengths and
weaknesses, and then identifying ways to correct management deficiencies, the
Quality Management Initiative enhanced and elevated the status of the agency. A
stronger Indian Health Service meant improved medical services and health
status for American Indians and Alaska Natives. The agency learned a painful
lesson: responsive and accountable management was an integral part of
improving American Indian and Alaska Native health status. Rhoades challenged
the agency. "More must be done and must be done better, with fewer
resources."[38]

## Enhancing Self-Determination

Restrictive procurement and administrative regulations by the Indian Health

Service skirted the Congressional intent of Indian self-determination. While tribes and tribal organizations viewed contracting as a means of achieving self-government, the Indian Health Service focused on contract administrative responsibilities. Consequently, in the first dozen years of 638 contracting, tribes experienced barriers impeding self-determination. Among these were inadequate funding, especially for tribal contractor indirect costs, burdensome contracting requirements, and issues regarding contractibility and divisibility of programs.[39]

The 638 self-determination contracting mechanism differed from typical federal contracting systems. For other contractors, the federal government required an "arm's length relationship" between it and the contractor. In such contracts, the federal government can unilaterally mandate changes in a contract and it may also unilaterally terminate a contract. Federal contractors also must comply with federal labor laws and equal employment opportunity laws. In self-determination contracts these requirements are modified or exempt. Changes in a 638 contract, for instance, can only be made with the consent of the contracting tribe or tribal organization, which may also retrocede contracts back to the federal government with a 120 day notice. Furthermore, 638 contractors are exempt from certain federal labor laws, and Indian preference laws have precedence over equal employment laws. Self-determination contracts are designed to foster the government-to-government relationship between tribes and the federal government, something not part of other federal contracts.[40]

Indian tribes expressed concern that federal agencies, including the Indian Health Service, retained restrictive administrative control over programs through the use of procurement regulations. Tribes voiced dissatisfaction regarding area office contract administrators who inconsistently interpreted federal contracting regulations. The National Indian Health Board identified "problems, delays and frustrations when dealing with the [638] procurement process." Inadequate funding levels frustrated tribes, resulting in cash-flow challenges stemming from delays in IHS's voucher reimbursement system.[41]

Because the Indian Health Service viewed contracting as extensions of itself, the agency maintained that it was responsible for administering contracts according to federal contracting and procurement laws, limiting the "flexibility of 638 contractors to modify the scope of services they have agreed to deliver." Tribes needed "flexibility in program financial management (and perhaps some limitation of financial risk)." Given such flexibility, tribes were more inclined to assume responsibility for controlling comprehensive health programs. Tribes also were concerned over the lack of technical assistance provided by the Indian Health Service. The National Indian Health Board encouraged the agency to provide greater technical assistance to tribes, especially in the areas of healthcare planning, infrastructure capacity, contract administration, and healthcare service delivery.[42]

In response to tribal concerns, the 100th Congress amended the Indian Self-Determination Act four times, marking a Congressional desire to fulfill the intent of the law. The new provisions and mandates required the Indian Health Service to use 638 contracting as an "intergovernmental activity to be actively fostered and encouraged." While the amendments reinforced the intent of Congress, they clearly and deliberately marked a departure from the way in which the Indian Health Service implemented the law. Congress explicitly defined the intent of self-determination: Indian tribes must participate on an equal basis with the Indian Health Service in assuming control over programs developed for them, with the Secretary of Health and Human Services encouraging self-determination activities.[43]

The amendments provided key departures that enhanced self-determination. The federal government clarified its responsibilities not only to American Indians but also to tribal governments. Congress pledged support to assist tribes in developing "strong and stable tribal governments, capable of administering quality programs." To strengthen tribal control of programs, the amendments provided "that no contract entered into pursuant to this Act (other than construction contracts) shall be construed to be a procurement contract." Non-construction contracts were no longer subjected to federal procurement regulations.

Section 201 of Public Law 100-472 enhanced tribal rights to contract for and plan, conduct, or administer programs or portions of programs authorized under the Johnson-O'Malley, Snyder, and Indian Health Transfer acts, as amended. This authority allowed tribes to contract for any program administered by the secretary, even if appropriations were made to other federal agencies. The purpose of the amendment was to ensure that the Indian Health Service did not "consider any program or portion thereof to be exempt from Self-Determination contracts." Tribes were entitled to contract for IHS service unit functions and any area office function, including program planning and statistical analysis, technical assistance, administrative support, financial management (including third party health benefits billing), clinical support, training, contract health services administration, and other program or administrative function. Tribes could also redesign management and field office functions to better meet their needs.[44]

The Indian Health Service continued to interpret the law cautiously, holding that the agency did not have authority to enter into any contract that could impair the trust responsibility or reduce program funding for one tribe in order to make contracting available to another tribe. The Indian Health Service used a service population of 1,800 as the minimum for the establishment of a clinical program. The National Indian Health Board, recognizing the legitimate legal concerns of the agency, encouraged it to adopt a "case-by-case approach" to divisibility and to negotiate "practical solutions on a local level." In 1990, the federal district court, in *Southern Indian Health Council, Inc., v. Otis R. Bowen, et al.* held that IHS was legally obligated to divide programs if a tribe or consortium of tribes desired to operate their share of a particular program.[45]

The amended self-determination act required the secretary of Health and

Human Services, on a non-reimbursable basis and subject to appropriations, to provide technical assistance to tribes and tribal organizations to develop and modify proposals to assume control of any program, or provide for the assumption of any program, operated for American Indians and Alaska Natives. Tribes were given the option of using grants to secure technical assistance from providers of their choice. To overcome the difficulty tribes had in staffing facilities (including fringe benefits), the amended act made permanent a provision that allowed tribal contractors to acquire IHS employees under the Intergovernmental Personnel Act but only if tribal governments agreed to pay the employer's share of such costs. By so doing, tribes made better use of their federal resources and were in a better position to recruit and retain employees, both of which were important in developing tribally controlled facilities. Congress also authorized tribes to acquire federal property, including property secured with 638 contracts or grants, if such property was used for the purpose of the contract.

To counteract long-standing tribal concerns over indirect costs, the amended act provided that upon the approval of a 638 contract, and if requested by an Indian tribe or organization, the secretary could add the indirect cost into the contract for the first year. Subsequent year indirect costs would then be funded subject to adjustments in direct program costs. The secretary was prohibited from reducing funds required for 638 contracts, except pursuant to reduced appropriations, completion of contract, changes in funds needed for contract maturity, tribal resolution, or legislative directive. Although the law did not prescribe it, the Senate Select Committee on Indian Affairs requested the departments of Interior and Health and Human Services to develop a uniform and consistent set of regulations for all 638 contracts and ensure that tribes participated in the promulgation of regulations governing the amendments.[46]

## Relocation West?

As tribes increased their management sophistication and assumed greater control over IHS programs, Congress considered moving portions of the agency to a centralized site in the West, where technological assistance would be closer to the American Indian population center. The Office of Management and Budget recommended relocating the Indian Health Service headquarters to the West, although with passage of the self-determination amendments, Congress directed the agency to conduct a feasibility study first. At a centralized site in the West, the Indian Health Service could provide program and management assistance in the areas of procurement, financial management, third party reimbursements, billing, and program development. Because the Indian Health Service operated with limited resources, Rhoades demanded the most effective utilization of resources to assist the tribes, even if it was necessary to relocate or restructure headquarter functions.[47]

The Indian Health Service evaluated its internal organizational structure and geographical diversity in a November 1989 "Report to Congress: Preliminary Findings of the IHS Relocation Study." In it, Rhoades concluded that headquarter functions located in Rockville, Maryland, that provided "program development and research, support, and technical assistance to Tribes, Area Offices, and Service Units would be more effective if located closer to Indian people in the Western States."[48]

Unlike the Office of Management and Budget, which recommended the relocation of the entire IHS headquarters to a site in the West, the IHS argued that the director and related staff should remain in the east. In Rockville, the director advised the secretary of Health and Human Services regarding Indian health issues, served as the health spokesperson for all American Indians and Alaska Natives, provided policy oversight, and acted as the principle line manager for the agency. Proximity to Congress and the national political infrastructure was a factor, in light of tribal concerns, for retaining the director and his staff in Rockville. The Indian Health Service agreed with the consolidation of various headquarter functions that were then located in Phoenix, Tucson, Santa Fe, and Albuquerque.

Most senior level administrators recognized the necessity of evaluating the geographical dispersion of headquarters functions. The dispersion of functions hindered communications, operational planning, and coordination between headquarters and the area offices. It also contributed to blurring organizational responsibilities for program and management oversight. The geographical fragmentation of headquarters among four western cities occurred haphazardly and resulted from the lack of organizational principles for determining where various functions might be carried out most effectively. Past decisions regarding the location of headquarter functions were unnecessarily influenced by professional staff, which was most egregiously illustrated by Erwin Rabeau.[49]

The decentralized nature of headquarter functions resulted in management challenges, especially in the Tucson Office of Health Program Research and Development, which struggled to plan, develop, and integrate "its activities in conjunction with other headquarters offices." Moreover, it failed to translate its "research and development activities into projects easily adapted by other headquarters components in the field." The consolidation of the Tucson research facility with other headquarters functions had potential disadvantages, including being used by headquarters to respond to "operational crises" that could divert it from its long-term objectives.[50]

Because of the dispersed headquarter functions and the realization that the agency served as an ombudsman on behalf of Indian tribes, the Indian Health Service recognized it needed to reconfigure its current organizational and geographical structure and co-locate all field-based functions to a centralized site closer to the Indian population in the West. Rhoades concurred that Albuquerque, New Mexico, should house the proposed IHS Center for Technical Support. In Albuquerque, the Indian Health Service could consolidate all headquarter functions and further program development, technical support, and technical assistance for both area offices and tribal governments. Bureaucratic lethargy and changing political crises, however, dashed the hopes of relocation and, despite millions of dollars of evaluation, none of the functions was consolidated as anticipated.[51]

## Sanitation and Housing

While the Indian Health Service faced a management crisis, its sanitation facilities program was an all-around success. Between 1960 and 1990, Congress appropriated nearly $900 million to provide Indian communities with essential sanitation facilities. While Congress did not appropriate the funds necessary to provide all tribal communities with services, it funded services that were widely recognized as having a most influential impact on Indian health. Two health indices pointed to the effectiveness of the program. Indian mortality rates from gastrointestinal diseases decreased from 15.4 per 100,000 to 1.6, and the Indian infant mortality rate decreased 85 percent during the first thirty years of the sanitation program. Both indices were lower among American Indians and Alaska Natives than among the general U.S. population.[52]

Specific examples of sanitation need still existed. In Alaska, only one-third of Alaska Natives had flush toilets and 14 percent still used a primitive haul system. Over 50 percent hauled water, with just four in ten having indoor water. The need for adequate housing with sanitation services remained acute in Alaska and contributed to a Hepatitis A epidemic in the late 1980s, when over 2,000 acute cases were reported. More than 300 cases were still reported in 1993.[53]

As was the case in rural America, solid waste collection and disposal remained a challenge in the 1980s. Many of the solid waste disposal sites in Indian Country conformed to health codes at the time they were constructed, but under new criteria established by the Environmental Protection Agency (EPA) in the 1970s and 1980s, many were considered open dumps in violation of federal environmental laws. Amendments to the Resource Conservation and Recovery Act led to the closure of open dump sites in the 1990s, with the Indian Health Service requesting $167 million to clean up solid waste dump sites.[54]

In 1987, members of the Oglala Sioux Tribe, residing in the Pine Ridge community of Wanblee, South Dakota, filed suit seeking injunctive and declaratory relief against the EPA, the Bureau of Indian Affairs, the Indian Health Service, and the Oglala Sioux Tribe. In *Blue Legs v. Environmental Protection Agency*, the United States District Court opined that the Oglala Sioux Tribe was responsible for regulating, operating, and maintaining fourteen open dumps on the Pine Ridge Reservation in conformity with the Resource Conservation and Recovery Act. Since the Bureau of Indian Affairs and the Indian Health Service were involved with solid waste management activities and contributed to open dumping on the reservation by allowing their solid waste to be disposed of in three of the tribe's open dumps, the Court ordered both federal agencies and the tribe to work in concert to clean up all fourteen sites.[55]

The Court of Appeals affirmed the ruling a year later, holding that the federal agencies were required to assist the tribe in cleaning up the sites based on the authority of the Snyder Act and the federal fiduciary relationship with tribal nations. In February 1990, the District Court, on remand from the Appellate Court, ordered the federal agencies and the tribe to implement a plan to clean up the dump sites. The Bureau of Indian Affairs was responsible for 50 percent of the $370,323 expense while the Indian Health Service and the Oglala Sioux Tribe were each responsible for 25 percent of the cost. As a result of the Court's ruling, the Indian Health Service restructured its priority system for constructing sanitation facilities. While prior to 1990 it focused on constructing water and sewage facilities, after 1990 it made solid waste disposal an immediate funding priority.[56]

## Bridging the Health Gap

In 1956, Congress directed the Public Health Service to answer three questions related to the status of American Indian health: 1) what was required to elevate it to an acceptable level? 2) How long would it take? and 3) What was the cost estimate? Thirty years later, George Lythencott, head of the Health Resources and Services Administration (then IHS parent organization) argued that the disparity between the American Indian and Alaska Native service population and the general U.S. population had increased. Between 1977 and 1984, the per-capita spending for the Indian service population declined from 75 percent to 69 percent of the national average. Lythencott expected this disparity to grow as budgets leveled off and the service population increased. A House Appropria-tions Committee responded by requesting the agency to identify the funds necessary to elevate Indian health status to a level enjoyed by the general population.[57]

The *Bridging the Gap: Report on the Task Force on Parity of Indian Health Services* study reported that, although the Indian Health Service made improvements in the delivery of Indian health services and conditions over the previous thirty years, "for the foreseeable future, IHS will continue to operate in an environment of steadily increasing demand." Unmet medical demand persisted due to funding shortfalls and a 10 to 15 percent understaffing rate at most health facilities. This posed concerns as the Indian Health Service faced a potential loss of accreditation and certification of its facilities. This in turn would make those facilities ineligible for Medicare and Medicaid reimbursements. Inadequate funding would also force the agency to use contract care funds exclusively for emergencies.[58]

Although the Indian Health Service experienced a per capita healthcare cost nearly 50 percent lower than the 1984 national average, per capita funding was not the most reliable indication of the disparate health status between American

Indians and the American population in general. IHS costs were lower than private health costs for several reasons. Since the Indian Health Service operated as a health maintenance organization, there were cost containment incentives built into the agency. Moreover, the agency had no malpractice insurance expenses because the federal government is its own insurer. And, finally, some American Indians utilized non-IHS facilities and treatment via private health insurance. The trade-off for this efficiency was the rationing of some services, especially contract medical care.

Regardless of these factors, disparities existed. Reduced budgets for scholarships and student loans diminished the number of American Indians in medical and health-related programs. Based on a national per capita expenditure of funds, the Indian Health Service required a 25 percent budget increase in 1984 to bring its level of hospital, medical, and dental care up to a parity level with the general population. "Carried to its logical, ethical conclusion," the Gap study reported, "parity of health status is achieved by maintaining demonstrably effective services and simultaneously targeting intractable health problems." Budgetary enhancements would not necessarily equate into health parity, but they would be a step in the right direction.[59]

The overall health status of American Indians and Alaska Natives improved after 1955, although it was not comparable with that of the general population. Despite general improvement, a sizeable percentage of the IHS user population remained in "poor health relative to the rest of the U.S." One means of measuring this "poor health" was in terms of productive years of life lost, or the difference between a person's age at death and age 65. Table 6.5 summarizes years of productive life lost and illustrates American Indians suffered from a disproportionate number of injury-related deaths.[60]

The patterns of morbidity and mortality among American Indians and Alaska Natives also shifted in the 1980s. While tuberculosis was no longer a leading cause of death, it was still four times more prevalent than among non-Indians. Likewise, gastroenteritis was twice as prevalent. Among the most significant indicators of health status in the 1990s was that American Indians and Alaska Natives did not live as long as other Americans. In 1982, 37 percent of all American Indian and Alaska Native deaths involved a person under the age of 45, while just 12 percent of all American deaths involved a similarly aged person. A birth rate nearly twice the non-Indian rate accounted for the disproportionately youthful American Indian and Alaska Native population.[61]

The leading causes of death among American Indians and Alaska Natives partially explained why they died at an earlier age than other Americans. More American Indians and Alaska Natives were vulnerable to social or external causes of death. Because of "long distances between destinations, poor roads, overcrowded and unsafe vehicles, and driving under the influence of alcohol," accidents, particularly motor vehicle accidents, led to an accidental death rate 3.4 times higher than the general U.S. population. Furthermore, American

Indians were twice as likely to die of homicide as non-Indians and nearly twice as likely to commit suicide. A 1992 study of 13,454 American Indian and Alaska Native youth demonstrated that these Americans were disproportionately represented in accidental, homicidal, and suicidal deaths. Students with positive attitudes toward school, self, and family were less likely to be injured in an accident, abused (sexually or physically), depressed, suicidal, or involved with substance abuse. While a majority of American Indian and Alaska Native youth were healthy, liked school, never rode with a driver who was drinking, were emotionally stable, and were free of abuse, the minority that experienced these risks was a much larger percentage than the national average.[62]

Table 6.5

*Mortality and Clinical Services Related to Select
Health Conditions: 1981-1983\**

|  | Productive Life Lost | |  | Hospital | Clinical |
|---|---|---|---|---|---|
|  | Years | Percent | Deaths | Days | Visits |
| IHS Total | 94,321 | 100.0 | 5,207 | 546,921 | 3,251,170 |
| Accidents | 31,050 | 32.9 | 957 | 76,277 | 198,221 |
| Infant Mortality | 22,295 | 23.6 | 343 | - | - |
| Violence | 12,704 | 13.5 | 363 | 12,015 | 14,664 |
| Cardiovascular | 6,620 | 7.0 | 1,362 | 32,780 | 143,723 |
| Alcoholism | 6,156 | 6.5 | 342 | 22,596 | 13,694 |
| Cancer | 4,036 | 4.3 | 615 | 17,051 | 6,213 |
| Respiratory Disease | 3,428 | 3.6 | 329 | 41,838 | 412,641 |
| Digestive Disease | 2,163 | 2.3 | 170 | 54,346 | 81,315 |
| Infectious Disease | 1,667 | 1.8 | 101 | 16,132 | 119,808 |
| Diabetes Mellitus | 882 | 0.9 | 165 | 16,398 | 121,071 |
| Chronic Renal Failure | 624 | 0.7 | 81 | 3,961 | 3,195 |
| Maternal Health | 75 | 0.1 | 2 | 73,634 | 239,404 |
| Musculoskeletal | - | - | - | 20,373 | 133,533 |
| All Other | 2,620 | 2.8 | 377 | 159,520 | 1,763,688 |

*Direct care only

(Source: *Bridging the Gap*, 1986)

A contributing factor to high rates of homicide was the paucity of mental health facilities and services. When Georgia White, a legal guardian for Florence Red Dog, sued Secretary of Health, Education and Welfare, Joseph Califano, in 1977 over the lack of mental health facilities, she secured a declarative judgment by the District Court of South Dakota, which ordered the Indian Health Service to provide for the mental health needs of American Indians based on the federal Indian trust relationship. Rhoades encouraged the agency to go a step further and bring Indian medicine men on staff to deal with health issues, including mental health.[63]

Rhoades recognized that despite the strengths of Indian communities, mental health issues were "pervasive and devastating." In 1988, Dr. Scott Nelson, Director of the IHS mental health program, initiated a National Mental Health Plan for American Indians and Alaska Natives that was designed to utilize community-based and culturally sensitive mental health services, with children given priority. Rhoades went a step beyond Congress and committed the Indian Health Service to strengthening mental health programs regardless of legislative enactments. The 1990 mental health budget of $21.5 million was an $8.5 million increase over the 1989 budget. The 1992 reauthorization of the Indian Health Care Improvement Act authorized $34 million for fiscal year 1995 and $36 million for fiscal year 1996.[64]

Table 6.6

*Comparison of Leading Major Congenital Malformations among American Indians and White Americans, 1981-1986*
(per 10,000 births)

| Malformation | American Indian Rate* | White Rate# |
|---|---|---|
| Patent ductus arteriosus | 33.5 | 26.5 |
| Hip dislocations (no CNS defects) | 31.4 | 32.3 |
| Fetal Alcohol Syndrome | 29.9 | 0.9 |
| Ventricular septal defect | 19.1 | 17.4 |
| Cleft lip | 17.5 | 9.7 |
| Hypospadias | 17.5 | 32.7 |
| Clubfoot without CNS defects | 15.5 | 27.5 |
| Hydrocephalus (no spina bifida) | 10.8 | 5.4 |
| Cleft palate (no cleft lip) | 9.8 | 3.2 |
| Down Syndrome | 6.7 | 8.5 |
| Rectal atresia and stenosis | 4.6 | 3.7 |
| Atrial septal defect | 4.1 | 2.1 |
| Spina bifida (no anencephaly) | 4.1 | 5.1 |
| Anencephaly | 3.6 | 3.0 |

*sample total 19,412
#sample total 3,361,963

(Source: *Congenital Malformations among Minority Groups*, 1989)

Corresponding with inadequate mental healthcare were other forms of injuries, including sexual abuse, which reached a crisis stage in the 1980s with widespread social ramifications in some areas of Indian Country. Sexual abuse of students at Indian boarding schools made national headlines but only touched the surface of the challenges. Child abuse and neglect also increased, with Congress in 1990 enacting the Indian Child Protection Act to combat the abuse of Indian children and family violence. The Indian Health Service, in cooperation with the Bureau of Indian Affairs, introduced Project Charlie and BABES (Beginning Alcohol Basic Education Studies) to provide children with opportunities to learn about themselves and strengthen their self-esteem despite living "under less than satisfactory conditions."[65]

To deal with substance abuse, Congress in 1986 enacted the Indian Alcohol and Substance Abuse Prevention and Treatment Act and authorized the Indian Health Service and the Bureau of Indian Affairs to attack Indian alcohol and substance abuse, particularly among youth. Two years later, after the Indian Health Service opened its first regional treatment program for youth suffering from alcohol and/or drug abuse, Congress amended the Indian Health Care Improvement Act and directed the Bureau of Indian Affairs, Indian Health Service, and tribal governments to coordinate these programs with existing mental health programs. This was no small endeavor due to poor coordination that undermined a continuum of care, high levels of staff turnover and burnout, differing missions, and the inability of the agencies to create tribal action plans (just 241 of 546 plans were completed).[66]

Alcohol and related deaths and/or injuries remained high in some American Indian and Alaska Native communities, with substance abuse a concern for both tribal communities and the Indian Health Service, with those fifteen to thirty-four years of age at the greatest risk. Owing to a largely rural and isolated population, the number of acquired immunodeficiency syndrome (AIDS) cases reported among American Indians and Alaska Natives (64) was low, although in the 1980s the rate doubled among American Indians.[67]

Another growing concern was the rising rate of Fetal Alcohol Syndrome (FAS). In 1979, the Indian Health Service established a Fetal Alcohol Syndrome Project to deal with the rapidly increasing rate of FAS deaths, particularly in the Southwest. By 1983, FAS was the second most frequently reported cause of mental retardation in children. The National Institutes of Health estimated that one out of every 750 live births in the United States represented a baby with FAS. Among Southwestern tribes, the FAS incident rate was one in every 633 births, with some tribes as high as one in 100. Due to difficult socioeconomic conditions, American Indian women from the northern plains were statistically more likely to deliver FAS or FAE (fetal alcohol effect) children, with those in the Aberdeen Area twelve times more likely to die of cirrhosis, and those in the Billings Area fifteen times more likely to die of alcoholism than women in the general population.[68]

The Fetal Alcohol Syndrome Project, located in Albuquerque, New Mexico, terminated in 1985 when program funding expired. In 1991, the Indian Health Service sought to reestablish the project by allocating discretionary funds for health education and prevention/awareness programs, and coordinating these programs with state projects. Data indicate that the incidence rate continued to grow, with 1.5 cases of FAS per 1,000 live births in the Navajo Area and 15.6 per 1,000 live births in the Billings Area. Birth defects related to FAS were responsible for one-quarter of American Indian and Alaska Native neonatal deaths. Congress authorized the creation of the Office of Women's Indian Health Care in 1992 to deal with FAS, FAE, and related birth defects. American Indian and Alaska Native children remained thirty times more likely than white Americans to experience the effects of FAS. Table 6.6 shows the rates of various congenital malformations among American Indians and white Americans.[69]

While the Indian Health Service traditionally provided acute care services, its preventive and educational programs became more widely accepted and successful by the 1980s, leading to a shift in the focus of medicine. As American Indians lived longer—their life expectancy increased to 71.6 years of age vs. 75.0 for the general population—chronic diseases such as cancer, heart disease, and diabetes increased. Non-insulin dependent diabetes (type II) reached a crisis level in Indian Country. Between 1971 and 1983 the number of outpatient visits related to diabetes nearly tripled from 55,000 to 154,000. By 1983, 76 percent of all American Indian lower extremity amputations were on patients with diabetes, more than 50 percent higher than the general population. Renal failure among American Indians with diabetes was nearly 4 times the non-Indian rate. The incidence of diabetes-induced blindness was also higher among American Indians. Table 6.7 illustrates the prevalence of non-insulin dependent diabetes among select minority groups.[70]

Table 6.7

*Prevalence of Non-Insulin Dependent Diabetes by Age Groups, 1990*
(Per 100,000)

| Age | Black | Hispanic | Indian/Alaska Native |
|-----|-------|----------|----------------------|
| 0-24 | 1.5 | 1.0 | 2.0 |
| 24-44 | 21.6 | 30.0 | 27.0 |
| 45-54 | 85.3 | 74.0 | 142.0 |
| 55-64 | 118.1 | 129.0 | N/A |
| 65-74 | 129.3 | 133.0 | 193.0 |
| 75+ | 130.9 | 118.0 | 146.0 |

(Source: *Indian Health Care Act Amendment Hearing*, 1992)

No tribal nation experienced a diabetes rate comparable to the Pima of the Gila River Indian Community in Arizona, where a longitudinal study of the disease began in 1965. Pima children of diabetic pregnancies tended to suffer "excessively high rates of diabetes as adolescents and young adults." Medical theories suggested that diabetes afflicted American Indians more severely than non-Indians possibly due to the presence of a thrift gene which, over the centuries prior to European contact and prior to the displacement of traditional diets, allowed calories to be stored during times of plenty to be used in times of famine. With sedentary lifestyles and diets high in processed foods, those with the thrift gene may have been prone to both obesity and diabetes.[71]

In response to the high rate of diabetes in the Southwest, the Indian Health Service initiated the Zuni Diabetes Project in 1983, encouraging the use of aerobic exercise, education, and diet in an effort to reduce the prevalence of the disease. In 1988, the agency established the "Year of the Foot" by expanding its goal of preventing amputations due to diabetes, providing training for physicians, and developing educational programs for service users. Rhoades appointed diabetes control officers to the Phoenix, Nashville, and California Area Offices, and Centers of Excellence were established in Alaska, Northern Minnesota, and southern Arizona. Diabetes struck American Indians and Alaska Natives at a rate 3.5 times greater than the U.S. general population rate, as shown in Table 6.8.[72]

Reflective of an increasing life expectancy, American Indians faced a rising rate of heart disease, which by the 1990s became the leading cause of death among American Indians. High levels of unemployment, coupled with a sedentary life and foods high in carbohydrates and fat, contributed to obesity and diabetes. Hypertension, a high risk factor of heart disease, was often overlooked because the Indian Health Service too often remained acute-care oriented.[73]

Table 6.8

*Age-Adjusted Diabetes Mortality Rates, 1990*

| *IHS Area* | *Rate/100,000* | *IHS Area* | *Rate/100,000* |
|---|---|---|---|
| Tucson | 68.0 | Nashville | 40.6 |
| Phoenix | 49.6 | Oklahoma | 24.2 |
| Albuquerque | 47.9 | California | 20.8 |
| Bemidji | 47.0 | Billings | 20.6 |
| Aberdeen | 44.1 | Alaska | 6.1 |
| IHS (All Areas) | 35.8 | U.S. (all populations) | 9.8 |

(Source: *Indian Health Care Act Amendment Hearings*, 1992)

Malignant neoplasms were the second leading cause of death for American Indians over the age of forty-five. While American Indians and Alaska Natives experienced a lower incidence rate for cancer than did the general population, their survival rate was also lower, suggesting that malignancies affected American Indians and Alaska Natives differently than they did non-Indians. In the 1980s, Rhoades established both cervical and breast cancer screening programs to mitigate these concerns. In 1983, as part of Surgeon General C. Everett Koop's anti-smoking campaign, the Indian Health Service became the first national health organization to become smoke-free, with smoking cessation projects initiated in all tribal communities.[74]

## Facilities and Personnel

In the 1980s, the Indian Health Service constructed eleven new hospitals and remodeled or constructed a score of new health clinics and health centers.[75] This enabled the agency to deliver additional services, although it continued to face challenges in staffing hospitals with nurses, especially registered and specialty nurses. By 1990, the combined nursing staff (registered, practical, nurse's aides) represented nearly one-quarter of the Indian Health Service work force and, as Table 6.9 indicates, remained in short supply.[76]

Table 6.9

*IHS Specialty Nursing Vacancy Rates, 1990*

| Area Office | Total Positions | Vacancies | Vacancy Rate Percent |
|---|---|---|---|
| Overall | 2,430 | 338 | 14 |
| Aberdeen | 272 | 47 | 17 |
| Alaska | 305 | 30 | 10 |
| Albuquerque | 201 | 34 | 17 |
| Bemidji | 64 | 9 | 14 |
| Billings | 147 | 17 | 12 |
| California | 3 | 0 | 0 |
| Nashville | 30 | 1 | 3 |
| Navajo | 568 | 109 | 19 |
| Oklahoma | 328 | 44 | 13 |
| Phoenix | 433 | 42 | 10 |
| Portland | 49 | 4 | 8 |
| Tucson | 33 | 1 | 3 |

(Source: *Indian Health Service Nursing Shortage*, 1990)

The Indian Health Service continued to struggle in its efforts to attract physicians, increasingly relying on the National Health Service Corps (NHSC). Throughout the 1980s the agency secured an average of 130 to 150 physicians a year from the NHSC. But such physicians, like those under the Doctor-Dentist draft law, had just a two-year commitment and most rarely stayed beyond their required tenure. While NHSC physicians filled a critical need, the Indian Health

Service preferred volunteer physicians rather than those fulfilling a buy-back commitment. But this required active recruitment, an activity the Indian Health Service struggled with due to its limited recruitment office. Adding to the difficulty of attracting physicians in the 1980s was the fact that the Public Health Service was no longer viewed as a place of stable employment, having closed nine hospitals in 1983 alone. The Plains tribes felt the physician shortage most acutely, with a vacancy rate of 50 percent. Even the Phoenix Area Office experienced a 9 percent vacancy rate.[77]

The Indian Health Service also faced difficulties in attracting American Indian physicians. While the Association of American Indian Physicians encouraged American Indians and Alaska Natives to enter the field of medicine, Congressional parsimony hampered their efforts. Programs such as INMED required financial resources, despite the fact that between 1976 and 1983 the program turned out thirty-nine American Indian physicians. Medical schools, such as the University of Minnesota and Dartmouth College, continued to recruit American Indians. Most American Indians and Alaska Natives who entered medical school entered the field of family medicine or psychiatry, rather than internal medicine.[78]

The 1980s were challenging years for the Indian Health Service. While new goals were established and more restrictive eligibility requirements were adopted, budget reductions and a growing service population required new approaches to healthcare. While the Indian Health Service continued to provide preventive services, it remained crisis care–oriented. Consequently, ill-health remained a part of Indian Country, although its sources increasingly stemmed from behavioral risks rather than pathogens. Nonetheless, Congress charged the Indian Health Service with elevating Indian healthcare to comparable level with the rest of the American population. Budget shortfalls, however, plagued the agency and undermined the desire of tribal nations to control their own health destiny.[79]

# Notes

1. Between June 21 and December 9, 1985, Rhoades was on assignment to the Health Resources and Services Administration, during which time Dr. Gerald Ivey served as director of the program. Rhoades was reassigned pending an investigation into alleged actions that he inappropriately secured a college scholarship for his daughter, actions for which he was later exonerated. Emery Johnson called the accusations an attempt by bureaucrats to discredit Rhoades because he was an advocate for American Indians. Rhoades, along with Congress and President Reagan, faced a hostile Indian health bureaucracy that did not want to see the health program transferred to Indian control. Marsha F. Goldsmith, "American Indian Medicine Aims to Add Physicians, Improve Health," *Journal of the American Medical Association* (254:14) October 11, 1985, 1873-

1876. Todd, *Interview with Dr. Everett R. Rhoades*.

2. Rhoades argued that the Indian Self-Determination Act should have been called the Indian Contracting Act because tribes believed they were "fully competent domestic nations" with the passage of the law. When tribes realized they were not prepared to assume control over the programs, they blamed the Indian Health Service for failed expectations. "Indian Health," *Hearing before the Select Committee on Indian Affairs United States Senate*, 96th Congress, 1st session, August 2, 1979, 33. The IHS service population increased 2.7 percent per year, excluding the impact of new tribes. While the IHS per-capita spending rate in 1984 was $879.00, the non-Indian per capita expenditure was $1,378.00.

3. Ronald Reagan's address on Reservation Economies, *Public Papers of the Presidents of the United States, Ronald Reagan 1983* vol. 1, (Washington, D.C.: Government Printing Office, 1984), 96-100. "Indian Health Care: An Overview of the Federal Government's Role," *A Staff Report for the Use of the Select Committee on Health and the Environment of the Committee on Energy and Commerce United States House of Representatives*, 98th Congress, 2d session, April 1984. *Indian Health Relocation Study: Report to Congress* (Indian Health Service, November 1, 1989), 9.

4. "Indian Health Care Amendments of 1984," *HR 98-763* (Washington, D.C., Government Printing Office, 98th Congress, 2nd Session, May 21, 1984), 47. Graham argued Indian Health Service budgeting would become centralized and would lose the input of tribes, area offices, and service units. Emery Johnson advocated such an elevation, believing the agency would become more accountable and better able to increase collections of Medicare and Medicaid. Furthermore, the elevation would help the Indian Health Service secure policy decisions more quickly. "Reauthorization of the Indian Health Care Improvement Act," *Hearing before the Select Committee on Indian Affairs United States Senate on S. 2166*, Washington, D.C., 98th Congress, 2d session, February 29, 1984, 48-52, 100-101, 106-107.

5. "Indian Health Care Amendments of 1984," *House Report 98-763* part 2, 98th Congress, 2d session, May 21, 1984, 70. The House argued elevation would unnecessarily increase the direct supervision responsibilities of the Assistant Secretary for Health. *Indian Health Service Accomplishments*, fiscal year 1988 (Department of Health and Human Services, Public Health Service, Indian Health Service, 1989), 2. "Indian Health Care Act Amendments of 1987," *House Report 100-222* part 2, 100th Congress, 1st session, December 8, 1987, 27. The Indian Health Service retained its eleven area offices (excluding the Tucson Program Office) that administered direct care to American Indians and Alaska Natives, as well as contract care through tertiary contracting methods. Although each area office carried out its own programmatic functions and activities unique to its constituency, there were core functions they all had in common, including general administrative functions (resource allocation); program planning, analysis and evaluation; tribal assistance and community development; management of the provisions for routine clinical and health services and IHS health facilities; management of environmental health and sanitation services; and management of data, information, and communication resources. Included within the headquarters office was the Office of the Director, which was responsible for establishing policies and priorities for the delivery of services and coordinating activities and resources with other

federal and local agencies to promote and develop tribal control of programs; the Office of Administration and Management, which advised and supported the Director in developing and implementing management policy; the Office of Planning, Evaluation and Legislation, which advised and supported the Director in program policy and legislative affairs; the Office of Tribal Affairs, which advised the Director on policy matters regarding tribal activities, including the concept of Indian Self-Determination; the Office of Health Programs, which formulated program objectives, healthcare standards, policies and priorities regarding the allocation of resources and the development and management of IHS programs; the Office of Environmental Health and Engineering, which administered the environmental health and sanitation facilities programs by providing consultation and technical assistance to the Director, Area Offices and Tribal governments and Alaska Native corporations; the Office of Information Resources Management, which administered the agency's information technology and services; and the Office of Health Program Research and Development, which developed and demonstrated methods and techniques for the improvement of operations and management of healthcare delivery systems.

6. Everett Rhoades, Luncheon Address at the Third Annual Research Conference, Tucson, Arizona, March 20, 1990.

7. *Indian Health Care*, 232.

8. "Indian Health Service Oversight and Reauthorization of the Indian Health Care Improvement Act," *Hearing before the Select Committee on Indian Affairs United States Senate*, 96th Congress 2nd session, March 28, 1980, 103-104.

9. *Rincon Band of Mission Indians v. Harris*, 618 F2d 569 (1980) provides an overview of the funding mechanism.

10. *Rincon Band of Mission Indians v. Califano*, 464 F. Supp. 934 (1979).

11. *Rincon Band of Mission Indians v. Harris*, 618 F2d 569 (1980).

12. The General Accounting Office reported in the summer of 1982 ("Report to the Chairman, Committee on Appropriations United States Senate") that the Indian Health Service had not yet distributed its funds to the neediest tribes and that the agency needed a more equitable approach to distributing its total appropriations. GAO also alleged that the agency did not completely or consistently identify all funds available to help meet the needs of California tribes in particular. "Indian Health Service Not Yet Distributing Funds Equitably among Tribes," *House Document 82-54*, July 2, 1982, 5, 9 and 15.

13. *Allocation of Resources in the Indian Health Service*, A Handbook on the Resource Allocation Methodology (Department of Health and Human Services, Public Health Service, Indian Health Service, 1988), 25.

14. *Allocation of Resources in the Indian Health Service*, 33.

15. *Indian Health Care*, 155.

16. *Indian Health Care*, 156. Personal Interview with Dr. Jennie Joe, Native American Research and Training Center, University of Arizona, Tucson, April 5, 1990.

17. *Code of Federal Regulations*, Chapter 42, section 36.12 (1988 edition).

18. *Code of Federal Regulations*, Chapter 42, section 36.23, (1988 edition).

19. "Eligibility for Health Care Services Provided by the Indian Health Service," *Hearing before the Select Committee on Indian Affairs United States Senate*, Sacramento, California, 100th Congress, 2d session, June 30, 1988, 212.

20. *McNabb v. Bowen* 829 F. 2d 787, (1987).

21. *McNabb v. Heckler*, 628 F. Supp. 549 (1986).

22. Congress authorized such reimbursements in the 1992 Indian Health Care Improvement Act amendments (106 stat. 4526). These amendments allowed tribal or IHS facilities to retain 80 percent of the collected Medicare and Medicaid funds with such funds not considered when determining health appropriations for the facility. This was done as an incentive for facilities to collect and report all such funds (many had underreported such collections for fear of having collections charged against their annual appropriation). Tribal rights of recovery from private insurance carriers were also provided in the 1992 amendments. Many tribes complained that insurance companies refused to pay for services in tribally operated facilities even though they would in an IHS facility. *Senate Report 102-392 on S. 2481*, August 27, 1992 in *U.S Code and Administrative News* Vol. 6, 102d Congress, 2d session, 3943-4037.

23. *Morton v. Ruiz*, 415 US 231 (1974).

24. "Department of the Interior and Related Agencies Appropriations Bill, 1983," *House Report 97-942*, House of Representatives, 97th Congress, 2d session, December 2, 1982, 108. *Indian Health Service Contract Health Services Final Report*, Macro Systems, Inc., April 1984 (in "Fiscal Year 1985 Budget," *Hearings before the Select Committee on Indian Affairs United States Senate*, Washington, D.C., 98th Congress, 2d session, February 21/23, 1984, 286-332. "Indian Health Oversight," *Hearing before the Select Committee on Indian Affairs United States Senate*, Washington, D.C., 98th Congress, 1st session, July 28, 1983, 1-128. *Federal Register* (48:109), June 6, 1983, 25,274.

25. *Federal Register* (51:111), June 10, 1986, 21,119.

26. "Delaying the Implementation of a Certain Rule Affecting the Provision of Health Services by the Indian Health Service," *Senate Report 100-493*, 100th Congress, 2d session, August 25, 1988, 5-9. The blood quantum requirement would have dropped 125,000 Indians from the eligibility rolls for health services. By retaining a simple tribal membership requirement, Rhoades estimated an additional 125,000 Indians would be eligible for contract health services. *Federal Register* (52:179), September 16, 1987, 35,044.

27. Rhoades, Luncheon address. *Federal Register* (55:5), February 9, 1990, 4609. Direct and contract health services are currently provided if an individual is 1) a member of a federally recognized Indian tribe; 2) a resident within a Health Service Delivery Area; and 3) a non-member of a federally recognized tribe if a minor child and if residing within a Health Service Delivery Area. Care may be provided to other Indians (funds and resources allowing) if a person meets criteria 1 and 3 above but does not live in a Health Delivery Service Area but formerly did. Contract care will not be provided for these individuals. Services to non-Indian women pregnant with an eligible Indian's child will be provided but only during the time of pregnancy and through post-partum. Non-Indian members of an eligible Indian's household are eligible only if the care rendered is necessary to control an acute infectious disease or public health hazard. Services are also provided to an otherwise eligible member for up to 90 days after the person ceases to reside in a Health Service Delivery Area when the service unit director has been notified of the move. *Code of Federal Regulations*, volume 42, section 36.12 (1994 edition). "Delaying the Implementation of a Certain Rule Affecting the Provision of Health

Services by the Indian Health Service," 10.

28. "Oversight of BIA and IHS 1983 Budget Submissions," *Hearing before the Select Committee on Indian Affairs United States Senate*, Washington, D.C., 97th Congress, 2d session, May 26, 1982, 57. Meriam, *The Problem of Indian Administration*, 189. In 1985, retired director Emery Johnson blamed the agency's bureaucracy for some of the management troubles, arguing that the "self-perpetuating bureaucracy" resisted supporting Rhoades because of its opposition to turning programs over to tribal governments. Goldsmith, "American Indian medicine aims to add physicians, improve health," 1876. "Final Report and Legislative Recommendations," *A Report of the Special Committee on Investigations of the Select Committee on Indian Affairs United States Senate*, 101st Congress, 1st session, November 20, 1989, 162.

29. Rhoades, Luncheon Address. "Reauthorization of the Indian Health Care Improvement Act," 48-52.

30. *Indian Health Care*, 251.

31. In May 1985, the Senate conducted an investigation of the Billings Area Office for alleged unlawful expenditure of funds ($400,000). The Senate Select Committee found too many physicians in administrative positions, detracting from the healthcare in Montana. "Investigation of Indian Health Services," *Hearing before the Select Committee on Indian Affairs United States Senate*, Billings, Montana, 99th Congress, 1st session, May 30, 1985. "Final Report and Legislative Recommendations," 155-157. The Aberdeen, Albuquerque, Bemidji, and Oklahoma City area offices had questionable management practices.

32. "Federal Government's Relationship with American Indians," *Hearings before the Special Committee on Investigations of the Select Committee on Indian Affairs United States Senate on Mismanagement of Indian Health Service (IHS), Department of Health and Human Services* part 8, Washington, D.C., 101st Congress, 1st session, May 15, 1989, 31, 157-159.

33. *Hearings before the Special Committee on Investigations of the Select Committee on Indian Affairs United States Senate*, part 8, 161. Rhoades acknowledged weaknesses in the Indian Health Service but argued that Congress had never provided adequate funds for the agency to establish a strong management structure despite creating over $200,000,000 in new programs. "Addendum to the Statement by Everett R. Rhoades, MD, Director Indian Health Service before the Select Committee on Indian Affairs Special Committee on Investigations, United States Senate, May 15, 1989," in *Hearings before the Special Committee on Investigations of the Select Committee on Indian Affairs United States Senate*, part 8, 161-176.

34. "A Plan for Quality Management in the Indian Health Service," draft copy, (Department of Health and Human Services, Public Health Service, Indian Health Service, September 18, 1989), 1.

35. There was some criticism of the agency for using a "Project USA" program, a referral system operated in conjunction with the American Medical Association that provided short-term doctors while regular physicians were on leave or vacation. The criticism was that these physicians were too old and not as up-to-date on current practices. "Federal Government's Relationship with American Indians," part 8, 23-25.

36. "A Plan for Quality Management in the Indian Health Service," (Department of Health and Human Services, Public Health Service, Indian Health Service, October 31,

1989), 5.

37. "A Plan for Quality Management in the Indian Health Service," October 31, 1989, 9. The specific strategic, financial, and administrative changes targeted by the Quality Management Initiative included: 1) Federal Direct Care Programs: make critical improvements in administrative systems and ensure competence and professional integrity among key area office administrative staff; 2) Medicare and Medicaid: Ensure compliance with state and collections federal regulations and close the gap on uncollected earnings; 3) Other Third Party Collections: ensure appropriate oversight and close the gap on uncontrolled earnings; 4) Tribal Direct Care: establish processes for assisting Programs and tribes in staffing and managing healthcare services and for overseeing those services; 5) Contract Health Services: improve financial management and predictability and develop and install methods for negotiating the best rate; 6) Relationships with External Authorities: Improve responsiveness and anticipate needs; 7) Senior Management Staff: organize senior managers to participate in agency decision making and agenda-setting and instill in senior managers a shared set of professional values, a shared sense of direction, and shared responsibility for agency strategy and performance.

38. Rhoades, Luncheon Address.

39. Indirect costs such as liability insurance, which tribes were forced to pay out of program funds, were burdensome and infringed on the responsibility of the federal government, which also carried liability insurance as part of the federal Indian trust responsibility. "Indian Self Determination and Education Assistance Act Amendments of 1987," *Senate Report no. 100-274*, 100th Congress, 1st session, December 22, 1987, 26.

40. *Code of Federal Regulations* vol. 42, section 271.51 (April 1, 1995, edition). *Indian Health Care*, 222.

41. *Indian Health Care*, 223. *Evaluation Report: The Indian Health Service's Implementation of the Indian Self-Determination Process*, 89.

42. *Indian Health Care*, 228.

43. 102 stat. 1329 (PL 100-202); 102 stat. 1817 (PL 100-446); 102 stat. 2285 (PL 100-472); and 102 stat 2940 (PL 100-581). *Summary Report of the NIHB Self-Determination Act Committee*, National Indian Health Board Memorandum, December 27, 1988, 1.

44. "Indian Self-Determination and Education Assistance Act Amendment of 1987," 23.

45. "Implementation of Amendments to the Indian Self-Determination Act," *Hearings before the Select Committee on Indian Affairs, United States Senate*, 101st Congress, 1st session, June 9, 1989, 320. *Summary Report of the NIHB Self-Determination Act Committee*, 16. *Southern Indian Health Council v. Otis Bowen, et al.* Civil 88-0240-EJG (1990).

46. "Indian Self-Determination and Educational Assistance Act Amendments of 1987," 38-39. PL 100-472, 102 Stat. 2295, section 207.

47. *Report to Congress: Indian Health Service Relocation Study*, 8. "Budget Views and Estimates for Fiscal Year 1989," *A Report Submitted to the Budget Committee Prepared by the Select Committee on Indian Affairs United States Senate* 100th Congress, 2d session, March 1988. The Senate Select Committee opposed the relocation

until it could solicit tribal involvement and input. The committee requested a study to determine the feasibility and results of such a movement. The House proposed a $2.5 million appropriation for a feasibility study. "Department of the Interior and Related Agencies Appropriations for 1989," part 8, *Hearing before a Select Committee of the Committee on Appropriations House of Representatives*, 100th Congress, 2d session, March 9, 1988.

48. *Report to Congress: Indian Health Service Relocation Study*, 3.

49. *Report to Congress: Indian Health Service Relocation Study*, 3 and 19.

50. *Report to Congress: Indian Health Service Relocation Study*, 4.

51. The Relocation study argued that such a facility in the West would not only consolidate all functions into a cohesive package for area offices, tribes and tribal contractors, but would also be more conducive for American Indian and Alaska Native recruitment into headquarters administrative positions. The high costs of living in the Washington, D.C., area and the distance from tribal activities traditionally made recruitment of Native Americans in Rockville difficult. Better access by tribal governments to program support and technical assistance, sensitization of IHS professionals to the needs of the Indian people, and greater opportunity for medical professionals to practice clinical medicine on behalf of American Indians were all benefits to relocation. The primary mission of the proposed Center for Technical Support was to "establish and maintain a response mechanism to help IHS fulfill the requirements of the 93-638 amendments regarding the provisions of technical assistance to the tribes, serve as a comprehensive program development, research, and support resource for Area Offices and Tribes and establish and maintain a field-based focus for the creation, integration and transfer of knowledge throughout IHS and to the tribes." *Report to Congress: Indian Health Service Relocation Study*, 1.

52. Despite its success, President Reagan sought to transfer the program out of the Indian Health Service so the agency could focus strictly on medicine. "Indian Health Protection and Disease Prevention Act of 1983," *Hearing before the Select Committee on Indian Affairs United States Senate on S. 400*, Gallup, New Mexico, 99th Congress, 1st session, June 1, 1985, 158. In 1992, the IHS listed a $594,238,000 sanitation facilities deficiency (95,569 water units, 69,217 sewer units, 113,267 solid waste units). This did not include an estimated $1 billion for water and sewer needs for the 2 to 5 percent of existing American Indian and Alaska Native homes and communities that were not considered economically feasible at the time. *Trends in Indian Health 1992*, 105. A recent study on the Warm Springs Reservation (Oregon) showed that Indian infant mortality rates may have been misleading because of the use of identifying race from death certificates rather than from the use of birth certificates. If death rates were calculated based on birth certificate identification, the rate may have been 15.8 per 1,000 live births rather than the reported 10.2. Warm Springs had an infant death rate 2.6 times the national average in the 1980s. Risk factors identified included Sudden Infant Death Syndrome, a high teen birth rate (three times the state average), the number of deliveries to unwed mothers (40 percent), and the number of pregnant mothers known to use drugs and/or alcohol (30 percent) and smoke cigarettes (26 percent). Data show the median age of death on Warm Springs at 44 years, compared with 75 for the state average. Roy M. Nakamura, Richard King, Ernest H. Kimball, Robert K. Oye and Steven D. Helgerson, "Excess Infant Mortality in an American Indian Population, 1940-1990," *Journal of the*

*American Medical Association* (266:16) October 23/30, 1991, 2244-2248.

53. "Subsistence, Health Care, and Housing of Alaska Natives," *Hearings before the Select Committee on Indian Affairs United States Senate* Bethel, Alaska, 102d Congress, 2d session, May 24, 1992. "Water and Sanitation Problems in Alaska," *Hearings before the Select Committee on Indian Affairs United States Senate*, 103rd Congress, 1st session, May 5, 1993, 3. Nearly half of all Alaska Natives had privies (37 percent have flush toilets) and less than half had a water source at home. High rates of hepatitis B were also present. While funding for housing declined, Congress maintained the Indian housing program because of the continuing high unemployment in Indian Country, geographic isolation, and the trust status of most Indian land, which restricts credit. "Indian Housing Act," *Hearings before the Committee on Interior and Insular Affairs House of Representatives on H.R. 1928* 98th Congress, 1st session, April 12/19, 1983, 36-38.

54. "Administration of Indian Programs by the Environmental Protection Agency," *Hearing before the Select Committee on Indian Affairs United States Senate, Oversight Hearing on the Administration of Indian Programs by the Environmental Protection Agency* Washington, D.C., 101st Congress, 1st session, June 23, 1989.

55. *Blue Legs v. United States Environmental Protection Agency* 668 F. Supp. 1329 (1987).

56. *Blue Legs v. United States Bureau of Indian Affairs* 867 F2d 1094 (1989); *Blue Legs v. United States Environmental Protection Agency* 732 F. Supp. 81 (1990).

57. *Health Services for American Indians*, iv. *Bridging the Gap: Report of the Task Force on Parity of Indian Health Services* (Department of Health and Human Services, Public Health Service, Indian Health Service, May 1986), 25. "Department of the Interior and Related Agencies Appropriations Bill, 1985," *House Report no. 98-886* 98th Congress, 2d session, June 29, 1984, 103.

58. "Department of Interior and Related Agencies Appropriations for Fiscal Year 1984," part 9. *Bridging the Gap*, 15.

59. *Bridging the Gap*, 26.

60. *Indian Health Care*, 19.

61. The American Indian and Alaska Native birth rate was 28.1 births per 1,000 while the U.S. general rate was 16.7 per 1,000. There may be no better statistic showing the youthfulness of the Indian population than two additional statistics: 12.8 percent of American Indians and Alaska Natives were under the age of five while just 7.4 percent of the general population was, and just 5.5 percent of the American Indian and Alaska Native population was older than 65 while 12.6 percent of the general population was. *Regional Differences in Indian Health 1994*, (Department of Health and Human Services, Public Health Service, Indian Health Service, 1994) 24 and 29.

62. "Federal Government's Relationship with American Indians," part 8, 60. Robert W. Blum, Brian Harmon, Linda Harris, Lois Bergeisen and Michael D. Resnick, "American Indian-Alaska Native Youth Health," *Journal of the American Medical Association* (267:12), March 25, 1992, 1637-1644. The report did not address the needs of those most at risk—school dropouts—because it was a school-based study. Due to the unique geographic and cultural characteristics of Alaska Native youth, they were one and a half times more likely to have attempted suicide, more than one and a half times as

likely to have experienced abuse, and were twice as likely to smoke daily (as compared with American Indians in the study sample). There was no difference in perceived health status, drugs used, pregnancy history, body image, or sexual intercourse experiences. The sample was compared to a group of rural white youths in Minnesota who were part of a larger youth study undertaken in 1987.

63. *White v. Califano* 437 F. Supp. 543 (1977). The district court ruling was subsequently affirmed by the appellate court (581 F2d 697) in 1978. The court ordered the Indian Health Service to provide services but in accordance with regulations concerning priorities when funds, facilities, or personnel were insufficient. The Indian Health Service denied responsibility because no federal statute ever required it to provide services. The agency assumed any services provided should be discretionary. The court disagreed based on the trust responsibility and the general pronouncements of Congress, which the court interpreted as requiring the agency to provide Indians with health services. "Indian Health," *Hearing before the Select Committee on Indian Affairs United States Senate*, 46. Rhoades interpreted the *Califano* case as mandating the IHS to start a mental health program (p. 43).

64. "Indian Health Care," *Hearing before the Committee on Interior and Insular Affairs United States House of Representatives*, 101st Congress, 2d session, March 29, 1990, 1. "Indian Health Amendments," 106 stat. 4526. *Senate Report 102-392*, 79-81.

65. "Child Abuse and Neglect," *Hearing before the Select Committee on Indian Affairs United States Senate* Flagstaff, Arizona, 101st Congress, 2d session, November 22, 1988. "Final Report and Legislative Recommendations," 89-104. Title IV, Indian Child Protection, PL 101-630, 104 stat. 4594. "Child Abuse on North Dakota Reservations and Implementation of the Indian Child Protection and Family Violence Prevention Act," *Hearing before the Select Committee on Indian Affairs United States Senate*, Bismarck, North Dakota, 103rd Congress, 2d session, June 3, 1994. Between October 1, 1992 and May 26, 1994, there were 69 reported cases of child sexual abuse among North Dakota's Indian population. Just fourteen cases ended in conviction, with thirty-six declining prosecution and sixteen pending. The Indian Health Service had about a dozen youth treatment centers across the western United States. With regards to alcohol and drug abuse, Rhoades told the Senate Committee on Indian Affairs in 1991 that no program would be successful unless non-Indians changed their attitudes about Indians and substance abuse. "A major goal of the IHS," Rhoades told the Committee, "is to correct the deeply held alienation, self-dissatisfaction and negative self-image possessed by so many Indian people, especially youth." "Indian Anti-Drug Abuse Amendment of 1991," *Hearing before the Select Committee on Indian Affairs United States Senate on S. 290*, 102d Congress, 1st session, May 23, 1991, 60. Rhoades estimated that 95 percent of all Indians and Alaska Natives were affected directly or indirectly by a family member's substance abuse.

66. Title IV Demand Reduction (Public Law 99-570), 100 Stat. 3207. Congress ordered coordinated alcohol and substance abuse programs according to one IHS official because prior to the law "BIA washed their hands of substance abuse because it's a disease. IHS would not treat people with law and order problems because it was not their jurisdiction." "BIA and IHS Inspector General Reports on Indian Alcohol and Drug Abuse Programs," *Hearing before the Select Committee on Indian Affairs United States Senate*, 102d Congress, 2d session, July 30, 1992, 105. *Indian Alcohol and Substance*

*Abuse: Legislative Intent and Reality*, draft copy of the Department of Health and Human Services Office of the Inspector General, May 1992, 3 and 17. Rhoades pointed out the difficulties of the mental health program, including the fact that 95 percent of the alcoholism programs were contracted to the tribes themselves with whom Rhoades took the government-to-government relationship "very seriously." In light of the Inspector General's finding that the counselors were not certified, Rhoades argued that although most of the counselors were tribal members, the high Indian high school dropout rates hindered the Congressional requirement of certification. "We will get this done," the director told the Committee. But "not as fast as many people would like."

67. M. M. Gallaher, D. W. Fleming, L. R. Berger and C. M. Sewell, "Pedestrian and Hypothermia Deaths among Native Americans in New Mexico Between Bar and Home," *Journal of the American Medical Association* (267:10) March 11, 1992, 1345-1348. Blum, "American Indian-Alaska Native Youth Health," and C. Schlife, "Smokeless Tobacco Use in Rural Alaska," *Journal of the American Medical Association* (257:14), April 10, 1987, 1861-1865. Sylvia G. Simpson, Raymond Reid, Susan Baker and Stephen Teret, "Injuries Among the Hopi Indians," *Journal of the American Medical Association* (249:14) April 8, 1983, 1873-1876. Leads from the MMWR, "Distribution of AIDS Cases, by Racial/Ethnic Group and Exposure Category, United States, June 1, 1981-July 4, 1988," *Journal of the American Medical Association* (261:2) January 13, 1989, 201. The Indian and Alaska Native cases were broken down as follows: homosexual or bisexual men (40); heterosexual men (10); women (10); and children under age 13 (4).

68. Philip A. May, Karen J. Hymbaugh, Jon A. Aase and Jonathan M. Samet, "Epidemiology of Fetal Alcohol Syndrome Among American Indians of the Southwest," *Social Biology* (30:4) 1983, 374-387. The original study was conducted in the four corners region of Arizona, Utah, Colorado and New Mexico. Of 243 children examined, 31.3 percent had FAS, 16 percent had FAE, 5.3 percent were considered suspicious and 47.4 percent were diagnosed as normal (p. 378). The Navajo and the Pueblos had the lowest rate while the Apache and Ute had the highest. "The Indian Health Promotion and Disease Prevention Act of 1985," 206. "Senate Report 102-392," 36.

69. 106 stat. at 4559. "Department of the Interior and Related Agencies Appropriations for fiscal year 1991," *Hearing before the Select Committee on Indian Affairs United States Senate*, 101st Congress, 2d session, October 16, 1990, 13. Cindy Duimstra, Darlene Johnson, Charlotte Kutsch, Belle Wang, Miriam Zentner, Scott Kellerman, and Thomas Welty, "A Fetal Alcohol Syndrome Surveillance Pilot Project in American Indian Communities in the Northern Plains," *Public Health Reports* (108:2) March-April 1993, 225. Leads from MMWR, "Leading Major Congenital Malformations among Minority Groups in the United States, 1981-1988," *Journal of the American Medical Association* (261:2) January 13, 1989, 207.

70. "Prevention and Control of Diabetes among Native Americans," *Hearing before the Select Committee on Indian Affairs United States Senate* 99th Congress, 2d session, April 15, 1986, 112.

71. "Prevention and Control of Diabetes among Native Americans," 126. Of 21 Pima children examined for congenital anomalies, 38 percent were born of diabetic mothers whose disease was diagnosed before the age of 25. Just 3.7 percent of children

born to other mothers suffered anomalies. L. J. Comess, "Congenital Anomalies and Diabetes in the Pima Indians of Arizona," 471-477. Robert E. Windom, Assistant Secretary for Health and Human Services, wrote in 1988 that the Pima diabetes research presented a unique opportunity to study the effects of non-insulin dependent diabetes and heart disease (the Pimas have a very high rate of diabetes but a very low rate of heart disease). "From the Assistant Secretary for Health," *Journal of the American Medical Association* (260:10) September 9, 1988, 1346. "Prevention and Control of Diabetes among Native Americans," 111-112. "Indian Health Protection and Disease Prevention Act of 1985," 181.

72. "Indian Health Protection and Disease Prevention Act of 1985," 165. The Zuni began with two classes per week and soon were offering forty-six classes per week. "Indian Health Care Act Amendments of 1992," *Hearing before the Select Committee on Indian Affairs United States Senate*, 102nd Congress, 2d session, April 1, 1992, 155.

73. Kimberly Glasbrenner, "Seeking 'Indian-acceptable' ways to fight hypertension," *Journal of the American Medical Association* (254:14) October 11, 1985, 1877.

74. William L. Heyward, Anne Lanier, Brian J. McMahan, Mary Anne Fitzgerald, Steven Kilkinny and Thaddeus R. Paprocki, "Early Detection of Primary Hepatocellular Carcinoma," *Journal of the American Medical Association* (254:21), December 6, 1985, 3052-3054.

"Indian Health Service Facilities Become Smoke-Free," *Journal of the American Medical Association* (258:2) May 1985, 185.

75. "Indian Health Facilities," *Hearing before the Select Committee on Indian Affairs United States Senate* 101st Congress, 2d session, March 22, 1990, 109. Hospitals were constructed in the following communities and years: Bethel, Alaska (1980) at a cost of $34,100,000 to serve a user population of 23,773; Ada, Oklahoma (1980) at a cost of $14,374,000 to serve a user population of 20,962; Red Lake, Minnesota (1981) at a cost of $9,566,000 to serve a user population of 4,207; Cherokee, North Carolina (1981) at a cost of $10,341,000 to serve a user population of 6,423; Chinle, Arizona (1982) at a cost of $19,758,000 to serve a user population of 25,394; Tahlequah, Oklahoma (1983) at a cost of $21,334,000 to serve a user population of 31,295; Browning, Montana (1985) at a cost of $15,086,000 to serve a user population of 8,724; Crownpoint, New Mexico (1987) at a cost of $17,734,000 to serve a user population of 13,967; Kanakanak, Alaska (1987) at a cost of $16,578,000 to serve a user population of 8,724; Sacaton, Arizona (1988) at a cost of $15,735,000 to serve a user population of 10,910; and Rosebud, South Dakota (1989) at a cost of $20,700,000 to serve a user population of 9,253.

76. "Indian Health Service Nursing Shortage," *Hearing before the Select Committee on Indian Affairs United States Senate*, 101st Congress, 2d session, June 14, 1990, 160-163. The shortage was attributed to the usual problems: lack of continuing education, lower pay than other federal agencies, and the heavy workloads (48 hour weeks and/or 7 day a week shifts were not uncommon). A wide variety of tasks kept nurses from completing their "critical need nursing care," which was also cited as a reason for leaving the agency. In the 1992 amendments to the Indian Health Care Improvement Act Congress provided for continuing educational allowances for nurses and a retention bonus (25 percent of all IHS retention bonuses) as a means of attracting more nurses to the Indian Health Service. Section 1 of Title I "Health Manpower" of PL 102-573. Under section 110, the secretary was authorized to use grants to establish an INMED program

for Indian nurses. "Reauthorizing and Amending the Indian Health Care Improvement Act and for other Purposes," *House Report 98-763*, part 1, 26-27.

77. *Clinical Staffing in the Indian Health Service*, Special Report Prepared by the Health Program, Office of Technology Assessment, United States Congress, February, 1987, 6. "Department of the Interior and Related Agencies Appropriations for Fiscal Year 1984," part 9, 393.

78. "Indian Health Issues Grand Forks, North Dakota," *Hearing before the Select Committee on Indian Affairs United States Senate*, Grand Forks, North Dakota, 98th Congress, 1st session, June 2, 1983, 3-61. PL 102-392, Title I, section 110. Many American Indians and Alaska Natives had cultural taboos restricting experimentation on live bodies, animal or human, and dissecting cadavers, animal or human. "American Indian medicine aims to add physicians, improve health," 1871.

79. The Clinton budget in 1995 did not propose any new funds for sanitation facilities or other health facilities and no new funds were factored into the budget based on population increases. The Senate Select Committee on Indian Affairs requested that Clinton restore cut funds. "Health Care Reform in Indian Country oversight of the Indian Health Service," *Hearing before the Select Committee on Indian Affairs United States Senate*, 103rd Congress, 2d session, April 6, 1994, 78-82.

# CHAPTER SEVEN

## Into the Twenty-First Century

In the fall of 1993, President Bill Clinton nominated Michael Trujillo of Laguna Pueblo (New Mexico) to replace Everett Rhoades as the sixth director of the Indian Health Service. Trujillo, an internal medicine specialist, was the first director to require the consent of the Senate before taking office and was confirmed on March 22, 1994. He was reconfirmed to a second four-year term on June 18, 1998, and set a vision for the Indian Health Service and tribal nations to put their "heads together and come up with solutions for our people." In such a spirit of collaboration, tribal nations could "take responsibility" for their own well-being while at the same time promote partnerships with state and private healthcare organizations. Trujillo's partnerships became known as the "Friends of the Indians," and included a consortium of thirty-one professional organizations that advocated with the Indian Health Service on behalf of the health needs of American Indians and Alaska Natives.[1]

Trujillo guided the agency as it entered the twenty-first century and was followed by Charles W. Grim (2002-2007), Robert McSwain (2007-2009), and Yvette Roubideaux, who was appointed by President Barack Obama in March 2009 and confirmed by the Senate on May 6, 2009. Grim, a member of the Cherokee Nation of Oklahoma, McSwain, a member of the North Fork Rancheria of Mono Indians of California, and Roubideaux, a member of the Rosebud Sioux tribe and the first female director of the Indian Health Service, advocated for modernization of the agency, greater accountability, improved collaboration with state and local health organizations, and health promotion and disease prevention.[2]

## Refocusing Healthcare

The arrival of the twenty-first century ushered in an era of health promotion and disease prevention. Grim argued that the leading causes of death among American

Indians and Alaska Natives were preventable "if people choose to have a lifestyle that promotes health and prevents disease." The changing health challenges required new paradigms and new approaches to medicine. With the Indian Health Service funded at just 55 percent of minimum needs, fiscal resources remained a concern, especially as the service population continued to grow. Today there are 1.9 million American Indians and Alaska Natives residing on or near reservations and 600,000 living in urban areas dependent on the agency for all or most of their healthcare needs.[3]

Providing meaningful care to eligible patients is challenging and Congressional parsimony adds to these challenges. In 2003, the national per capita expenditure for Medicare totaled $5,915; the IHS per capita spending totaled just $1,914—and $800 within the Navajo Nation. Just nineteen of forty-nine IHS and tribal hospitals have surgery programs, resulting in lack of services for patients who often travel great distances for specialized care. Turnover rates remain high within the Indian Health Service, with nurses (23 percent), physicians (18 percent) and pharmacists (11 percent) experiencing the highest vacancy rates, making program continuity difficult. While the Indian Health Service no longer operates under the theory that the Indian Medical Service did a century ago when it was assumed "the Indians would ultimately all die of epidemic diseases," it still faces the same chronic shortages of professional staff and fiscal resources.[4]

After fifty years of IHS services, tribes still face difficult public health challenges that result from low socioeconomic status, geographic and social isolation, low educational attainment, poor community and spiritual wellness, limited economic opportunities, poverty, and discrimination. Some people assume that since American Indians and Alaska Natives receive "free" healthcare they should have fewer, not more, health concerns than other Americans. But while medical services may be "free" to many American Indians and Alaska Natives, "access to timely and appropriate care" necessary to well-being is influenced by availability of services, proximity to facilities, insurance coverage, particular health concerns, and healthcare resources. These factors, along with insufficient funding, are exacerbated by "the lack of a strong, comprehensive federal Indian health care policy." But beyond policy concerns, the "connection between poverty and poor health cannot be broken just by access to health services or treatment alone." As Grim argued in 2003, "It [also] requires behavioral changes."[5]

## A Need for New Research Protocols

New challenges for the Indian Health Service loom on the horizon, including adopting appropriate medical research protocols in Indian Country. Since the allegations of forced sterilizations in the 1970s, the Indian Health Service and tribal communities have grappled over the role of research and patient/tribal privacy rights. In the 1990s, the issue of ownership and confidentiality of medical research pointed to the need for updating protocols. Issues such as intellectual property rights and cultural sensitivities are central to research, including ethno-botanical and bio-medical research. In the 1990s, the Navajo Tribal Council halted all research involving the Navajo due to cultural insensitivities on the part of researchers. In order for medical research to proceed, the Navajo Tribal Council must be convinced that the Navajo people will benefit from such research and that it will be conducted in a culturally appropriate manner. The focus must be on healing, not simply research.[6]

The decision of the Navajo Nation to limit medical research stemmed from several factors, including the 1993 Hantavirus epidemic that broke out in several locations in the United States, including most severely in the Four Corners region of Arizona, Utah, Colorado, and New Mexico. When the Centers for Disease Control and Prevention (CDCP) visited the Navajo Nation and began researching the origin of the virus, many Navajo were enraged when the CDCP violated cultural protocols. Violations included interviewing relatives of the deceased during the four day mourning period and using placebos on some Navajo patients while others were given the anti-viral drug ribaviran. Other *faux pas* included examining umbilical cords to determine if a placental blood transfusion would be effective as a bone-marrow transplant in fighting severe combined immune deficiency in violation of Navajo cultural beliefs that the umbilical cord "contains the spirit of the newborn."[7]

More recently, the Havasupai Tribe sued Arizona State University, the Arizona Board of Regents, and three ASU researchers over violations of protocol agreements. ASU researchers collected more than 400 blood samples from tribal members between 1990 and 1994 to study the incidence of diabetes among the Havasupai. Without Havasupai approval or knowledge, however, the researchers used the samples to study inbreeding, schizophrenia, and North American migration theories. An independent investigation discovered "numerous unauthorized studies, experiments and projects" by universities across the United States leading to dozens of scholarly papers, dissertations, and articles that were unrelated to diabetes. In 2004, the Havasupai Tribe filed a $50 million lawsuit against ASU and the Board of Regents; 52 tribal members also filed their own $25 million lawsuit.[8]

While these *faux pas* are external to the Indian Health Service, the agency is not immune to such issues. As it entered the new millennium, it, too, considered new delivery and research paradigms. Research remains essential to furthering individual and community well-being and mitigating the effects of centuries of ill-health. But such paradigms must extend beyond simple cures and corrective measures and must consider what is culturally relevant if it is to be meaningful and successful. Paradigms that relegate culture to a secondary status must be supplanted with those that respect and adhere to cultural norms. New paradigms are needed that enable the Indian Health Service to broadly determine regional and local differences in tribal health attitudes, knowledge, and beliefs. These issues are essential, as some American Indians and Alaska Natives live on reservations or trust lands, while others live in cities; some maintain their indigenous language, others do not; some observe traditional spiritual practices and beliefs, while others do not. A standard clinical disease model, while simple and easy to use, does not factor in cultural norms, customs, and traditions.[9]

What is needed is a social conservation model of research. Such a model considers the life circumstances of the local community and the salient features of community norms and behaviors. These can then be integrated into research and medical paradigms. In so doing, statistics such as causes of death, which are easily identifiable but provide little in terms of guiding research in combating health challenges, can play a more significant role in determining courses of action that lead to solving difficult challenges. The medical research community must closely examine the relationship between quality of care, health promotion, and disease prevention. Research that reinforces the distribution of resources to support secondary and tertiary care rather than the primary cause of ill-health leaves unchallenged the root causes of poor health.

While the Indian Health Service has made significant progress in advancing healthcare, the health status of American Indians and Alaska Natives remains inferior to that of other Americans, not only in incidence of disease but also in severity. While the mission of the Indian Health Service is to "raise the physical, mental, social, and spiritual health of American Indians and Alaska Natives to the highest level," the task has become increasingly difficult as population increases, demand for services, medical costs, recruitment and retention challenges, lag times for referral services, and chronic diseases strain the agency, with the result that it continues to operate as a crisis-oriented healthcare organization.[10]

In 2006, Secretary of Health and Human Services Michael Leavitt outlined nine health priorities for Health and Human Services agencies, including the Indian Health Service. Director Charles Grim adapted these to the Indian Health Service to focus on the need for a social conservation model. Under long-term healthcare goals, Grim directed the agency to support American Indian elders and their families by keeping them together and within the community for as long as possible. The goal is to create emotionally and mentally healthy families and provide a "sense of structure and cultural identity." This emphasis on "self-direction" increases community-based care in a manner that encourages and supports the traditional role of family within American Indian and Alaska Native communities and, therefore, serves a conservation role in healthcare delivery.[11]

Healthcare providers and medical institutions can and must learn to recognize and appreciate the cultural uniqueness of tribal communities and the relevance of local mores and attitudes. Utilizing such a paradigm implies that medical researchers, anthropologists, and policy analysts, all of whom seek to improve Indian healthcare and well-being, are willing to involve the local community in the process and recognize its unique contributions in discovering solutions to complex challenges.

## Eligibility and Eligibility Concerns

Another important issue that will surface again is the issue of eligibility for services. In the final decades of the twentieth century there was an effort on the part of the Congress and administration to modify eligibility for health services by redefining blood quantum requirements. Any redefinition of eligibility that increases blood quantum will result in the denial of services and care to a segment of the American Indian and Alaska Native population and has the potential to effectively terminate Indian health services. Based on current projections, less than 3 percent of American Indians will be full-blooded in 2080, while the number with less than one-quarter Indian blood will rise dramatically. These people may find themselves threatened with the loss of services. While the Indian Health Service considered redefining eligibility in terms of blood quantum, tribal nations argued that culture, not blood, should define eligibility. Such a definition better correlates with federal policies encouraging Indian self-determination and self-governance. Policies that do not support self-governance will have a devastating impact on indigenous healthcare.[12]

Restrictive eligibility requirements will not only deny an increasing number of American Indians of care, but they may also force those ineligible for services to leave their reservation communities simply because they may be unable to compete with those who are eligible. This could be the ultimate form of program termination, since services will be reduced as the eligible population declines. Conditions may eventually warrant a cessation of health services; restrictive eligibility will then have accomplished its objective of terminating health services.

Some tribal leaders continue to fear termination of services, while others fear loss of control over such programs. Trujillo called for tribes to "put their heads together and come up with a solution for our people." Consequently, a growing sentiment among tribes is to develop and control their own health programs via self-governance compacts. In the 1990s and continuing into the first decade of the twenty-first century, tribal leaders expressed concerns over the Indian Health Service being absorbed into a larger national healthcare system. Foremost among these concerns are the protection of tribal sovereignty and the fulfillment of the federal trust responsibility. During the George W. Bush administration the Indian Health Service worked to strengthen its partnership with tribes. Grim and McSwain each met with tribal leaders to discuss reforming the agency as a distinct component of the larger national healthcare reform efforts. Tribal consultation focused on how to better meet the needs of American Indian and Alaska Native patients within the broader context of reform efforts and availability.[13]

Tribal leaders lobbied President Clinton to remain true to his pledge that nationalized healthcare would not require American Indians and Alaska Natives to forgo IHS services. The president went on record in a Bernalillo, New Mexico, meeting with tribal leaders that he supported tribes having the option of utilizing IHS services or seeking care from a provider of their choice. While President Obama pledged to modernize and strengthen the Indian Health Service and include an American Indian policy advisor so that tribes have direct access at the highest level of his administration, Congress, at the president's request, introduced H.R. 676 in January 2009 to nationalize healthcare. Under the bill, the Indian Health Service would have five years before it would be folded into the national health plan. The ongoing debate over healthcare has important implications for American Indians and Alaska Natives. Should too many opt out of the Indian Health Service, there could be a systematic effort to reduce services further and ultimately terminate Indian-only services.[14]

Former director Everett Rhoades, while not opposed to reform, opposed all attempts to nationalize healthcare if they included the Indian Health Service, viewing nationalization as a means of denying health services. The Indian Health Service has never been adequately funded, meaning eligible patients have been denied services. How would nationalized healthcare "be any different?" Rhoades asked. Rhoades was not alone, as tribal leaders from across the nation testified before the Senate Select Committee on Indian Affairs. The Red Lake Chippewa tribal council, for instance, voted unanimously to oppose nationalized healthcare based on political considerations. Bemidji Area Office director Kathy Annette shared the concerns of tribal leaders when she expressed fear over the loss of the federal trust responsibility and the subjection of tribal health to state jurisdiction. The Navajo Tribal Council expressed similar concerns. Grim shared tribal concerns, opining tribal health programs were at "great risk of being lost or forgotten if they are absorbed into larger organizations and programs."[15]

As healthcare costs increase and as more American Indians and Alaska Natives are able to provide for their own healthcare via better education, economic opportunities, or tribal revenues from gaming, eligibility standards will undoubtedly be revisited. When they are, questions related to criteria will be important. Another issue likely to surface is, if tribes are to exercise self-government, should they not be expected to assume more financial responsibility for their own healthcare? And if so, what is the proper role of the federal government and how would this impact the federal Indian trust relationship? Policy questions aside, there are political considerations that tribal nations must consider. These include the legacy of transfer politics, which some tribal leaders viewed as setting up termination. State barriers and tribal responses to them, urban versus reservation-based services, and the future of healthcare are other considerations.

## Impediments to Healthcare

With the transfer of healthcare responsibility and the idea of integrating Indian-only services into the Public Health Service in 1955, there was a presumption that American Indians and Alaska Natives would have access to a wider array of services and providers than had been previously available. But despite the establishment of the Indian Health Service a half century ago, American Indians and Alaska Natives "suffer disproportionately from a variety of illnesses and disease," with "poor health a community characteristic." Consequently, ill-health is a drain on tribal communities and contributes to a cycle of poor health.[16]

While the presumption of greater access to services is accurate, there remain social and cultural barriers that influence American Indian and Alaska Native access to health services. While Americans enjoy the best medical care in the world, the services available to American Indians and Alaska Natives are impacted by socio-cultural factors that contribute to health disparities. These include bias and discrimination. "Too often, a physician's perception of a patient's race and ethnicity . . . is . . . used by the health-care team to make clinical decisions and medical and social judgments about the patient." In addition, healthcare providers often communicate "lower expectations" for American Indian and Alaska Native patients, and frequently use a "less participatory decision-making style" of communication. Since American Indian and Alaska Native patients tend to ask fewer questions and are unlikely to "speak out against mistreatment," they are "vulnerable to unfair treatment."[17]

Cultural misunderstanding and language barriers also influence care. Too many healthcare providers are unwittingly insensitive to or reject traditional healing methods and medicine, raising additional barriers. If health services are not provided in a culturally sensitive manner and in an appropriate language, "treatment will remain ineffective." The Association of American Indian Physicians in 2002 unanimously approved a resolution supporting American Indian and Alaska Native traditional healing and medicine as one component of healthcare. To its credit, the Indian Health Service is making traditional medicine available and accessible in all of its clinics and hospitals, and is constructing all new facilities with space for traditional healing practices.[18]

Language barriers continue to impact well-being, as limited English proficiency speakers receive less information about their medical condition and treatment and understand less of the instructions related to their treatment. As a result, they are less likely to keep appointments and receive preventive services and tend to make more emergency room visits. Nearly 25 percent of reservation-based American Indians and Alaska Natives speak their indigenous language and a similar percentage has limited language proficiency. Many such speakers take family members along to translate, which encumbers its own set of challenges, including confidentiality and appropriate translations. The Indian Health Service currently does not provide any formal language assistance to its patients. The challenge is exacerbated at non-IHS (i.e., contract) facilities.[19]

Socioeconomic conditions influence overall levels of health. Low levels of education and income impact well-being—25.9 percent of American Indians and Alaska Natives live in poverty, the highest rate of all ethnic groups in the United States—so health disparities remain. Lack of housing or substandard housing also impact American Indian and Alaska Native health. Lower socioeconomic levels tend to result in higher levels of smoking, alcohol abuse, risky behavior, and overall lower levels of well-being. These behaviors directly influence well-being. The Indian Health Service reports that "behavioral issues contribute to about 70 percent of the diseases that occur at a higher rate in Indian Country." Grim initiated a Behavioral Health Initiative to address the fact that one-third of the demand on IHS facilities is related to mental health, alcoholism, and substance abuse, each of which is preventable. "Effective behavioral health techniques can be used side-by-side with tribal traditions and customs," Grim opined, to reduce demand for chronic disease management and make existing services more effective.[20]

Grim also advocated a health promotion and disease prevention initiative to enable American Indian and Alaska Native communities to "take responsibility for their health by exercising, eating right, taking advantage of medical screenings, and avoiding risky behaviors." Increased risk-taking by American Indian and Alaska Native males is correlated with "loss of cultural identity, anomie, loss of traditional roles for males, failure of primary socialization, and unresolved grief from historical trauma." Health promotion and disease prevention is crucial, as "to continue on a treatment track alone [will] bankrupt the nation's health system, including the Indian Health Service."[21]

Beyond social and cultural factors, there are structural barriers that impact American Indian and Alaska Native access to healthcare and contribute to health disparities. These are internal to the Indian Health Service and include management issues, geographic location of facilities, aging facilities, wait time for services, retention and recruitment of professional staff, and misdiagnosis of disease. While the Indian Health Service is not an insurance program for eligible patients, it is a federally funded agency that provides health services to American Indians and Alaska Natives. It is a program of universal eligibility operating with limited availability. Funds are discretionary, not an entitlement. Eligible American Indians too often are denied state services and fall back to IHS facilities because state agencies assume the agency is the primary caregiver for Indians. In reality, the Indian Health Service is a residual provider, encouraging American Indians and Alaska Natives to first seek services from other agencies before utilizing its facilities. The Indian Health Service collaborates with federal entitlement programs such as Medicare and Medicaid, and with state and local agencies, including private insurance providers to ensure adequate care is provided.[22]

But while the Indian Health Service provides direct and contract services, and contracts with tribes and tribal groups to operate and manage their own facilities, there are additional structural barriers that limit the efficiency of services. Many facilities are located in remote locations where the climate can be inhospitable, roads impassable, and transportation difficult. It is common for Navajo patients, for instance, to travel over unpaved roads for nearly 100 miles to access facilities. On the Cheyenne River Sioux Reservation, patients might travel ninety miles to Pierre to reach the nearest obstetric services. Lack of transportation means either American Indians and Alaska Natives rely on others for transportation or they do not make the trip. Many are "unable to plan ahead and make appointments at the IHS facilities; thus many [patients] show up without appointments, leading to long wait times." At the Cherokee Nation (Oklahoma) IHS hospital, diagnostic tests are provided only on specific days each month, and if a patient is unable to utilize the time available, he must wait until the following month. This rationing of healthcare is "not a good way to practice medicine."[23]

To its credit, the Indian Health Service utilizes telemedicine to reduce the geographic barriers. Such technology enables the agency to provide or support health-related activities, including professional education, community health education, public health research, and health service administration from a distance. It also enables remote villages and facilities to send and receive digital images of certain medical conditions and communicate with larger, better equipped hospitals. Unfortunately, telemedicine is infrequently used due to high patient demands and high turnover rates, which require constant training for new employees to become proficient in using such technology.[24]

Aging and antiquated facilities represent yet another barrier. The average age of IHS facilities is thirty-six years, compared nine years for the private sector. The old Pawnee Health Clinic at 103 years is the oldest facility. In 2003, Grim encouraged modernization and replacement efforts via collaborative projects between tribes and the Indian Health Service. The agency in 2009 identified a backlog of $506 million in repairs. Without adequate funding for repairs and replacements, some hospitals have used third party collections to make repairs, taking funds away from patient care. Due to challenges associated with antiquated facilities and inefficient use of space, IHS and tribal facilities operate at lower productivity rates that result in patient delays and extended wait times.[25]

The ability to recruit and retain healthcare providers remains a challenge for the agency and impacts the overall quality of care American Indians and Alaska Natives receive. Retention issues stem not only from medical personnel leaving for greener pastures in the private sector, but also because of the frustration due to their inability to provide care at the level they are trained to do. High demands lead to overworked staff, which in turn leads to burnout. High turnover rates leave gaps in service and disrupt continuity of care. In 2001, the vacancy rate for dentists was 21 percent and for optometrists 14 percent. The average length of service for IHS physicians remains just 8.1 years.[26]

The challenges for providers is not unlike those of fifty years ago: long hours in remote locations, lack of modern amenities, disparities in compensation, inadequate housing, lack of employment opportunities for spouses, limited community activities for children, lack of continuing education, and substandard educational systems for their children. A winter 2002 example from the Cheyenne River Sioux illustrates the effects of provider shortages.

> The Eagle Butte Service Unit . . . has been swamped with children with Influenza A, RSV [Respiratory Syntactical Virus], and one fatal case of meningitis. There are only three doctors on duty, one Physician Assistant, and one Nurse Practioner. The only pediatrician is the Clinical Director who will not see any patients, even though there is a serious need for services of a pediatrician. Several of the children have presented with breathing problems, high fever, and severe vomiting. The

average waiting time at the clinic has been four and six hours. The average time at the emergency room is similar. Most babies have been sent home without any testing to determine what they have and with nothing but cough syrup, only to be life-flighted soon thereafter because the child could not breathe. The children were all diagnosed by the non-IHS hospital with RSV.[27]

While the Indian Health Service has utilized bonuses and allowances, as well as scholarships and loan repayment programs, for physicians in an effort to retain them, it has been unable to stem the drain of healthcare providers. Between 1983 and 2003, the Indian Health Service used scholarships and loan repayments to increase its professional staff by 51 percent and its American Indian and Alaska Native staff by 230 percent, but still failed to fill all vacant positions. By 2003, 36 percent of the IHS professional staff was American Indian or Alaska Native, as compared to just 16 percent 20 years earlier. Training American Indian and Alaska Native staff, however, is not a panacea for provider shortages. While there are 300 members of the Association of American Indian Physicians, with 200 having served in an IHS facility at one time, just 69 were with the agency in 2000. Most leave the agency because of "symptoms of burnout" and "frustration . . . [in] provid[ing] quality health care."[28]

A final structural obstacle is the misdiagnosis or late diagnosis of disease. While often associated with frequent staff turnover and the inconsistent care provided, misdiagnosis can lead to fatalities. In stories eerily reminiscent of the pre-1950s era, numerous American Indian patients have been misdiagnosed and died as a result.

Valerie Dupris Curley [explained] that many doctors at her IHS facility are temporary providers. Consequently, during each visit for her husband who has a chronic medical condition, they have to repeat his medical history for the providers. [Another] woman explained that for two years she was seen by different providers and misdiagnosed repeatedly. She was finally diagnosed with cancer. She expressed that "there should be doctors at IHS facilities that can stay and help people."

Another patient sought relief for back pain for two years without proper diagnosis. After two years of pain medication, he was diagnosed with cancer and died three weeks later. A woman from Rosebud Sioux complained of persistent stomach pain and was diagnosed with heartburn. She later discovered she had terminal stomach cancer. High turnover rates among health providers contribute to this inconsistent care. Furthermore, providers often are not trained in disease detection, especially cancer. A failure to screen for preventable diseases adds to the misdiagnosis or late diagnosis. Grim encouraged American Indian patients to "go back . . . and ask questions of their providers." A failure to properly diagnose disease is "an indicator of a lack of quality care [that has] a detrimental effect on [the] overall health" of American Indians and Alaska Natives.[29]

As limiting as social and structural barriers are, there are financial impediments that impede patient access to and the success of the Indian Health Service. Broadly speaking, per-capita expenditures for the Indian Health Service are not only less than other federal health programs, but such expenditures fail to keep pace with inflation and population growth.

The Indian Health Service was authorized by the Indian Health Care Improvement Act in 1976 to receive Medicare and Medicaid reimbursements, with such third party collections used to supplement the appropriated revenue of the agency and tribal health facilities. The Indian Health Service in 2007 received $650 million in reimbursements (excluding unreported tribal reimbursements). The Congressional intent was for these reimbursements to be used to supplement appropriated dollars and ensure adequate medical services were available to American Indians and Alaska Natives. Too often, however, these revenues are used to ensure that agency facilities meet safety standards and that all hospitals and clinics remain accredited.[30]

But while third party collections have increased over the past fifteen years, the lack of appropriated dollars results in the Indian Health Service "defer[ring] and den[ying] payment for medical services that are thought to be of lower priority." Congress clearly intended "that any Medicare and Medicaid funds received by the Indian Health Service program be used to supplement—and not supplant—current IHS appropriations." In 2004, the Indian Health Service relied upon third party collections for 16 percent of its funding.[31]

In 2003, critics of the Indian Health Service charged that the agency was funded at just 52 percent of the appropriate level of need, with an unmet healthcare need of over $3 billion. This level of unmet need hearkens back to the 1970s and the Rincon Band of Mission Indians lawsuit against the Indian Health Service in which the tribe sought redress for disparate levels of funding. In 1980, the U.S. Supreme Court ordered the Indian Health Service to establish what came to be known as the Indian Health Care Improvement Fund to provide additional funding for tribes in California and elsewhere where disparities existed. From this, the Federal Employee Health Benefit Program Disparity Index, or FDI, was established to measure unmet Indian healthcare needs for specific service units and/or areas relative to the benchmark cost for the average American. In essence, the lower the ratio the greater the healthcare need. In 2000, the federal benchmark was $2,980; for the IHS user population the amount was $1,728, for an FDI ratio of .58. Three years later the ratio slipped to .52.[32]

Inflation also diminishes the buying power of appropriated dollars. While the IHS user population is increasing at an annual rate of 1.8 percent, federal appropriations increases are just 1.6 percent. Consequently, while the dental budget increased $5,700,000 in 2005, the Indian Health Service provided 92,000 fewer services. Public health nursing budget increases of $3,000,000 resulted in 13,000 fewer services. In 2004, the Indian Health Service received a 2.6 percent increase in appropriations, far short of the 5.5 percent increase for Medicaid and 10.9 percent for Medicare.[33]

Contract care services are especially impacted by the loss of purchasing power. In some instances, American Indians and Alaska Natives in need of contract medical services are denied care unless life or limb is at risk. More often than not, contract services are curtailed mid-year if funding thresholds are surpassed. In addition to denying services, contract care is subject to inflationary pressures. Between 1998 and 2003, billed costs per visit increased 69 percent to $614; during that same period, outpatient care visits declined 38 percent to 128,571. Despite a 27 percent increase in contract health service funding during this same period, the number of services provided decreased. Despite gaming revenue and the availability of private insurance, American Indians and Alaska Natives are less likely to have health insurance. The Kaiser Foundation reports that 49 percent of American Indians have access to insurance (83 percent for all Americans) but just 22.9 percent of the IHS user population has insurance.[34]

Another 17 percent of American Indians and Alaska Natives have insurance through Medicare or Medicaid, State Children's Health Insurance Program, or the Veteran's Administration, leaving more than one-third of American Indians without any insurance (the overall U.S. rate of uninsurance is 12 percent). For a majority of American Indians without insurance, the Indian Health Service is their only healthcare provider. Some American Indians believe that federal treaties signed by their ancestors ceding land and resources in the eighteenth and nineteenth centuries guaranteed healthcare and exempts them from having to access Medicare and Medicaid and their burdensome regulations.[35]

One result of these barriers to healthcare is the potential for intra- and inter-tribal feuds over the increasingly scarce Indian health resources. The ramifications of declining budgets among various Indian health organizations and communities has the potential to divide Indian Country into the health services *haves* and *have nots*. An example from the Billings, Montana, IHS Area Office and urban programs from Missoula, Montana, demonstrates this potential for strife and divisiveness between reservation and urban Indians. When urban Indian health programs were first established, they were independent of the Indian Health Service. By the 1980s, Congress authorized the Indian Health Service to consolidate urban programs and placed them under its control. In Billings, the Missoula Indian Alcohol and Drug Services Program and the Native American Services Agency were placed under IHS control in 1983 and, by 1987, were targeted for elimination.[36]

Urban Indians sought to delay and prevent any changes in the status of their programs while the neighboring Confederated Salish and Kootenai Tribes resisted the added responsibility for urban Indian healthcare in Missoula, where the Indian Health Service desired the Salish and Kootenai to assume all responsibility for the Missoula urban programs. Both sides objected, with the Indian Health Service eventually withdrawing any changes in eligibility standards. Nonetheless, the Missoula example suggests that there will be future conflicts among urban and reservation Indians based on the growing demand for scarce resources. With just 1 percent of the IHS budget set aside for urban programs, but with more than 600,000 urban American Indians and Alaska Natives—37 percent of these Indians live in urban areas with no urban or IHS facilities—the potential for urban versus rural conflict remains a distinct possibility. Such conflicts have the potential to negatively impact urban Indian healthcare. And with urban Indians at a greater risk for mental health, substance abuse, gang activity, teen pregnancy, abuse, and neglect than their reservation counterparts, denial of services will have grave implications.[37]

## A Vision for the Twenty-First Century

Beyond these struggles there remain unresolved issues that must be addressed by Roubideaux and future IHS and tribal leaders. These include issues such as: What is the proper role of tribal nations in the delivery of services? How can federal, state, and tribal governments work together to accomplish the good of the whole? How will responsibilities be defined in the future? And who should be responsible and to what extent for services? Definitive answers to these questions are necessary if meaningful care and services are to be delivered to American Indians and Alaska Natives.

What is needed in Indian Country is a new approach in the delivery of services, one that gives voice to American Indian concerns in developing programs that fit the needs of local tribal communities. As tribal nations exercise their inherent sovereign powers they may be in a better position to ensure that healthcare providers adjust their "skills to the special problems connected with improving the health of American Indians" and make them suitable and acceptable to the consumers of those services. IHS physicians and healthcare providers must not only be cognizant of the *science* of medicine, but they must also consciously promote the *art* of their practice by adapting to local norms.[38]

In the 1990s, and continuing into the twenty-first century, the Indian Health Service struggled to define its core goals and purpose. Everett Rhoades outlined his vision in 1987 when the Indian Health Service established a series of goals designed to change personal and community behaviors. Among these goals were health awareness through the use of seat belts, stressing the dangers of smoking, the importance of stress reduction, healthy lifestyles, immunizations and screenings, and community monitoring. Trujillo targeted nine health initiatives that focused on traditional medicine, children and adolescent health, elder care, women's health, injury prevention, domestic violence and child abuse prevention, healthcare financing, state health initiatives, and sanitation facilities. Grim established three additional goals: health promotion and disease prevention, behavioral health, and chronic care management. McSwain advanced collaborative efforts with the Boys and Girls Clubs of America, Nike Corporation, the Mayo Clinic, and Harvard University. Most recently, Roubideaux identified four priority areas in her confirmation hearings: strengthening partnerships with tribes, reforming the agency by reviewing the delivery of services in terms of quality and quantity, improving access to care, and making the Indian Health Service more transparent and accountable to its constituents.[39]

Indian healthcare in the twenty-first century requires the utilization of traditional Indian medicine in concert with Western medicine, a concept that is by no means novel. This requires healthcare providers not only to consider the relationship of the patient and his cultural surroundings without overlooking the importance of ceremony (since illness is seen as the result of disharmony) but also to understand the local philosophy of illness, respect that philosophy, and work within the local support system in the healing process. These principles were expressed at the Annual Meeting of the Association of American Indian Physicians in the late 1990s when Mescalero Apache medicine woman Meredith Begay urged Western doctors to examine more than just the physical side of ill-health. Western medicine, Begay asserted, looks only at the physical side of ill-health but Indian medicine deals with the physical, emotional, and the spiritual aspects of ill-health. Physician Verlyn Corbett reinforced this point by noting the more Western medicine understands community health concepts, "the more trusting Indians will be with seeking treatments."[40]

## Twenty-First-Century Health Indices

The 1957 Public Health Service-sanctioned studies of American Indian and Alaska Native health focused almost exclusively on environmental (poverty, poor housing, geographical isolation) or inheritable (social and cultural) issues as the root cause of disease and ill-health. Between 1955 and the 1970s, when *esprit de corps* was at its peak, the Indian Health Service made strides in eliminating environmental deficiencies via sanitation improvements and the implementation of community health programs. While the Indian Health Service was successful in eliminating or reducing many of the environmental causes of ill-health, it was less successful in changing behaviors associated with poor health. Consequently, today's health challenges require social, rather than exclusively medical, solutions.[41]

Broad quality of life factors, such as lower life expectancy (72.3 years for American Indians and Alaska Natives vs. 76.9 for the overall U.S. population in 2001) result from inadequate education, disproportionate levels of poverty, discrimination, and cultural differences. These social and economic conditions resulted in 2003 American Indian and Alaska Native mortality rates from tuberculosis that were 750 percent higher; alcoholism rates 550 percent higher; diabetes rates 190 percent higher; unintentional injury rates 150 percent higher; homicide rates 100 percent higher; and suicide rates 70 percent higher. The American Indian and Alaska Native service population is younger than the overall U.S. population partially due to high mortality rates. Table 7.1 illustrates the mortality rates for major health factors as of 2003.

Seven of the top ten morbidity and mortality rates for American Indians and Alaska Natives are directly related to behavioral issues and lifestyle choices.

Diabetes remains the most serious health challenge today, with more than 50 percent of all American Indian and Alaska Native adults diabetic. Type II diabetes, the most common form of diabetes in Indian Country, can be managed with proper exercise and diet. Nonetheless, the disease is ravaging tribal communities and maiming and killing American Indians and Alaska Natives. And it is not just adults at risk; the incidence rate among children in rapidly increasing. Treating diabetes could consume 40 percent of the IHS budget if appropriate behavioral changes are not made. The only practical way of reducing diabetes is prevention, which must begin within tribal communities.[42]

Table 7.1

*Mortality Disparity Rates, 2003\**

| Category | American Indian/Alaska Native | U.S. All Races | Ratio to U.S. |
|---|---|---|---|
| All Causes | 1027.2 | 832.7 | 1.2 |
| Alcohol | 43.6 | 6.7 | 6.5 |
| Breast Cancer | 21.0 | 25.3 | 0.8 |
| Cerebrovascular | 50.9 | 53.5 | 1.0 |
| Cervical Cancer | 4.7 | 2.5 | 1.9 |
| Diabetes | 74.2 | 25.3 | 2.9 |
| Heart Disease | 231.1 | 232.2 | 1.0 |
| HIV Infection | 3.1 | 4.7 | 0.7 |
| Homicide | 12.2 | 6.0 | 2.0 |
| Infant Deaths (per 1000 live) | 11.7 | 6.9 | 1.7 |
| Malignant Neoplasm | 180.7 | 190.1 | 1.0 |
| Maternal Deaths | 11.1 | 12.1 | 0.9 |
| Motor Vehicle Crashes | 51.2 | 15.3 | 3.3 |
| Pneumonia/Influenza | 32.3 | 22.0 | 1.5 |
| Suicide | 17.9 | 10.8 | 1.7 |
| Tuberculosis | 1.7 | 0.2 | 8.5 |
| Unintentional Injuries | 94.8 | 37.3 | 2.5 |

* American Indian/Alaska Native rates are from 2002-2004 and U.S. all races rates are from 2003

(Source: *Indian Health Service*, 2009)

High risk behaviors among American Indian youth also affect health status, leading to high rates of accidental deaths, homicides, and suicides. Adding in social factors, such as isolation, limited opportunities, and cultural stresses, American Indian and Alaska Native youth face numerous risks. Many of these are preventable and include behavioral changes such as using seat belts and contraceptives, practicing abstinence, increasing social activities, preventing high school dropout, etc. American Indian youth experience twice the risks for dropping out of high school, living in poverty, and experiencing an early death. But they are half as likely to use contraceptives. The result is that some youth are less healthy than their non-Indian counterparts.[43]

American Indians and Alaska Natives remain at a higher risk for mental health challenges, as well. Budget constraints restrict the Indian Health Service to providing emergency services only. Substance abuse, depression, anxiety, violence, and suicide remain significant concerns today. Lack of resources often mandate American Indians and Alaska Natives go without services. With alcohol tied to nearly 12 percent of American Indian deaths, the need for mental health services is apparent. Unintentional injuries also strike American Indians and Alaska Natives at 1.5 times the U.S. rate. These injuries are usually associated with alcohol and drug abuse. Such injuries result in 46 percent of the Years of Potential Life Lost. Motor vehicle death rates are twice the national rate, pedestrian-related vehicle death rates are three times the rate, drownings are twice the national rate, and fire-related deaths are three times the rate.[44]

As American Indians and Alaska Natives live longer they are increasingly experiencing higher rates of death from heart diseases, which today is the number 1 cause of death in Indian Country, with the rate for American Indians double the national rate. While American Indians experience a lower stroke rate, as their life expectancy rises so, too, does their likelihood of stroke. While cancer incidence and death rates are lower among American Indians and Alaska Natives than the national averages, the rate of American Indian cancer deaths to new cancer cases is higher than non-Indians. American Indians also have the lowest cancer survival rates of any ethnic group in the United States.[45]

AIDS remains a silent killer in some American Indian and Alaska Native communities. Transmitted largely via needles and unprotected sex (along with high levels of sexually transmitted diseases), AIDS now affects American Indians and Alaska Natives at a 40 percent higher rate than Caucasians. The Indian Health Service fears that because American Indians and Alaska Natives are "already sicker" than the U.S. population as a whole, AIDS may "exact a greater toll" among them and cause untold suffering.[46]

Not surprisingly, the history of healthcare among American Indians since European contact is somewhat of "an unnatural history of disease." More than any other ethnic group in the United States, American Indians and Alaska Natives experience a lower level of well-being. And their well-being is more intimately associated with the "social, economic, and political conditions" under which these Americans live. As these conditions change, so, too, will American Indian and Alaska Native health conditions. Some providers fear that while American Indian health has improved, relative to the improvement in overall American health the real status of American Indian health has reached a plateau. Critics fear that "the lower frequency at which American Indians access care will erode the previous health status improvements." Particularly at risk are the elderly, disabled, and infants, largely because of transportation limitations, social disadvantages, and language barriers.[47]

Some gains in health status may be illusional. A reduction in infant mortality among the Warms Springs (Oregon) Klamath and Modoc tribes may not be nearly as dramatic as initially reported. According to the Indian Health Service, the infant mortality rate at Warm Springs was lower than the national average. But when a team of researchers evaluated the methodology used by the Indian Health Service they discovered that the rate has actually increased due to "frequent misclassification of race on death certificates." The Indian Health Service used death certificates with designation of race to determine infant death rates and, by so doing, established a rate of 10.2 deaths per 1,000 live births. Using birth certificates to determine infant death rates increased it to 15.8 deaths per 1,000 live births. While lower than the 62.7 deaths per 1,000 live births in the 1950s, the Warm Springs example illustrates the data management of the Indian Health Service can be manipulated.[48]

Other studies point to a rise in fetal alcohol syndrome (FAS) and fetal alcohol effect (FAE) among some tribal nations. While the Indian Health Service funds an FAS project in the Northern Plains, it has not yet discovered a way to track substance abuse among prenatal patients. In the interim, tribes have assumed this responsibility and are jailing prenatal abusers in an attempt to protect the unborn, an effort many experts criticize as ignoring the root cause of alcohol abuse.[49]

To stem the national tide of changing health needs and to ensure a healthy nation in the twenty-first century, the Department of Health and Human Services issued a series of national health objectives in 1990 entitled "Healthy People 2000." Twenty-two of these objectives were specific to American Indians and Alaska Natives, and were designed to reduce behavioral health risks. These objectives are important as they set guidelines to assist the Indian Health Service in raising the health status of American Indians and Alaska Natives to a level equal that of the rest of the nation, a goal that will be difficult to cure without social and behavioral changes among American Indians and Alaska Natives and substantive changes in federal Indian health policy.

## Future Challenges

As the Indian Health Service entered the twenty-first century, challenges remained. The question is: Have American Indians and Alaska Natives received better care over the past half century since the Indian Health Service was established in 1955? In the years immediately following the Indian Health Transfer Act there was a high level of *espirit de corps* within the agency. Healthcare providers like Ray Shaw and Carruth Wagner had a clear vision of what was required to combat ill-health and improve Indian health status. There was a united effort on the part of healthcare providers throughout Indian Country. As the years passed, the level of *espirit de corps* diminished and the agency lost sight of its vision while at the same time it matured into a federal bureaucracy. While there were improvements in healthcare, changing conditions, such as social and behavioral causes of disease and a booming youth population, required new approaches in the delivery of services. Epidemic diseases such as AIDS, diabetes, cancer, and violent deaths continue to increase and remain a fact of life in Indian Country.

It is also prudent to consider the success of community-based programs in providing a culturally relevant and community-oriented approach to well-being. While community hospitals were constructed, sanitation facilities installed, and community health workers trained and employed, much remains to be done. Tribal nations continue to assume control over their own hospitals and clinics via 638 contracts or self-governance compacts (now over 50 percent of the Indian Health Service) and hire their own healthcare professionals. In much of Indian Country, however, there is still a lack of continuity in providing health services. Turnover rates for physicians, nurses, pharmacists, and other providers remain high. Chronic shortages result in the Indian Health Service hiring temporary physicians, which does not lend itself to continuity and community-oriented medicine.

While there are more American Indian and Alaska Native health professionals than ever before employed by the Indian Health Service, the agency continues to struggle in developing a community-based program that is relevant to the unique and distinct American Indian and Alaska Native communities. This may be due to the inability of federal agencies finding the ways and means of adapting programs to fit the needs of 564 distinct tribal communities. Culturally relevant programs are not likely until tribal nations assume broader control over their own health services and the federal government fully funds healthcare services. As importantly, American Indians and Alaska Natives must adopt appropriate social and behavioral changes.

Finally, in the twenty-first century can tribal nations expect Congress to fully fund a program that they purchased at the great expense of their land and resources? Is health parity attainable? While there have been funding increases since the Indian Health Transfer Act, and a budget that surpassed $4 billion in 2009, the agency continues to struggle to secure adequate funding. The Congress since the 1990s has sought to reduce program funding and/or transfer respon-sibilities to the states, subjecting tribal nations to state authority. Congress has never made Indian healthcare a priority, with such parsimony leading to tribal feuds over scarce resources. These feuds include reservation versus urban, and estab-lished tribes versus recently recognized tribes. As the agency has matured, Con-gress has failed to provide it with the resources necessary to operate efficiently. If history is an indicator, Congress is unlikely to fulfill its legal and moral obligation to American Indians and Alaska Natives.

The Indian Health Service has made important gains in the past half century. More American Indians and Alaska Natives today are living a less harsh life than their forefathers and mothers. Yet, the ultimate question is: Has the United States made good on its moral and legal pledge to tribal nations by ensuring them of a reasonable standard of health? Despite impressive gains since 1955, health parity remains an elusive goal, leading to the conclusion that the nation has not yet fulfilled its legal and moral fiduciary responsibility to American Indians and Alaska Natives by providing them healthcare parity.

# Notes

1. Trujillo was nominated as director by several Alaska Native organizations. Born in the old Santa Fe Indian Hospital on April 11, 1944, Trujillo earned 2 bachelor's degrees and a master's degree at the University of New Mexico and a medical degree from the University of Minnesota. He received a clinical fellowship at the prestigious Mayo Clinic in Rochester, Minnesota, and became the first American Indian trained in internal medicine at Mayo Clinic. He also received training as a family practitioner, but spent most of his career with the Indian Health Service developing and implementing health programs. *Hearings before the Select Committee on Indian Affairs United States Senate*, 103rd Congress, 2d session, January 27, 1994. *Congressional Record* (140:33), March 22, 1994, S3445. Trujillo was a member of the American College of Physician Executives, the Association of American Indian Physicians, the Association of Military Surgeons of the United States, the National Rural Health Care Association, the Western Canadian/American Health Council, and the American Public Health Association. He served on numerous committees within the Indian Health Service. "IHS Head Sees Unification Needed to Solve Problems," *Indian Country Today* (September 22, 1993), A1-2. "Michael Trujillo Begins Second Term as Indian Health Service Director," www.hhs.gov/news/press/1998.

2. Grim holds a doctorate in dental surgery and a master's degree in health services administration. He is a career Commissioned Corps Officer in the United States Public Health Service (Rear Admiral). He was appointed by President George W. Bush and was subsequently reappointed to a second term as director in September 2007, but withdrew his name from consideration after the Office of Management and Budget "excised comments referring to laws . . . requir(ing) the federal government to provide healthcare for American Indians." "Nomination Withdrawn," *Journal of the American Medical Association*, October 10, 2007, (298:14), 1631. McSwain served as acting director from September 2007 until he was confirmed by the Senate on April 29, 2008. He holds a bachelor's degree in business administration and a master's degree in public administration. Roubideaux was Assistant Professor in Family and Community Medicine at the University of Arizona at the time of her appointment. She served as Medical Officer and Clinical Director at the San Carlos Apache Hospital and at the Huhugam Memorial Hospital in the Gila River Indian Community, where she conducted extensive research on diabetes. She holds a master's degree in Public Health from the Harvard School of Public Health and an MD from Harvard Medical School.

3. Charles W. Grim, "Former Director of the Indian Health Service," aianhealthcareers.org. p.1. "Barack Obama: Principles for Stronger Tribal Communities," barakobama.com, May 23, 2009.

4. *Broken Promises: Evaluating the Native American Health Care System* (Washington, D.C.: United States Commission on Civil Rights, September 2004), 98. Gregg, *The Indians and the Nurse*, 38.

5. Jennie Joe, "The Delivery of Health Care to American Indians: History, Policies and Prospects," in Donald E. Green and Thomas V. Tonnesen, Eds. *American Indians: Social Justice and Public Policy* (Milwaukee: University of Wisconsin System Institute on Race and Ethnicity, 1991), 150. "Department of Health and Human Services, Statement of Charles W. Grim, D.D.S., M.H.S.A. Interim Director, Indian Health Service, before the Senate Committee on Indian Affairs, June 11, 2003" (Washington, D.C.: GPO, 2003), 11.

6. Kelly Bannister, "Indigenous Knowledge and Traditional Plant Resources of the Secwepemc (Shuswa) Nation," in Mary Riley, ed., *Indigenous Intellectual Property Rights: Legal Obstacles and Innovative Solutions* (Altamira Press, 2004), 288. "Navajos Curtail Health Studies," *The Arizona Republic* (106:172, November 6, 1995), A-1.

7. "Navajos Curtail Health Studies." After birth, the Navajo hold a ceremony and bury the cord "in a secret place on the reservation."

8. As of April 2009, the suit had not yet been resolved and is being reviewed by the Arizona Supreme Court.

9. John Red Horse, Troy Johnson and Diane Weiner, "Commentary: Cultural Perspectives on Research among American Indians," *American Indian Culture and Research Journal* (13:3-4, 1989).

10. "Opening Statement: Indian Health Service Director Designate Yvette Roubideaux before the Senate Committee on Indian Affairs," United States Senate, Committee on Indian Affairs (Washington, D.C., Government Printing Office, April 23, 2009), 2.

11. Charles W. Grim, "Indian Health Service Tackles New Priorities in Health Care," *U.S. Medicine: The Voice of Federal Medicine* (Washington, D.C., January 2007), 3.

12. Rashid Bashshur, William Steeler and Tim Murphy, "On Changing Indian Eligibility for Health Care," *American Journal of Public Health* (77:6, June 1987). "Statement of Grim," 9. Grim adds that increased political influence by tribal governments is having a positive impact on health.

13. *Federal Register* (52:179, September 16, 1987), 35044. "Opening Statement from Director Designate Yvette Roubideaux." "Statement of Grim," 18.

14. "National Health Care Reform and Its Implications for Indian Health Care," *Hearings before the Committee on Indian Affairs United States Senate*, 103rd Congress, 2d session, May 9, 1994. "Principles for Strong Tribal Communities," 1. H.R. 676, a bill "To provide for comprehensive health insurance coverage for all United States residents, improved health care delivery, and for other purposes," in Section 401(b) of Title IV states that "This Act provides for health programs of the Indian Health Service to initially remain independent for the 5-year period that begins on the date of the establishment of the [United States National Health Insurance] program, after which such programs shall be integrated into the USNHI program."

15. "National Health Care Reform and Its Implications for Indian Health Care," May 9, 1994. "Health Care Reform in Indian Country: Oversight of the Indian Health Service." "Statement of Grim," 18.

16. *Broken Promises*, 7.

17. Venice L. Bonham, "Race, Ethnicity, and Pain Treatment: Striving to Understand the Causes of Disparities in Pain Treatments," *Journal of Law, Medicine and Ethics*, Vol. 29 (Spring 2001), 52. Ann Garwick and Sally Auger, "What Do Providers Need to Know about American Indian Culture? Recommendations for Urban Indian Family Caregivers," *Families, Systems and Health*, Official Journal of Collaborative Family Healthcare Association, Vol. 18, (2002), 177.

18. *Broken Promises*, 32-33.

19. *Broken Promises*, 37.

20. U.S. Census Bureau, Public Information Office, "Nation's Household Income

Stable in 2000, Poverty Rate Virtually Equals Record Low," *Census Bureau Reports*, September 25, 2001, CB01-158. James Krieger and Donna L. Higgins, "Housing and Health: Time Again for Public Health Action," *American Journal of Public Health*, vol. 92 (2002) 758. Grim, "Former Director," 2.

21. Grim, "Former Director," 3. Everett Rhoades, "The Health Status of American Indian and Alaska Native Males," *American Journal of Public Health*, vol. 93 (2003), 777, "Statement of Grim," 6.

22. Rhoades, "Barriers to Health Care."

23. *Broken Promises*, 70-71. Dr. Craig Vanderwagen, acting Chief Medical Officer of the Indian Health Service, quoted in *Broken Promises*, 66.

24. *Broken Promises*, 74-75.

25. "Statement of Grim," 15. *Broken Promises*, 76.

26. *Broken Promises*, 77. The Registered Nurse vacancy rate among the Navajo is 25 percent per annum.

27. *Broken Promises*, 70.

28. U.S. Department of Health and Human Services, Indian Health Service, Fiscal Year 2005 Budget Justifications, Indian Health Professionals, IHS-119.

29. *Broken Promises*, 81-83.

30. Indian Health Service Factsheet accessed at *www.info.ihs.gov*.

31. Health and Human Services, Indian Health Service Justification of Estimates for Appropriations Committees, IHS-2. *House Report 94-1194*, 2746. *Broken Promises*, 100.

32. *Broken Promises*, 90, 92-93. Not everyone agreed that the FDI index is accurate. The Alaska Native Health Board noted the index failed to consider small and extremely isolated facilities "where medical conditions and comparisons simply do not apply."

33. *Broken Promises*, 99.

34. *Broken Promises*, 103. Henry J. Kaiser Family Foundation, "American Indian and Alaska Native Health Coverage and Access to Care," (February 2004).

35. *Broken Promises*, 110-111.

36. Rodney L. Brod and Ronald Ladue, "Political Mobilization and Conflict among Western Urban and Reservation Indian Health Service Programs," *American Indian Culture and Research Journal* (13:3-4, 1989).

37. *The Health Status of Urban American Indians and Alaska Natives: An Analysis of Select Vital Records and Census Data Sources*, Urban Indians Health Institute, (Seattle, Washington, 2004).

38. John L. Schultz, *White Medicine Indian Lives...As Long As the Grass Shall Grow* (Colorado State University, 1976).

39. Everett R. Rhoades, John Hammond, Thomas K. Welty, Aaron O. Handler and Robert W. Amler, "The Indian Burden of Illness and Future Health Interventions," *Public Health Reports* (102:4, July-August 1987). "Michael Trujillo begins Second Term as IHS Director, *www.ihs.gov/1998press*. Grim, "Former Director of the Indian Health Service," 2. "Statement by Robert G. McSwain, Director of the Indian Health Service, on nomination to Director of the Indian Health Service before the Committee on Indian Affairs, United States Senate," dated February 7, 2008, 2. Roubideaux, "Opening Statement," 3-5.

40. "Tribes Urge Western Doctors to Be More Open to 'Old Ways'," *The Arizona Republic* (104:84, August 9, 1993), A-1.

41. Gregory R. Campbell, "The Changing Dimension of Native American Health: A Critical Understanding of Contemporary Native American Health Issues," *American Indian Culture and Research Journal* (13:3-4, 1989).

42. The Pima Indians of Arizona now have the highest rate of diabetes of any people group in the world, with rates approaching 70 percent. Carolyn Smith-Morris, *Diabetes among the Pima* (Tucson: University of Arizona Press, 2006). For forty years the Pima have been the most-studied diabetic population in the world.

43. Blum et al. "American Indian-Alaska Native Youth Health."

44. *Broken Promises*, 14-15.

45. *Broken Promises*, 15, 17-18. "Arizona group gets $4 million to fight Indian cancer disparities," *Arizona Republic*, October 29, 2005, B-8. Arizona Indians have the lowest five year survival rate for all forms of cancer.

46. "AIDS Takes a Growing Toll on Native Americans," *Arizona Republic*, Special Report, July 3, 2005, A-1, 16-17.

47. Campbell, "The Changing Dimension of Native American Health: A Critical Understanding of Contemporary Native American Health Issues."

48. Nakamura et al., "Excess Infant Mortality in an American Indian Population, 1940-1990."

49. Duimstra et al., "A Fetal Alcohol Syndrome Surveillance Pilot Project in American Indian Communities in the Northern Plains." "Tribes Using Jail, Birth Control, to Fight FAS Abuse," *Indian Country Today* Southwest Edition (15:16, October 16, 1995).

# BIBLIOGRAPHY

## The National Archives of the United States

*Ratified Treaties 1854-1855*. National Archives, Record Group 75, T-494, Rolls 5-6, Indian Records Office.

*Ratified Treaties 1856-1863*. National Archives, Record Group 75, Indian Records Office.

*Official Letters of W. J. McConnell*. National Archives, Record Group 48, Secretary of the Interior Records Office.

*Indian Inspection Reports*. National Archives, Record Group 48, Office of the Secretary of the Interior, Indian Division.

*Office of Indian Affairs, Circulars*. National Archives, Record Group 75, M1121, Rolls 9, 10, 11, Educational Circulars.

## Articles

"A Truly Remote Place," *Journal of the American Medical Association* (230:6) November 11, 1974.

Abramowitz, J. "A Children's Dental Program for American Indians," *Journal of the American Dental Association* (81:8) August 1970.

"AIPRC's Report on Indian Health," *American Indian Journal* (3:2) Spring 1977.

"American Indians Trained as Physician Assistants," *Health Services and Mental Health Administration Health Reports* (86:7) July 1971.

"Awards, Honors," *Journal of the American Medical Association* (192:7) May 17, 1965.

Bannister, Kelly P. "Indigenous Knowledge and Traditional Plant Resources of the Secwepemc (Shuswa) Nation," in Mary Riley, editor, *Indigenous Intellectual Property Rights: Legal Obstacles and Innovative Solutions* (California: Altamira Press, 2004).

Bartha, Gregory W., Thomas A. Burch and Peter H. Bennett. "Hyperglycemia in Washoe and Northern Paiute Indians," *Diabetes* (22:1) January 1973.

Bashshur, Rashid, William Steeler and Tim Murphy. "On Changing Indian Eligibility for Health Care," *American Journal of Public Health* (77:6) June 1987.

Bathke, Jerry. "The Community Health Medic in Indian America," *World Health Association Public Health Paper No. 60* (Geneva, Switzerland), 1974.

Bean, L. J. and Corrine Wood, "The Crisis in Indian Health: A California Example," *The Indian Historian* (2:3) Fall 1969.

Benson, Otis O. "Conditions in the Indian Medical Service," *Journal of the American Medical Association* (81:16) 1923.

Blue Spruce, George. "American Indians as Dental Patients," *Public Health Reports* (76:12) December 1961.

———. "Needed: Indian Health Professionals," *Health Services Reports* (88:8) October 1973.

Blum, Robert W., Brian Harmon, Linda Harris, Lois Bergeisen and Michael D. Resnick. "American Indian-Alaska Native Youth Health," *Journal of the American Medical Association* (267:12) March 25, 1992.

Bonham, Venice L. "Race, Ethnicity, and Pain Treatment: Striving to Understand the Causes of Disparities in Pain Treatments," *Journal of Law, Medicine and Ethics*, Vol. 29 (Spring 2001).

Braasch, W. F., B. J. Branton and A. J. Chesley. "Survey of Medical Care Among the Upper Midwest Indians," *Journal of the American Medical Association* (139:4) January 22, 1949.

Brod, Rodney L. and Ronald Ladue. "Political Mobilization and Conflict among Western Urban and Reservation Indian Health Service Programs," *American Indian Culture and Research Journal* (13:3-4) 1989.

Brodt, William. "Implications for Training Curriculum from a Task Inventory Survey of Indian Community Health Representatives," *Public Health Reports* (90:6) December 1975.

Bronner, Felix. "Fluoridation—Issue or Obsession?" *The American Journal of Clinical Nutrition* (22:10) October 1969.

Brown, James E. and Chris Christiansen. "Biliary Tract Disease among the Navajo," *Journal of the American Medical Association* (202:11) December 11, 1967.

Brown, Virginia B., William B. Mason and Michael Kaczmarski. "A Computerized Health Information Service," *Nursing Outlook* (19:3) March 1971.

Campbell, Gregory R. "The Changing Dimension of Native American Health: A Critical Understanding of Contemporary Native American Health Issues," *American Indian Culture and Research Journal* (13:3-4) 1989.

Castillo, David D. "The Impact of Euro-American Exploration and Settlement," in *Handbook of North American Indians: California* (Washington, D.C.: Smithsonian Institution, 1978).

Castro, Tony. "Crisis of the Urban Indian," *Human Needs* (1:2) August 1972.

Chelikowsky, Bruce. "Half of the 1983 Plague Cases Reported in the United States Occurred in Indians," *Public Health Reports* (99:1) January-February 1984.

Cobb, John C. and Chandler R. Dawson. "Trachoma among Southwestern Indians," *Journal of the American Medical Association* (175:5) November 1961.

Comess, L. J., P. H. Bennett, M. B. Man, T. A. Burch and Max Miller. "Congenital Anomalies and Diabetes in the Pima Indians of Arizona," *Diabetes* (18:7) July 1969.

"Committee on Legislation," *Journal of the American Medical Association* (149:3). May 17, 1952.

"Committee on Legislation," *Journal of the American Medical Association* (151:9). February 28, 1953.

"Committee on Legislation," *Journal of the American Medical Association* (152:2). May 9, 1953.

"Committee on Legislation," *Journal of the American Medical Association* (155:8) June 19, 1954.

"Council on Medical Service," *Journal of the American Medical Association* (186:4) November 26, 1963.

"Council on Medical Service," *Journal of the American Medical Association* (190:4) October 26, 1964.

Cowen, Ron. "Seeds of Protection: Ancestral Menus May Hold a Message for Diabetes-Prone Descendants," *Science News* (137) June 2, 1990.

De Geyndt, Willy. "Health Behaviors and Health Needs of Urban Indians in Minneapolis," *Public Health Reports* (88:4) April 1973.

Deuschle, Kurt W. "Training and Use of Medical Auxiliaries in a Navajo Community," *Public Health Reports* (78:6) June 1963.

Dillingham, Brint. "Indian Health Service and the Health Information System," *American Indian Journal* (3:4) Fall 1977.

———. "Indian Women and IHS Sterilization Practices," *American Indian Journal* (3:1) January 1977.

———. "Sterilization of Native Americans," *American Indian Journal* (3:7), July 1977.

———. "Sterilization Update," *American Indian Journal* (3:9) September 1977.

"Distribution of AIDS Cases, by Racial/Ethnic Group and Exposure Category, United States, June 1, 1981-July 4, 1988," *Journal of the American Medical Association* (261:2) January 13, 1989.

Duimstra, Cindy, Darlene Johnson, Charlotte Kutsch, Belle Wang, Miriam Zentner, Scott Kellerman and Thomas Welty. "A Fetal Alcohol Syndrome Surveillance Pilot Project in American Indian Communities in the Northern Plains," *Public Health Reports* (108:2) March-April 1993.

Emerson, Haven. "Morbidity of the American Indians," *Science* (68:1626) 1926.

Fahy, Agnes and Carl Muschenheim. "Third National Conference on American Indian Health," *Journal of the American Medical Association* (194:10) December 6, 1965.

Fleming, Arthur. "Indian Health," *Public Health Reports* (74:6) June 1959.

Foard, Fred T. "The Federal Government and American Indians' Health," *Journal of the American Medical Association* (142:5) February 4, 1950.

Foster, Ashley, Alice M. Haggerty and Edwin O. Goodman. "Use of Health Services in Relation to the Physical Environment of an Indian Population," *Health Services Reports* (88:8) October 1973.

Foster, Stanley O. "Trachoma in an American Indian Village," *Public Health Reports* (80:9) September 1965.

"From the Assistant Secretary for Health," *Journal of the American Medical Association* (260:10) September 9, 1988.

Gallaher, M. M., D. W. Fleming, L. R. Berger and C. M. Sewell. "Pedestrian and Hypothermia Deaths among Native Americans in New Mexico Between Bar and Home," *Journal of the American Medical Association* (267:10) March 11, 1992.

Garwick, Ann and Sally Auger. "What Do Providers Need to Know about American Indian Culture? Recommendations for Urban Family Caregivers," Families, Systems and Health, Official Journal of Collaborative Family Healthcare Association (18) 2002.

"Genetic Lag Plagues Indian Survival," *Journal of the American Medical Association* (205:3) July 15, 1968.

Glasbrenner, Kimberly. "Seeking 'Indian-Acceptable' Ways to Fight Hypertension," *Journal of the American Medical Association* (254:14) October 11, 1985.

Goldsmith, Marsha F. "American Indian medicine aims to add physicians, improve health," *Journal of the American Medical Association* (254:14) October 11, 1985.

"Government Services" *Journal of the American Medical Association* (152:14) August 1, 1953.

"Government Services: Public Health Service" *Journal of the American Medical Association* (160:7) February 18, 1956.

Grim, Charles W. "IHS Tackles New Priorities in Health Care," *U.S. Medicine: The Voice of Federal Medicine* Washington, D.C., January 2007.

Gunn, Sisvan W. A. "Totemic Medicine and Shamanism Among the Northwest American Indians," *Journal of the American Medical Association* (196:8) May 23, 1966.

Harrison, Thomas J. "Training for Village Health Aides in the Kotzebue Area of Alaska," *Public Health Reports* (80:7) July 1965.

"Healthier Indian Mothers and Babies," *Public Health Reports* (79:6) June 1964.

Henry, R. E., Thomas A. Burch, Peter H. Bennett and Max Miller. "Diabetes in the Cocopah Indians," *Diabetes* (18:7) July 1969.

Hesse, Frank. "A Dietary Study of the Pima Indian," *American Journal of Clinical Nutrition* (7:5) September-October 1959.

———. "Incidence of Cholecystitis and Other Diseases among the Pima Indians of Southern Arizona," *Journal of the American Medical Association* (170:15) August 8, 1959.

Heyward, William L., Anne P. Lanier, Brian J. McMahan, Mary Anne Fitzgerald, Steven Kilkinny and Thaddeus R. Paprocki. "Early Detection of Primary Hepatocellular Carcinoma," *Journal of the American Medical Association* (254:21) December 6, 1985.

Hill, Charles A. "Measure of Longevity of American Indians," *Public Health Reports* (85:3) March 1970.

Hoffman, Frederick L. "Conditions in the Indian Medical Service," *Journal of the American Medical Association* (75:7) 1920.

———. "Conditions in the Indian Medical Service," *Journal of the American Medical Association* (81:10) 1923.

Hostetter, C. L. and J. D. Felsen. "Multiple Variable Motivators Involved in the Recruitment of Physicians for the Indian Health Service," *Rural Health* (90:4) July-August 1975.

Hrdlicka, Ales. "The Vanishing Indian," *Science* (46:1185) 1917.

Iba, B. Y., J. D. Niswander and L. Woodville. "Relation of Prenatal Care to Birth Weight, Major Malformations, and Newborn Deaths of American Indians," *Health Services Reports* (88:8) October 1973.

"Indian Aide Helps Reservation Physician," *Journal of the American Medical Association* (224:8) May 21, 1973.

"Indian Healing Ceremonies Get New Lease on Life," *Journal of the American Medical Association* (221:9) August 28, 1972.

"Indian Health Advisory Committee," *Journal of the American Medical Association* (161:6) June 9, 1956.

"Indian Health Service Facilities Become Smoke-Free," *Journal of the American Medical Association* (258:2) May 1985.

"Indian Health Service Modernizes Medical Care on Reservations," *Journal of the American Medical Association* (218:4) October 25, 1971.

"Infant Death Rate of American Indians Dropped 30% Since 1954," *Journal of the American Medical Association* (180:11) March 17, 1962.

Irvine, John. "The Navajo," *Journal of the American Medical Association* (213:1) July 6, 1970.

Joe, Jennie. "The Delivery of Health Care to American Indians: History, Policies and Prospects," in Donald E. Green and Thomas V. Tonnesen, *American Indians: Social Justice and Public Policy* (Milwaukee: University of Wisconsin System Institute on Race and Ethnicity, 1991).

Jonz, Wallace W. "Staffing Health Education Programs for American Indians," *Public Health Reports* (81:7) July 1966.

Kane, Robert L. "Community Medicine on the Navajo Reservation," *Health Services and Mental Health Administration Health Reports* (86:8) August 1971.

Karsten Larson, Janet. "And Then There Were None: Is Federal Policy Endangering the American Indian 'Species?'" *Christian Century* (94) January 26, 1977.

Keneally, Henry J. "The Philosophy of Good Tribal Relations," *Journal of American Indian Education* (1:3) May 1962.

Kost-Grant, Brian L. "Self-Inflicted Gunshot Wounds Among Alaska Natives," *Public Health Reports* (98:1) January-February 1983.

Krieger, James and Donna L. Higgins. "Housing and Health: Time Again for Public Health Action," *American Journal of Public Health* (92) 2002.

Kunitz, Stephen J. and John C. Slocumb. "The Use of Surgery to Avoid Childbearing among Navajo and Hopi Indians," *Human Biology* (48:1) February 1976.

Lasersohn, William. "Acute Diarrheal Disease in a Zuni Village," *Public Health Reports* (80:5) May 1965.

"Leading Major Congenital Malformations among Minority Groups in the United States, 1981-1988," *Journal of the American Medical Association* (261:2) January 13, 1989.

Lemon, Frank R. "Health Problems of the Navajos in Monument Valley, Utah," *Public Health Reports* (75:11) November 1960.

Leupp, Frances, "Outlines of an Indian Policy," *Outlook* (79) 1909.

Liberty, Margot, David V. Hughney and Richard Scaglion. "Rural and Urban Omaha Indian Fertility," *Human Biology* (48:1) February 1976.

"Life on an Isolated Indian Reservation Not Perfect, but," *Journal of the American Medical Association* (230:6) November 11, 1974.

Mail, Patricia D. "Hippocrates Was a Medicine Man: The Health Care of Native Americans in the Twentieth Century," *The Annals of the American Academy* (436:3) March 1978.

Martin, Morgan. "Native American Medicine: Thoughts for Posttraditional Healers," *Journal of the American Medical Association* (245:2) January 9, 1981.

Matthews, Washington. "Consumption among the Indians," *Transactions of the American Climatological Association* 1886.

———. "Further Contribution to the Study of Consumption among the Indians," *Transactions of the American Climatological Association* 1886.

May, Philip A., Karen J. Hymbaugh, Jon A. Aase and Jonathan M. Samet. "Epidemiology of Fetal Alcohol Syndrome Among American Indians of the Southwest," *Social Biology* (30:4) 1983.

McCreary, C., C. Deegan and D. Thompson. "Indian Health in Minnesota," *Minnesota Medicine* (2:56), October 1973.

McDermott, Walsh, Kurt W. Deuschle, and Clifford R. Barnett. "Health Care Experiment at Many Farms," *Science* (175:1) January 7, 1972.

"McGibony Named Director of Health of Indian Service," *Journal of the American Medical Association* (117:2) 1941.

"Medical News" *Journal of the American Medical Association* (150:16) December 20, 1952.

"Medical News," *Journal of the American Medical Association* (195:5) January 31, 1966.

"Medical News: Progress Report: Some Gains, But a Lot Remains to Be Done," *Journal of the American Medical Association* (218:4) October 25, 1971.

"Medicine's Door Opens Wider to Indians," *Journal of the American Medical Association* (218:5) November 1, 1971.

"Metabolic Research Unit for Phoenix Medical Center," *Public Health Reports* (82:4) April 1967.

Miller, M., T. A. Burch, P. H. Bennett and A. G. Steinberg. "Prevalence of Diabetes Mellitus in American Indians: Results of Glucose Tolerance Tests in the Pima Indians of Arizona," *Diabetes* (14) July 1965.

Mortimer, E. A. "Indian Health: An Unmet Problem," *Pediatrics* (51:6) June 1973.

Nakamura, Roy M., Richard King, Ernest H. Kimball, Robert K. Oye and Steven D. Helgerson. "Excess Infant Mortality in an American Indian Population, 1940-1990," *Journal of the American Medical Association* (266:16) October 23/30, 1991.

"Navajo Health Authority Is Planning Pan-Indian Medical School," *Health Services Reports* (89:5) September-October 1974.

"Nearly 100 Indians in Medical School," *Journal of the American Medical Association* (230:6) November 11, 1974.

"New Director Appointed for Indian Medical Service," *Indians at Work* (8:10) 1941.

Niswander, Jerry D. and Morton S. Adams "Oral Clefts in the American Indian," *Public Health Reports* (82:9) September 1967.

"Nomination Withdrawn," *Journal of the American Medical Association* (298:14) October 10, 2007.

Oakland, L., and R. L. Kane. "The Working Mother and Child Neglect on the Navajo Reservation," *Pediatrics* (51:5) May 1973.

Odgen, Michael, Mozart I. Spector and Charles A. Hill. "Suicide and Homicide among Indians," *Public Health Reports* (85:1) January 1970.

"Organizational News," *Journal of the American Medical Association* (149:3) May 17, 1952.

Owens, Arthur. "The New Surge in Physicians' Earnings and Expenses," *Medical Economics* (46:12) December 1969.

Owens, Mitchell V. "Graduate Education Program in Public Health for American Indians," *Public Health Reports* (94:3) May-June 1979.

Owens, Mitchell V., Charles M. Cameron, Jr., and Patti Hickman. "Job Achievements of Indian and Non-Indian Graduates in Public Health: How Do They Compare?" *Public Health Reports* (102:4) July-August 1987.

Portney, G. L. and S. B. Portney. "Epidemiology of Trachoma in the San Xavier Papago Indians," *Archives of Ophthalmology* (86:9) September 1971.

"Presidential Medal of Freedom Awarded to Annie D. Wauneka," *Public Health Reports* (78:10) October 1963.

Rabeau, Erwin S. and Angel Reund. "Evaluation of PHS Program Providing Family Planning Services for American Indians," *American Journal of Public Health* (59:8) August 1969.

Red Horse, John, Troy Johnson and Diane Weiner. "Commentary: Cultural Perspectives on Research among American Indians," *American Indian Culture and Research Journal* (13:3-4) 1989.

Rhoades, Everett R. "Barriers to Health Care: The Unique Problems Facing American Indians," *Civil Rights Digest* (10:1) Fall 1977.

————. "The Health Status of American Indian and Alaska Native Males," *American Journal of Public Health* (93) 2003.

Rhoades, Everett R., John Hammond, Thomas K. Welty, Aaron O. Handler and Robert W. Amler. "The Indian Burden of Illness and Future Health Interventions," *Public Health Reports* (102:4) July-August 1987.

Rubenstein, A., J. Boyle, C. L. Odoroff and S. J. Kunitz. "Effects of Improved Sanitary Facilities on Infant Diarrhea in a Hopi Village," *Public Health Reports* (84:12) December 1969.

Ruggera, Gary. "Diet Counseling to Improve Hematocrit Values of Children on the Blackfeet Reservation," *Health Services Reports* (88:8) October 1973.

"Satellite Helps to Bring Health Care to the Indians," *Journal of the American Medical Association* (230:6) November 11, 1974.

Schlafman, Irving. "Health Systems Research to Deliver Comprehensive Services to Indians," *Public Health Reports* (84:8) August 1969.

Schlife, C. "Smokeless Tobacco Use in Rural Alaska," *Journal of the American Medical Association* (257:14) April 10, 1987.

Senese, Guy. "Self-Determination and American Indian Education: An Illusion of Control," *Educational Theory* (36:2) Spring 1986.

Sievers, Maurice L. "Disease Patterns Among Southwestern Indians," *Public Health Reports* (81:12) December 1966.

————. "Cigarette and Alcohol Usage by Southwestern American Indians," *American Journal of Public Health and the Nation's Health* (58:1) January 1968.

Sievers, Maurice L. and Jeffrey R. Fisher. "Diseases of North American Indians," in Henry Rothschild, ed., *Biocultural Aspects of Disease* (New York: Academic Press, 1981).

Sievers, Maurice L. and James R. Marquis. "The Southwestern American Indian's Burden: Biliary Disease," *Journal of the American Medical Association* (182:5) November 3, 1962.

Simpson, Sylvia G., Raymond Reid, Susan P. Baker and Stephen Teret. "Injuries Among the Hopi Indians," *Journal of the American Medical Association* (249:14) April 8, 1983.

Stevenson, Albert H. "Sanitary Facilities Construction Program for Indians and Alaska Natives," *Public Health Reports* (76:4) April 1961.

"Substitute Doctors Are on the Way to Aid the Indian Health Service," *Journal of the American Medical Association* (218:5) November 1, 1971.

Taylor, Carl W. Jr., and Armin L. Saeger, Jr. "Maternal Health and Socioeconomic Status of Non Reservation Indians," *Public Health Reports* (83:6) June 1968.

Temkin-Greener, Helena, Stephen J. Kunitz, David Broudy and Marlene Haffner. "Surgical Fertility Regulation among Women on the Navajo Indian Reservation, 1972-1978," *American Journal of Public Health* (71:4) April 1981.

"The Indians' Health and Public Health," *American Journal of Public Health* (44:11), November 1954.

Trennert, Robert. "White Man's Medicine v. Hopi Tradition: The Smallpox Epidemic of 1899," *Journal of Arizona History* (33:4) Winter 1992.

Uhrich, Richard B. "Tribal Community Health Representatives of the Indian Health Service," *Public Health Reports* (84:11) November 1969.

"Undergraduate Medical Education," *Journal of the American Medical Association* (234:13) December 29, 1975.

Wagner, Carruth J. and Erwin S. Rabeau. "Indian Poverty and Indian Health," *Health, Education and Welfare Indicators* (Department of Health, Education and Welfare), March 1964.

Wallace, Helen M. "Childhood Tuberculosis with Reference to the American Indian," *Public Health Reports* (82:1) January 1967.

———. "The Health of American Indian Children," *Health Services Reports* (87:9) November 1972.

———. "The Health of American Indian Children," *American Journal of Disabled Children* (125:3) March 1973.

———. "The Health of American Indian Children: A Survey of Current Problems and Needs," *Clinical Pediatrics* (12:2) February 1973.

"Washington News," *Journal of the American Medical Association* (158:11) July 16, 1955.

"Washington News: Grants for Indian and Non-Indian Hospitals" *Journal of the American Medical Association* (163:16) April 20, 1957.

"Washington News," *Journal of the American Medical Association* (197:4) July 25, 1966.

Zimmerman, William Jr. "The Role of the Bureau of Indian Affairs," *The Annals of the American Academy of Political and Social Sciences* May 1957.

Zonis, R. D. "Chronic Otitis Media in the Arizona Indian," *Arizona Medicine* (27:6) June 1970.

## Books

Adair, John and K. W. Deuschle. *The People's Health: Medicine and Anthropology in a Navajo Community*. New York: Appleton-Century-Crofts, 1970.

Cahn, Edgar S. and David W. Hearne, editors. *Our Brother's Keeper: The Indian in White America*. New York: New American Library, 1969.

Crosby, Alfred W. *The Columbian Exchange*. Westport, CT: Greenwood Publishing Company, 1972.

DeJong, David H. *Plagues, Politics and Policy: The Indian Medical Service 1908-1955*. Lexington Books, 2008.

Dobyns, Henry F., and William R. Swagerty. *Their Number Became Thinned*. Knoxville: University of Tennessee Press, 1983.

Fixico, Donald L. *Termination and Relocation: Federal Indian Policy, 1945-1960*. Albuquerque: University of New Mexico Press, 1986.

Foreman, Grant. *Indian Removal*. Norman: University of Oklahoma Press, 1932.

Green, Donald E. and Thomas V. Tonnesen. *American Indians: Social Justice and Public Policy*. Milwaukee: University of Wisconsin System Institute on Race and Ethnicity, 1991.

Gregg, Elinor D. *The Indian and the Nurse*. Norman: University of Oklahoma Press, 1965.

*Health Status of Urban American Indians and Alaska Natives: An Analysis of Select Vital Records and Census Data Sources*. Seattle: Urban Indian Health Institute, 2004.

Kaiser Foundation. *American Indians and Alaska Native Health Coverage and Access to Care*. Kaiser Foundation, February 2004.

Kane, Robert and Rosalie Kane. *Federal Health Care (With Reservations!)*. New York: Springer Publishing Company, 1972.

Krauss, Bertram S. *Indian Health in Arizona: A Study of Health Conditions among Central and Southern Arizona Tribes*. Tucson: Bureau of Ethnic Research, University of Arizona, 1954.

LaFarge, Oliver, Ed. *The Changing Indian*. Norman: University of Oklahoma Press, 1942.

Meriam, Lewis. *The Problem of Indian Administration*. Baltimore: Johns Hopkins Press, 1928.

Moorhead, Warren K. *The American Indians in the United States: 1850-1914*. Freeport, NY: Books for Liberty Press, 1969 reprint.

Murphy, Joseph. "The Prevention of Tuberculosis in Indian Schools" in *Journal of the Proceedings and Addresses of the 47th Annual Meeting*. Winona, MN: National Education Association, 1909.

Parron, Thomas. *Alaska's Health: A Survey*. The Graduate School of Public Health, University of Pittsburgh, 1954.

Pierre, George. *American Indian Crisis*. San Antonio: The Naylor Company, 1971.

Prucha, Francis Paul. *The Great Father, The United States Government and the American Indians*. vol. 2. Lincoln: University of Nebraska Press, 1984.

Riley, Mary. *Indigenous Intellectual Property Rights: Legal Obstacles and Innovative Solutions*. Altamira Press, 2004.

Rothschild, Henry, ed. *Biocultural Aspects of Disease*. New York: Academic Press, 1981.

Schultz, John L. *White Medicine Indian Lives . . . As Long As the Grass Shall Grow*. Colorado State University, 1976.

Smith-Morris, Carolyn. *Diabetes Among the Pima*. Tucson: University of Arizona Press, 2006.

Sorkin, Alan. *American Indians and Federal Aid*. Brookings Institute, 1971.

Thornton, Russell. *American Indian Holocaust and Survival: A Population Study Since 1492*. Norman: University of Oklahoma Press, 1987.

Vogel, Virgil J. *American Indian Medicine*. Norman: University of Oklahoma Press, 1970.

Viola, Herman J. *Diplomats in Buckskin: A History of Delegations in Washington City*. Bluffton, NE: Rivilo Press, 1995.

# Court Decisions

*Blue Legs v. United States Environmental Protection Agency*. 668 F. Supp. 1329.

*Blue Legs v. United States Bureau of Indian Affairs*. 867 F2d 1094.

*Blue Legs v. United States Environmental Protection Agency*. 732 F. Supp. 81.

*Freeman v. Morton*. 499 F2d 497.

*McNabb v. Bowen*. 829 F. 2d 787.

*McNabb v. Heckler.* 628 F. Supp. 549.
*Morton v. Mancari.* 359 F. Supp. 585.
*Morton v. Mancari.* 417 U.S. 535.
*Morton v. Ruiz.* 415 U.S. 231.
*Rincon Band of Mission Indians v. Harris.* 618 F2d 569.
*Rincon Band of Mission Indians v. Califano.* 464 F. Supp. 934.
*Southern Indian Health Council v. Otis Bowen, et al.* Civil 88-0240-EJG.
*Tyndall v. United States.* Civil Action no. 77-0004.
*White v. Califano.* 437 F. Supp. 543.

# Unpublished Sources

Brands, Allen. *History of Pharmacy in the Indian Health Service.* Unpublished manuscript in the Commissioned Corps Centennial Archives, History of Medicine Division, National Library of Medicine, Bethesda, Maryland, 1981.

Johnson, Emery. "Indian Health Services and Indian Health Facilities." Health Services and Mental Health Administration. Indian Health Service mimeograph. March 1972.

McCammon, Charles S. "The Terms of Partnership: IHS and the Indian People." Presented at the 13th Annual Tribal Leaders Health Conference, Tucson, Arizona, April 24, 1970.

Rabeau, Erwin S. "The Division of Indian Health: Current and Future Program." Seminar on Indian Health, Tucson, Arizona, November 9-11, 1967.

Rucker, George W. "Indian Housing: A Background Paper." Presented to the 8th Annual Meeting of the Rural Housing Alliance. Rapid City, South Dakota, October 1973.

Schlafman, Irving. "Indian Management of Indian Health Programs." Presented at the Fifth Joint CS-COA Meeting, Washington, D.C., April 2, 1970.

Shaw, James R. "Historical Development of Indian Health Services." Unpublished history of the Indian Health Services, University of Arizona, October 18, 1982.

———. "Indian Health in Historical Perspective." Unpublished paper courtesy of the author, University of Arizona, Tucson, October 18, 1982.

———. Keynote Lunch Presentation. Seventh Annual Meeting of the National Council of Clinical Directors, Tucson, Arizona, 1982.

Thompson, G. P. Carlyle. "Coordination of Health Programs for American Indians and Alaska Natives." Presented at the Seminar on Indian Health, November 9-11, 1967.

Todd, John. "Interview with Dr. Ray Shaw." Unpublished manuscript in the Commissioned Corps Centennial Archives, History of Medicine, National Library of Medicine, Bethesda, Maryland.

———. "Interview with Dr. Carruth Wagner." Unpublished manuscript in the Commissioned Corps Centennial Archives, History of Medicine, National Library of Medicine, Bethesda, Maryland.

———. "Interview with Dr. Erwin S. Rabeau." Unpublished manuscript in the Commissioned Corps Centennial Archives, History of Medicine, National Library of Medicine, Bethesda, Maryland.

———. "Interview with Dr. Emery Johnson." Unpublished manuscript in the Commissioned Corps Centennial Archives, History of Medicine, National Library of Medicine, Bethesda, Maryland.

# Newspapers

*Indian Country Today.* (15:16) and (13:15).
*The Arizona Daily Star.* (135:291) and (135:292).
*The Arizona Republic.* (106:172) and (104:84).

# Interviews

Personal interview with Dr. Jennie Joe. Native American Research and Training Center, Tucson, Arizona, April 5, 1990.
Personal interview with Dr. Stanley Stitt. Tucson, Arizona, February 14, 1990.
Everett Rhoades. Luncheon Address at the Third Annual Research Conference, Tucson, Arizona, March 20, 1990.

## Government Printing Office Publications

"A First for Indian Citizens." *15th Annual Report of the Housing and Home Finance Agency, 1961.* Washington, D.C.: Government Printing Office, 1961.
"A Plan for Quality Management in the Indian Health Service." Department of Health and Human Services, Public Health Service, Indian Health Service, September 18, 1989.
"A Plan for Quality Management in the Indian Health Service." Department of Health and Human Services, Public Health Service, Indian Health Service, October 31, 1989.
*A Study of the Indian Health Service and Tribal Involvement in Health.* Urban Associates, Inc. Washington, D.C.: Government Printing Office, 1974.
*A Summary of the Initial System Designs.* Health Program Systems Center, Indian Health Service, 1969.
*Alaska Area Native Health Services: A Description of the Program.* Department of Health, Education and Welfare, Public Health Service, Indian Health Service, Alaska Area Native Health Service, 1978.
*Alcoholism a High Priority Health Problem: A Report of the Indian Health Service Task Force on Alcoholism.* Department of Health, Education and Welfare, Health Services and Mental Health Administration, Indian Health Service, 1972.
*Allocation of Resources in the Indian Health Service.* A Handbook on the Resource Allocation Methodology. Department of Health and Human Services, Public Health Service, Indian Health Service, 1988.
Andre, James M. *The Epidemiology of Alcoholism among American Indians and Alaska Natives.* Albuquerque: Indian Health Service, Office of Alcohol Programs, 1979.
*Annual Report.* Commissioner of Indian Affairs. Washington, D.C.. Government Printing Office, 1877, 1878, 1879, 1880, 1884, 1889, 1890, 1892, 1893, 1894, 1898, 1899, 1904, 1905, 1908, 1909, 1916, 1917, and 1955.
*Annual Report of the Department of Health, Education and Welfare.* Washington, D.C.: Government Printing Office, 1955, 1960, 1963, 1966 and 1968.
*Annual Report of the Secretary of the Interior.* Washington, D.C.: Government Printing Office, 1951, 1952, 1953, and 1955.

*Annual Statistical Review.* Department of Health, Education and Welfare, Public Health Service, Indian Health Service, 1969.

*Bridging the Gap: Report of the Task Force on Parity of Indian Health Services.* Department of Health and Human Services, Public Health Service, Indian Health Service, May 1986.

*Broken Promises: Evaluating the Native American Health Care Experience.* Washington, D.C.: United States Commission on Civil Rights, September 2004.

*Celebrating Thirty Years of Progress: The Indian Health Service and the Sanitation Facilities Construction Program.* Washington, D.C.: Indian Health Service, 1989.

*Commission on the Organization of the Executive Branch of Government: Functions and Activities of the National Government in the Field of Welfare.* Washington, D.C.: Government Printing Office, 1949.

*Congressional Record.* Washington, D.C.: Government Printing Office, (98, 100 and 140).

*Dental Services for American Indians and Alaska Natives.* Department of Health, Education and Welfare, Public Health Service, Indian Health Service, 1974.

*The Dentist in Indian Health.* Department of Health, Education and Welfare, Public Health Service, Indian Health Service, 1969.

Dizmang, Larry. "Suicide among the Cheyenne Indians.," In "Indian Education," *Hearings before the Special Subcommittee on Indian Education of the Senate Committee on Labor and Public Welfare United States Senate.* Part 5, 90th Congress, 1st and 2nd session, 1969.

*Evaluation Report: The Indian Health Service's Implementation of the Indian Self-Determination Process.* The National Indian Health Board and American Indian Technical Services, April 1984.

*The Federal Register.* Washington, D.C.: Government Printing Office, (40, 48, 51, 52 and 55).

*General Practice Residency Program.* Department of Health, Education and Welfare, Public Health Service, 1966.

Goldstein, Sol and Philip R. Trautmann. "Report on the Quinault Indian Consultation." In "Indian Education," *Hearings before the Special Subcommittee on Indian Education of the Senate Committee on Labor and Public Welfare United States Senate.* Part 5, 90th Congress, 1st and 2nd session, 1969.

Grim, Charles W. "Former Director of the IHS," aianhealthcareers.org.

*Health of the American Indian: Report of a Regional Task Force.* Department of Health, Education and Welfare, Public Health Service, Indian Health Service, April 1973.

*Health Services for American Indians.* Washington, D.C.: Government Printing Office, 1957.

Hrdlicka, Ales. "Tuberculosis among Certain Indian Tribes of the United States." *Bureau of American Ethnology.* Bulletin 42, Washington, D.C.: Government Printing Office, 1909.

*Indian Alcohol and Substance Abuse: Legislative Intent and Reality.* Department of Health and Human Services, Office of the Inspector General, May 1992.

Indian Health Service releases $500 million in Recovery Act Funds to Improve Health Care and Boost Economy in Indian Country, www.ihs.gov/publicaffairs.

*Indian Health Care.* Office of Technology Assessment. Washington, D.C.: Government Printing Office, 1986.

*Indian Health Highlights.* Washington: Division of Indian Health, 1964.

*Indian Health Relocation Study: Report to Congress.* Indian Health Service, November 1, 1989.

*Indian Health Service Accomplishments.* Fiscal Year 1988. Department of Health and Human Services, Public Health Service, Indian Health Service, 1989.

*Indian Health Service Alcoholism/Substance Abuse Prevention Initiative.* Department of Health and Human Services, Public Health Service, Health Resources and Services Administration, 1989.

*Indian Health Service Circular No. 77-2.* Washington, D.C., May 22, 1977.

*Indian Health Service Contract Health Services Final Report.* Macro Systems, Inc. Washington, D.C., April 1984.

*Indian Health Service Factsheet.* www.info.ihs.gov.

*Indian Health Service Office of Research and Development.* Department of Health, Education and Welfare, Health Services and Mental Health Administration, Public Health Service, Indian Health Service, 1973.

*Indian Housing in the United States.* A Staff Report on the Indian Housing Effort in the United States. Washington, D.C.: Government Printing Office, 1975.

*Indian Service Health Activities.* Office of Indian Affairs, Bulletin #11. Washington, D.C. :GPO, 1922.

*Justifications of Appropriation Estimates for Committee on Appropriations.* Indian Health Service. Fiscal Year 1966, 1967, 1968, 1970 and 1976.

Leon, Robert L. "Mental Health Considerations in the Indian Boarding School Program." In "Indian Education," *Hearings before the Special Subcommittee on Indian Education of the Senate Committee on Labor and Public Welfare United States Senate.* Part 5, 90th Congress, 1st and 2nd session, 1969.

*Making Health Resources Available to All Beneficiaries.* Washington, D.C.: United States Department of Health, Education and Welfare, Public Health Service, Division of Indian Health, January 9, 1967.

*Many Obstacles Remain to Be Overcome in Implementing the Indian Self-Determination Act.* Report to the Congress by the Comptroller General of the United States, January 1978.

*Michael Trujillo Begins Second Term as IHS Director.* www.ihs.gov/1998press.

Murphy, Joseph F. *Manual on Tuberculosis: Its Causes, Prevention and Treatment,* Washington, D.C.: GPO, 1910.

National Indian Health Board and American Indian Technical Services. *Evaluation Report: The Indian Health Service's Implementation of the Self-Determination Process.* Department of Health and Human Services, 1984.

Obama, Barack. *Principles for Stronger Tribal Communities.* Barackobama.com May 23, 2009.

*Plan for Medical Facilities Needed for Indian Health Services.* Washington, D.C.: Public Health Service, Division of Indian Health, 1958.

President Proposes 13 Percent Increase in FY 2010 Budget for Indian Health Service. www.ihs.gov/publicaffairs.

*Public Papers of the Presidents of the United States: Lyndon Baines Johnson, Containing the Public Messages, Speeches and Statements of the President 1963-1964.* Vol. 1. Washington, D.C.: Government Printing Office, 1965.

*Public Papers of the Presidents of the United States: Lyndon Baines Johnson, Containing the Messages, Speeches and Statements of the President 1968-1969.* Vol. 1. Washington, D.C.: Government Printing Office, 1970.

*Public Papers of the Presidents of the United States: Richard M. Nixon, Containing the Messages, Speeches and Statements of the President 1970.* Vol. 1. Washington, D.C.: Government Printing Office, 1971.

*Public Papers of the Presidents of the United States, Ronald Reagan 1983.* vol. 1. Washington, D.C.: Government Printing Office, 1984.

*Public Papers of the Presidents of the United States: William J. Clinton, 1993.* Book II. Washington, D.C.: Government Printing Office, 1994.

Raup, Ruth. *The Indian Health Program 1800-1955.* Washington, D.C.: Government Printing Office, United States Department of Health, Education and Welfare, Public Health Service, 1959.

*Regional Differences in Indian Health 1994.* Department of Health and Human Services, Public Health Service, Indian Health Service, 1994.

*Regulations for the Indian Department.* Office of Indian Affairs. Washington, D.C.: GPO, 1884.

Rund, Nadine. "Application of the Social Compass to the Study of Health." Health Program Systems Center, Indian Health Service, September 1968.

————. *Community Health Representative: A Changing Philosophy of Indian Involvement.* Washington, D.C.: Office of Program Development, Indian Health Service, 1970.

*Sanitation Facilities Construction: Project Administration Management.* Part I. Washington, D.C.: Indian Health Service, Division of Environmental Health, 1986.

*Summary Report of the NIHB Self-Determination Act Committee.* National Indian Health Board Memorandum, December 27, 1988.

*Task Force Six: Report on Indian Health.* American Indian Policy Review Commission. Washington, D.C.: Government Printing Office, 1976.

*Technical Comparative Analysis of Statutory, Regulatory, Jurisdictional Policy and Health Industry Entry Requirements Limiting Tribal Participation in Alternative Health Care Delivery Systems.* Systems Resource Management, Inc. Bethesda, Maryland, 1988.

*The Indian Health Program of the United States Public Health Service.* Department of Health, Education and Welfare, Public Health Service, Division of Indian Health, 1963 and 1969.

*The Indian Health Program.* Department of Health, Education and Welfare, Public Health Service, Indian Health Service, 1978.

*To the First Americans: First Annual Report on the Indian Health Program of the U.S. Public Health Service.* Washington, D.C.: Department of Health, Education and Welfare, Public Health Service, 1966.

*To the First Americans: Third Annual Report of the Indian Health Program of the U.S. Public Health Service.* Washington, D.C.: Government Printing Office, 1969.

"Towards an Indian Housing Delivery System." The Housing Assistance Council, Inc. November 1974, in *Indian Housing in the United States: A Staff Report on the Indian Housing Effort in the United States.* Washington, D.C.: Government Printing Office, 1975.

*Trends in Indian Health.* Department of Health and Human Services, Public Health Service, Indian Health Service, 1992, 1989, 1994, and 2001-2002.

*Tuberculosis among the North American Indians: Report of a Committee of the National Tuberculosis Association.* Washington, D.C.: Government Printing Office, 1923.

*United States Code of Federal Regulations.* Washington, D.C.: Government Printing Office, 1956 (Chapter 36), 1988 (Chapter 42), 1994 (Chapter 42) and 1995 (Chapter 42).

*United States Statutes at Large.* Washington, D.C.: Government Printing Office. (3, 4, 7, 12, 15, 35, 36, 42, 48, 50, 63, 67, 68, 71, 73, 78, 84, 87, 88, 90, 94, 100, 102, 104 and 106).

United States Census Bureau, Public Information Office. "Nation's Household Income Stable in 2000, Poverty Rate Virtually Equals Record Low," *Census Bureau Reports,* September 25, 2001.

*Urban Indian Health Programs Evaluative Report Fiscal Year 1983: A Report to the Director, Indian Health Service.* Indian Health Service, Office of Research and Development, Division of Health Systems Development, February 1984.

## U.S. Congress Committee Reports and Hearings

U.S. Congress. House. *Letter from the Secretary of War, Transmitting a Report of the Commissioner of Indian Affairs in relation to the execution of the act extending the benefit of Vaccination to the Indian Tribes, &c.* 22nd Congress, 2nd session, 1833. H. Doc. 82.

U.S. Congress. House. *Smallpox among the Indians, Letter from the Secretary of War upon the Subject of the Small Pox among the Indian tribes.* 25th Congress, 3rd session, 1838. H. Doc. 51.

U.S. Congress. House. *Report of the Joint Commission on Indian Tuberculosis Sanitarium and Yakima Indian Reservation Project.* 63rd Congress, 2nd session, 1915. H. Doc. 505.

U.S. Congress. House. Committee on Indian Affairs. *Letter from Secretary of the Interior to the House Committee on Indian Affairs.* 63rd Congress, 2nd session, 1915. H. Doc. 1254.

U.S. Congress. House. *Reorganizing the Indian Service.* 66th Congress, 3rd session, 1919. H. Rep. 1189.

U.S. Congress. House. *Hearings before the Committee on Indian Affairs House of Representatives on the Condition of Various. Tribes of Indians.* "Indians of the United States." 66th Congress, 1st session, September 29, 1919.

U.S. Congress. House. *Reorganizing the Indian Service: Report of the Committee of Indian Affairs.* 67th Congress, 1st session, 1921. H. Rep. 1278.

U.S. Congress. House. *Reorganizing the Indian Service: Report of the Committee of Indian Affairs.* 67th Congress, 1st session, 1921. H. Rep. 1228.

U.S. Congress. House. *Subcommittee of the Committee on Indian Affairs, Hearings before the Subcommittee on General Bills of the Committee on Indian Affairs.* 74th Congress, 1st session, 1935. House Bill 7781.

U.S. Congress. House. *Hearings before the Subcommittee of the Committee on Appropriations House of Representatives.* "Interior Department Appropriation Bill for 1950." 81st Congress, 1st session, part 1, January 26, 1949.

U.S. Congress. House. *House Report no. 797.* "Providing for Medical Services to Non-Indians in Indian Hospitals and for Other Purposes." 81st Congress, 1st session, June 14, 1949.

U.S. Congress. House. *House Report no. 641.* "Providing for Medical Services to Non-Indians in Indian Hospitals." 82d Congress, 1st session, June 25, 1951.

U.S. Congress. House. *House Report no. 870.* "Transfer the Maintenance and Operation of Hospitals and Health Facilities for Indians to the Public Health Service." 83rd Congress, 1st session, July 17, 1953, (serial 11667).

U.S. Congress. House. *House Report no. 2430.* "Transferring the Maintenance and Operation of Hospitals and Health Services for Indians to the Public Health Service." 83rd Congress, 2d session, July 21, 1954.

U.S. Congress. House. *House Report no. 228,* 84th Congress, 1st session, 1955.

U.S. Congress. House. *Hearings before the Subcommittee of the Committee on Appropriations House of Representatives.* "Department of Labor and Health, Education and Welfare Appropriation for 1958." 85th Congress, 1st session, February 18, 1957.

U.S. Congress. House. *Hearings before the Committee on Interstate and Foreign Commerce House of Representatives on HR 204 and HR 2380.*

U.S. Congress. House. "Construction of Indian Hospitals." 85th Congress, 1st session, April 9, 1957.

U.S. Congress. House. *Hearing before the Subcommittee on Health and Science of the Committee on Interstate and Foreign Commerce House of Representatives,* "Elko Indian Sanitation Facilities." 85th Congress, 1st session, April 10, 1957.

U.S. Congress. House. *House Report no. 574.* "Constructing Indian Hospitals." 85th Congress, 1st session, June 17, 1957.

U.S. Congress. House. *House Report no. 1052.* "Indian Hospitalization Payments to Bernalillo County, New Mexico." 85th Congress, 1st session, August 13, 1957.

U.S. Congress. House. *Hearings before a Subcommittee of the Committee on Appropriations House of Representatives.* "Department of the Interior and Related Agencies Appropriations for 1965." 88th Congress, 1st session, February 19, 1963.

U.S. Congress. House. *Hearing before the Subcommittee on Indian Affairs of the Committee on Interior and Insular Affairs House of Representatives.* "Review of the Indian Health Program." 88th Congress, 1st session, May 23, 1963.

U.S. Congress. House. *Hearings before a Subcommittee of the Committee on Appropriations House of Representatives.* "Department of the Interior and Related Agencies Appropriations for 1967." 89th Congress, 2d session, part 3, March 2, 1966.

U.S. Congress. House. *Hearings before a Subcommittee of the Committee on Appropriations House of Representatives.* "Department of the Interior and Related Agencies Appropriations for 1968." 90th Congress, 1st session, part 2, March 8, 1967.

U.S. Congress. House. *Hearings before the Subcommittee of the Committee on Appropriations House of Representatives.* "Department of the Interior and Related Agencies Appropriations for 1969." 90th Congress, 2nd session, Part III.

U.S. Congress. House. *Hearings before a Subcommittee of the Committee on Appropriations House of Representatives.* "Department of the Interior and Related Agencies Appropriations for 1970." 91st Congress, 1st session, part 3, March 24, 1969.

U.S. Congress. House. *Hearings before a Subcommittee of the Committee on Appropriations House of Representatives.* "Department of the Interior and Related Agencies Appropriations for 1974." 93d Congress, 1st session, part 4, April 11, 1973.

U.S. Congress. House. *Hearings before the Subcommittee on Indian Affairs of the Committee on Interior and Insular Affairs House of Representatives on S.B. 1017.* "Indian Self-Determination and Education Assistance Act." 93rd Congress, 2d session, May 20-21, 1974.

U.S. Congress. House. *Hearings before the Committee on Science and Technology, United States House of Representatives on H.R. 2931.* "1976 NASA Authorizations." 94th Congress, 1st session, February 4, 1975.

U.S. Congress. House. *Hearings before the Subcommittee on Indian Affairs of the Committee on Interior and Insular Affairs House of Representatives on H.R. 2525 and related bill.* "Indian Health Care Improvement Act." 94th Congress, 1st session, May 23-24, 1975, August 5, 1975 and September 25-26, 1975.

U.S. Congress. House. *Hearings before the Subcommittee on Health and the Environment of the Committee on Interstate and Foreign Commerce House of Representatives on H.R. 2525.* "Indian Health Care Improvement Act." 94th Congress, 2d session, April 27-28, 1976.

U.S. Congress. House. *House Report 94-1026.* "Indian Health Care Improvement Act." 94th Congress, 2d session, May 10, 1976.

U.S. Congress. House. *House Report 94-1026.* "Indian Health Care Improvement Act." Part 3. 94th Congress, 2d session, May 12, 1976.

U.S. Congress. House. *Hearings before a Subcommittee of the Committee on Appropriations House of Representatives.* "Department of the Interior and Related Agencies Appropriations for 1979." Part 4. 95th Congress 2d session, March 2-3, 1978.

U.S. Congress. House. *Hearings before a Subcommittee of the Committee on Appropriations House of Representatives.* "Department of Interior and Related Agencies Appropriations for 1982." Part 9. 97th Congress, 1st session, 1981.

U.S. Congress. House. *Hearings before a Subcommittee of the Committee on Appropriations House of Representatives.* "Department of the Interior and Related Agencies Appropriations for 1982." Part 9. 97th Congress, 1st session, March 2-3, 1981.

U.S. Congress. House. *House Document 82-54.* "Indian Health Service Not Yet Distributing Funds Equitably among Tribes." July 2, 1982.

U.S. Congress. House. *House Report 97-942.* "Department of the Interior and Related Agencies Appropriations Bill, 1983." 97th Congress, 2d session, December 2, 1982.

U.S. Congress. House. *Hearings before the Committee on Interior and Insular Affairs House of Representatives on H.R. 1928.* "Indian Housing Act." 98th Congress, 1st session, April 12/19, 1983.

U.S. Congress. House. *A Staff Report for the Use of the Select Committee on Health and the Environment of the Committee on Energy and Commerce United States House of Representatives.* "Indian Health Care: An Overview of the Federal Government's Role." 98th Congress, 2d session, April 1984.

U.S. Congress. House. *House Report 98-763.* "Reauthorizing and Amending the Indian Health Care Improvement Act and for Other Purposes." Part 1. 98th Congress, 2d session, May 14, 1984.

U.S. Congress. House. *House Report 98-763.* "Indian Health Care Amendments of 1984." Part 2. 98th Congress, 2d session, May 21, 1984.

U.S. Congress. House. *House Report no. 98-886.* "Department of the Interior and Related Agencies Appropriations Bill, 1985." 98th Congress, 2d session, June 29, 1984.

U.S. Congress. House. *House Report 98-1126.* "Indian Health Care Amendments of 1984." 98th Congress, 2d session, October 2, 1984.

U.S. Congress. House. *House Report 100-222.* "Indian Health Care Act Amendments of 1987." Part 2. 100th Congress, 1st session, December 8, 1987.

U.S. Congress. House. *Hearing before a Select Committee of the Committee on Appropriations House of Representatives.* "Department of the Interior and Related Agencies Appropriations for 1989." Part 8, 100th Congress, 2d session, March 9, 1988.

U.S. Congress. House. *Hearing before the Committee on Interior and Insular Affairs United States House of Representatives.* "Indian Health Care." 101st Congress, 2d session, March 29, 1990.

U.S. Congress. House. *Department of the Interior and Related Agencies Appropriations for 1984, Hearing before a Select Committee on Appropriations, House of representatives.* 98th Congress, 1st session, Part 9.

U.S. Congress. Senate. *Senate Report 156.* "Condition of the Indian Tribes: Report of the Joint Special Committee Appointed under Joint Resolution of March 3, 1865." 39th Congress, 2d session.

U.S. Congress. Senate. *Trachoma in Certain Indian Schools.* 60th Congress, 2nd session, 1909. S. Rep. 1025.

U.S. Congress. Senate. *Senate Document 1038.* "Contagious. and Infectious. Diseases among the Indians." 62d Congress, 3d session, 1913.

U.S. Congress. Senate. *Aspects of Indian Policy.* Senate Committee on Indian Affairs, Senate Committee Print. 79th Congress, 1st session. 1945.

U.S. Congress. Senate. *Senate Report no. 310: Analysis of the Statement of the Commissioner of Indian Affairs in Justification of Appropriations for 1944, and the Liquidation of the Indian Bureau.* "Survey of Conditions among the Indians of the United States." 78th Congress, 1st session, June 11, 1948.

U.S. Congress. Senate. *Senate Report no. 1095.* "Providing for Medical Services for Non-Indians in Indian Hospitals." 81st Congress, 1st session, September 20, 1949.

U.S. Congress. Senate. *Hearings before a Subcommittee of the Committee on Interior and Insular Affairs United States Senate on HR 303.* "Transfer of Indian Hospitals and Health Facilities to Public Health Service." 83rd Congress, 2nd session, 1954.

U.S. Congress. Senate. *Hearings before the Committee on Interior and Insular Affairs United States Senate.* "Hearings on the Proposed Transfer of Indian Hospitals and Health Facilities to the Public Health Service." 83rd Congress, 2d session, May 28 & 29, 1954.

U.S. Congress. Senate. *Senate Report no. 1530.* "Transfer the Maintenance and Operation of Hospitals and Health Facilities for Indians to the Public Health Service." 83rd Congress, 2d session, June 8, 1954.

U.S. Congress. Senate. *Senate Document 16.* "Proposed Provision-Department of Health, Education and Welfare, Communication for the President of the United States." 84th Congress, 1st session, March 23, 1955.

U.S. Congress. Senate. *Hearing before the Committee on Appropriations United States Senate on HR 9063.* "Urgent Deficiency Appropriation Bill, 1956." 84th Congress, 2d session, March 16, 1956.

U.S. Congress. Senate. *Senate Report no. 769.* "Authorizing Funds Available for

Construction of Indian Health Facilities to Be Used to Assist in the Construction of Community Hospitals Which Will Service Indians and Non-Indians." 85th Congress, 1st session, July 30, 1957.

U.S. Congress. Senate. *Senate Report no. 992.* "Indian Hospitalization Payments to Bernalillo County, New Mexico." 85th Congress 1st session, August 17, 1957.

U.S. Congress. Senate. *Hearings before the Subcommittee of the Committee on Appropriations United States Senate.* "Labor-Health, Education and Welfare Appropriations for 1959." 85th Congress, 2d session, April 1, 1958.

U.S. Congress. Senate. *Senate Report no. 1876.* "Amending the Act of August 5, 1954," 85th Congress, 2d session, July 22, 1958.

U.S. Congress. Senate. *Senate Report no. 244.* "Amending the Act of August 5, 1954." 86th Congress 1st session, May 11, 1959.

U.S. Congress. Senate. *Senate Report no. 589.* "Indian Sanitation Facilities." 86th Congress, 1st session, June 29, 1959.

U.S. Congress. Senate. *Senate Report no. 971.* "Interior Department and Related Agencies Appropriation Bill, 1965." 88th Congress, 2d session, April 4, 1964.

U.S. Congress. Senate. *Hearings before a Subcommittee of the Committee on Appropriations United States Senate.* "Department of the Interior and Related Agencies Appropriations for Fiscal Year 1967." 89th Congress, 2d session, March 8, 1966.

U.S. Congress. Senate. *Senate Report 233.* "Interior Department and Related Agencies Appropriations Bill, 1967." 90th Congress, 1st session, May 15, 1967.

U.S. Congress. Senate. *Hearings before a Subcommittee of the Committee on Appropriations United States Senate.* "Department of the Interior and Related Agencies Appropriations for Fiscal Year 1969." Part 2, 90th Congress, 2d session, March 6, 1968.

U.S. Congress. Senate. *Hearings before the Special Subcommittee on Indian Education of the Committee on Labor and Public Welfare United States Senate.* "Indian Education." Part 5, 90th Congress, 1st and 2d session, May 24, 1968.

U.S. Congress. Senate. *Senate Report 1269.* "Second Supplemental Appropriation Bill, 1968." 90th Congress, 2d session, June 19, 1968.

U.S. Congress. Senate. *Senate Report 1667.* "Supplemental Appropriations Bill, 1969." 90th Congress, 2d session, October 6, 1968.

U.S. Congress. Senate. *Hearings before a Subcommittee of the Committee on Appropriations United States Senate on H.R. 12781.* "Department of the Interior and Related Agencies Appropriations for Fiscal Year 1970." 91st Congress, 1st session, March 20, 1969.

U.S. Congress. Senate. *Hearings before the Special Subcommittee on Indian Education of the Senate Committee on Labor and Public Welfare United States Senate.* "Indian Education" Part 5, 90th Congress, 1st and 2nd session, 1969.

U.S. Congress. Senate. *Senate Report 92-1062.* "Emergency Health Personnel Act Amendment." 92d Congress, 2d session, August 16, 1972.

U.S. Congress. Senate. *Hearings before the Subcommittee on Indian Affairs of the Committee on Interior and Insular Affairs, United States Senate.* "Indian Health Recruitment Problems." November 19-20, 1972, 93rd Congress, 1st session.

U.S. Congress. Senate. *Hearings before the Subcommittee on Indian Affairs of the Committee on Interior and Insular Affairs United States Senate on SB 1017.* "Indian

Self-Determination and Education Program." 93rd Congress, 1st session, June 1 and 4, 1973.

U.S. Congress. Senate. *Hearings before the Subcommittee on Indian Affairs of the Committee on Interior and Insular Affairs United States Senate.* "Indian Health Care Improvement Act." 93rd Congress, 2d session, 1974.

U.S. Congress. Senate. *Senate Report 94-133.* 94th Congress, 1st session.

U.S. Congress. Senate. *Hearings before the Select Committee on Indian Affairs United States Senate.* "Indian Self-Determination and Education Assistance Act Implementation." 94th Congress, 1st session, 1977.

U.S. Congress. Senate. *Hearings before a Subcommittee of the Committee on Appropriations United States Senate.* "Department of the Interior and Related Agencies Appropriations for 1979." Part 2, 95th Congress, 1st session, March 23, 1978.

U.S. Congress. Senate. *Hearings before the Subcommittee of the Committee on Appropriations United States Senate.* "Department of the Interior and Related Agencies Appropriations for Fiscal Year 1978." Part 3 and Part 9, 95th Congress, 1st session.

U.S. Congress. Senate. *Hearings before the Select Committee on Indian Affairs United States Senate.* "Report on Indian Housing." 1979.

U.S. Congress. Senate. *Hearings before the Subcommittee of the Committee on Appropriations United States Senate.* "Department of the Interior and Related Agencies Appropriations for Fiscal Year 1979." Part 4, 95th Congress, 2nd session, 1978.

U.S. Congress. Senate. *Hearings before the Select Committee on Indian Affairs, United States Senate.* "Oversight Hearings on Indian Health." 96th Congress, 2d session, August 2, 1979.

U.S. Congress. Senate. *Hearing before the Select Committee on Indian Affairs United States Senate.* "Indian Health." 96th Congress, 1st session, August 2, 1979.

U.S. Congress. Senate. *Hearing before the Select Committee on Indian Affairs United States Senate.* "Indian Health Service Oversight and Reauthorization of the Indian Health Care Improvement Act." 96th Congress 2nd session, March 28, 1980.

U.S. Congress. Senate. *Hearings before the Select Committee of Indian Affairs United States Senate.* "Reauthorization of the Indian Health Care Improvement Act." 96th Congress, 2d session, April 21-22, 1980.

U.S. Congress. Senate. *Hearing before the Select Committee on Indian Affairs United States Senate.* "Oversight of BIA and IHS 1983 Budget Submissions." 97th Congress, 2d session, May 26, 1982.

U.S. Congress. Senate. *Hearing before the Select Committee on Indian Affairs United States Senate.* "Indian Health Issues Grand Forks, North Dakota." Grand Forks, North Dakota, 98th Congress, 1st session, June 2, 1983.

U.S. Congress. Senate. *Hearing before the Select Committee on Indian Affairs United States Senate.* "Indian Health Oversight." 98th Congress, 1st session, July 28, 1983.

U.S. Congress. Senate. *Hearings before the Select Committee on Indian Affairs United States Senate.* "Fiscal Year 1985 Budget." 98th Congress, 2d session, February 21/23, 1984.

U.S. Congress. Senate. *Hearing before the Select Committee on Indian Affairs United States Senate on S. 2166.* "Reauthorization of the Indian Health Care Improvement Act." 98th

Congress, 2d session, February 29, 1984.

U.S. Congress. Senate. *Hearing before the Select Committee on Indian Affairs United States Senate.* "Investigation of Indian Health Services." Billings, Montana. 99th Congress, 1st session, May 30, 1985.

U.S. Congress. Senate. *Hearing before the Select Committee on Indian Affairs United States Senate on S. 400.* "Indian Health Protection and Disease Prevention Act of 1985." Gallup, New Mexico. 99th Congress, 1st session, June 1, 1985.

U.S. Congress. Senate. *Hearing before the Select Committee on Indian Affairs United States Senate.* "Prevention and Control of Diabetes among Native Americans." 99th Congress, 2d session, April 15, 1986.

U.S. Congress. Senate. *Senate Report no. 100-274.* "Indian Self-Determination and Education Assistance Act Amendments of 1987." 100th Congress, 1st session, December 22, 1987.

U.S. Congress. Senate. *A Report Submitted to the Budget Committee Prepared by the Select Committee on Indian Affairs United States Senate.* "Budget Views and Estimates for Fiscal Year 1989." 100th Congress, 2d session, March 1988.

U.S. Congress. Senate. *Hearing before the Select Committee on Indian Affairs United States Senate.* "Eligibility for Health Care Services Provided by the Indian Health Service." Sacramento, California. 100th Congress, 2d session, June 30, 1988.

U.S. Congress. Senate. *Senate Report 100-493.* "Delaying the Implementation of a Certain Rule Affecting the Provision of Health Services by the Indian Health Service." 100th Congress, 2d session, August 25, 1988.

U.S. Congress. Senate. *Hearing before the Select Committee on Indian Affairs United States Senate.* "Child Abuse and Neglect." Flagstaff, Arizona. 101st Congress, 2d session, November 22, 1988.

U.S. Congress. Senate. *Hearings before the Special Committee on Investigations of the Select Committee on Indian Affairs United States Senate on Mismanagement of Indian Health Service (IHS), Department of Health and Human Services.* "Federal Government's Relationship With American Indians." Part 8. 101st Congress, 1st session, May 15, 1989.

U.S. Congress. Senate. *Hearings before the Select Committee on Indian Affairs, United States Senate.* "Implementation of Amendments to the Indian Self-Determination Act." 101st Congress, 1st session, June 9, 1989.

U.S. Congress. Senate. *A Report of the Special Committee on Investigations of the Select Committee on Indian Affairs United States Senate.* "Final Report and Legislative Recommendations." 101st Congress, 1st session, November 20, 1989.

U.S. Congress. Senate. *Hearing before the Select Committee on Indian Affairs United States Senate.* "Indian Health Facilities." 101st Congress, 2d session, March 22, 1990.

U.S. Congress. Senate. *Hearing before the Select Committee on Indian Affairs United States Senate.* "Indian Health Service Nursing Shortage." 101st Congress, 2d session, June 14, 1990.

U.S. Congress. Senate. *Hearing before the Select Committee on Indian Affairs United States Senate on S. 2645.* "Urban Indian Health Equity Bill." 101st Congress, 2d session, July 19, 1990.

U.S. Congress. Senate. *Hearing before the Select Committee on Indian Affairs United States Senate.* "Department of the Interior and Related Agencies Appropriations for Fiscal Year 1991." 101st Congress, 2d session, October 16, 1990.

U.S. Congress. Senate. *Senate Report 101-557.* "The Urban Indian Health Equity Act." 101st Congress, 2d session, October 26, 1990.

U.S. Congress. Senate. *Administration of Indian Programs by the EPA. Hearings before the Select Committee on Indian Affairs, United States Senate, Oversight Hearings on the Administration of Indian Programs by the EPA.* 101st Congress, 1st Session. June 23, 1989.

U.S. Congress. Senate. *Hearing before the Select Committee on Indian Affairs United States Senate on S. 290.* "Indian Anti-Drug Abuse Amendment of 1991." 102d Congress, 1st session, May 23, 1991.

U.S. Congress. Senate. *Hearing before the Select Committee on Indian Affairs United States Senate.* "Indian Health Care Act Amendments of 1992." 102nd Congress, 2d session, April 1, 1992.

U.S. Congress. Senate. *Hearing before the Select Committee on Indian Affairs United States Senate.* "BIA and IHS Inspector General Reports on Indian Alcohol and Drug Abuse Programs." 102d Congress, 2d session, July 30, 1992.

U.S. Congress. Senate. *Hearings before the Select Committee on Indian Affairs United States Senate.* "Water and Sanitation Problems in Alaska." 103rd Congress, 1st session, May 5, 1993.

U.S. Congress. Senate. *Hearings before the Select Committee on Indian Affairs United States Senate.* 103rd Congress, 2d session, January 27, 1994.

U.S. Congress. Senate. *Hearing before the Select Committee on Indian Affairs United States Senate.* "Health Care Reform in Indian Country Oversight of the Indian Health Service." 103rd Congress, 2d session, April 6, 1994.

U.S. Congress. Senate. *Hearings before the Committee on Indian Affairs, United States Senate.* "National Health Care Reform and Its Implications for Indian Health Care." 103rd Congress 2nd Session, May 9, 1994.

U.S. Congress. Senate. *Hearing before the Select Committee on Indian Affairs United States Senate.* "Child Abuse on North Dakota Reservations and Implementation of the Indian Child Protection and Family Violence Prevention Act." Bismarck, North Dakota. 103rd Congress, 2d session, June 3, 1994.

U.S. Congress. Senate. *Department of Health and Human Services, Statement of Charles W. Grim, DDS, M.H.H.A, Interim Director Indian Health Service before the Committee on Indian Affairs.* 108th Congress, 1st session, 2003.

U.S. Congress. Senate. *Statement by Robert G. McSwain, Director of the IHS, on Nomination to Director of the Indian Health before the Committee on Indian Affairs.* 110th Congress, 2nd Session, February 7, 2008.

U.S. Congress. Senate. *Opening Statement: IHS Director-Designate Yvette Roubideaux before the Committee on Indian Affairs.* 111th Congress, 1st session, April 23, 2009.

## Miscellaneous Government Reports

"A Statement Relative to the Past, Present and Future Medical Facilities Provided the Indians in the United States and the Natives of Alaska by the United States Government." Memorandum to John Collier from Dr. J.G. Townsend, September 23, 1936. *United States Code and Administrative News.* Vol. II. Washington, D.C.:

Government Printing Office, 1954.

*Appropriation Hearings for the Department of the Interior for Fiscal Year 1979.* H181-41, Part 4.

*Clinical Staffing in the Indian Health Service* Special Report. Office of Technology Assessment. United States Congress, February, 1987.

*Congressional Monitoring of Planning for Indian Health Care Facilities Is Still Needed.* Report to the Congress by the Comptroller General of the United States. April 16, 1980.

"Declaring the Sense of Congress on the Closing of Indian Hospitals." 86th Congress, 2d session, January 19, 1960.

"House Report 94-1026." *United States Code and Administrative News.* Vol. 3. Washington, D.C.: Government Printing Office, 1976.

"Indian Health Facilities-Funds." *United States Code and Administrative News.* Vol. II. Washington, D.C.: Government Printing Office, 1957.

*Indian Health Service: Contracting for Health Services under the Indian Self-Determination Act.* General Accounting Office Report. Washington, D.C.: Government Printing Office, 1986.

"Indians—Hospital and Health Facilities—Maintenance and Operation." *United States Code and Administrative News.* Vol. II. 83rd Congress, 2d session, 1954.

"Legislative History of the Indian Health Care Improvement Act." *United States Code and Administrative News.* Vol. 3. Washington, D.C.: Government Printing Office, 1976.

"Medical Research Using American Indians as Subjects." *Report of the Comptroller General of the United States to Senator James Abourezk.* Enclosure I. November 4, 1976.

*Programs and Problems in Providing Health Services to Indians.* Report to Congress by the Comptroller General of the United States. Washington, D.C.: Government Printing Office, 1973.

*Slow Progress on Eliminating Substandard Indian Housing.* Report to Congress by the Comptroller General of the United States. Washington, D.C.: Government Printing Office, 1971.

*Senate Report 102-392 on S. 2481. U.S Code and Administrative News.* Vol. 6. Washington, D.C.: Government Printing Office, 1992.

# INDEX

231

# ABOUT THE AUTHOR

**David H. DeJong** holds a PhD in American Indian policy studies from the University of Arizona. He is the author of five books, including *"If You Knew the Conditions:" A Chronicle of the Indian Medical Service and American Indian Healthcare, 1908-1955*, also published by Lexington Books. His interests in Indian health policy and history were heightened in the 1980s when he was selected via a national search to assist the Indian Health Service fulfill its statutory obligation to educate Indian Health Service employees about the history of the agency and unique political relationship that exists between tribal nations and the United States.

Dr. DeJong has written extensively on federal Indian health, education, and water policies and history. He is currently the Project Director of the U.S. Bureau of Reclamation–funded, tribally operated Pima-Maricopa Irrigation Project (P-MIP) on the Gila River Indian Reservation. The P-MIP is implementing the largest water rights settlement in North American history. He lives in Casa Grande, Arizona, with his wife of twenty-nine years and his five children.